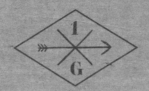

ONE GUN

RANCH
MALIBU

BIODYNAMIC RECIPES
FOR VIBRANT LIVING

ALICE BAMFORD
ANN EYSENRING

WITH RACHEL MARLOWE

Regan Arts.

Regan Arts.

65 Bleecker Street
New York, NY 10012

The information provided in this book is designed to provide helpful information on the subjects discussed. This book is not meant to be used, nor should it be used, to diagnose or treat any medical condition. For diagnosis or treatment of any medical problem, consult your own physician. The publisher and author are not responsible for any specific health needs that may require medical supervision and are not liable for any damages or negative consequences from any treatment, action, application, or preparation, to any person reading or following the information in this book.

First Regan Arts hardcover edition, April 2017.

Library of Congress Control Number: 2015946539

ISBN 978-1-941393-52-9

Interior design and hand-lettering by Laura Palese

Cover design by Richard Ljoenes

Printed in China

10 9 8 7 6 5 4 3 2 1

All cover photographs by Martin Löf, except front cover and second from bottom on back cover, which are by Jack Guy.

Photo by George Bamford, 8; Photo courtesy of Patrick Holden, 27; Photos by Jack Guy, 50-51, 52, 69, 88; Photo by Sherry Tessler, 56; Photo by George Auge, 57; Photo by Carlos Gonzalez Arnesto, 85; Photo courtesy of Leroy Hamilton, 91; Photo by Bela Hamilton, 128; Photo by Grey Rembert, 134-135.

All other photographs courtesy of Martin Löf.

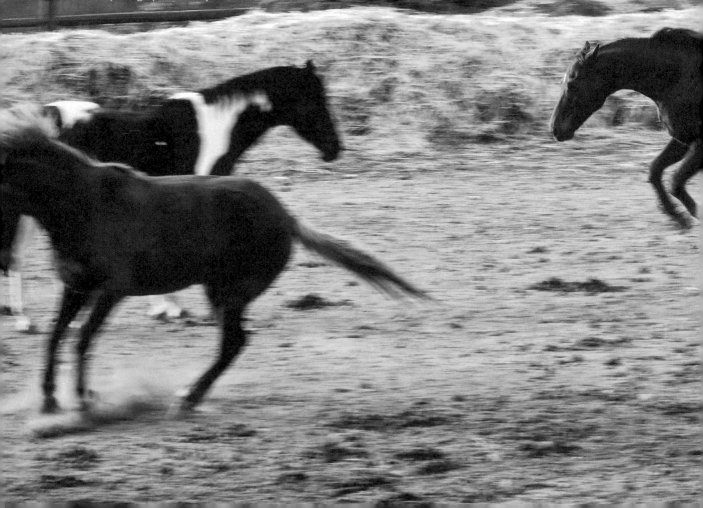

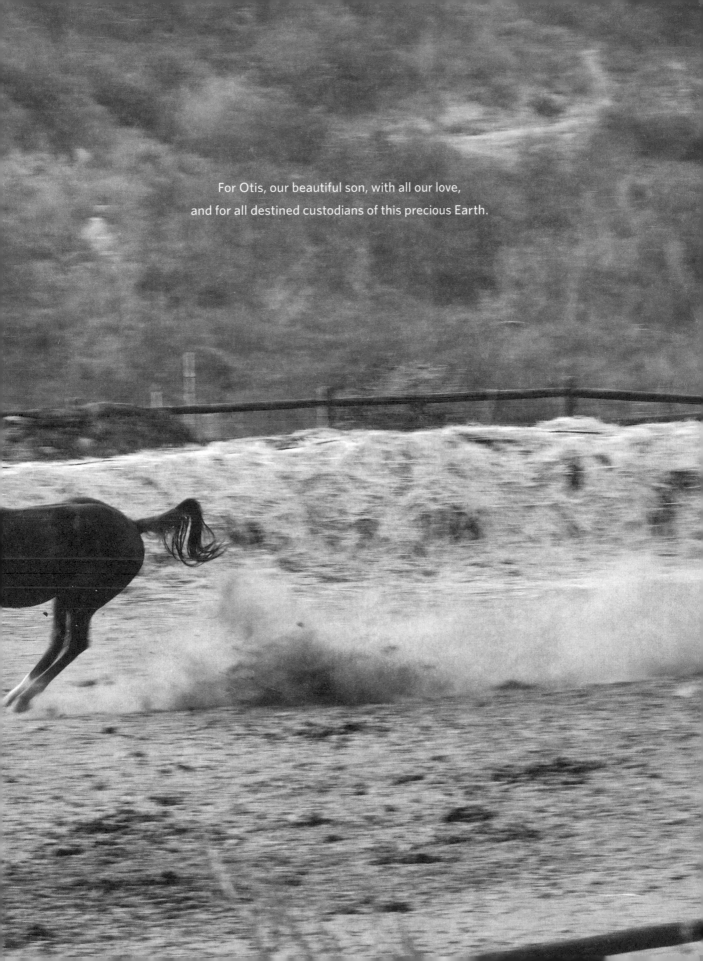

For Otis, our beautiful son, with all our love,
and for all destined custodians of this precious Earth.

Contents

— THE MALIBU BIODYNAMIC EATING PLAN —

130

THE MALIBU

Biodynamic DIET

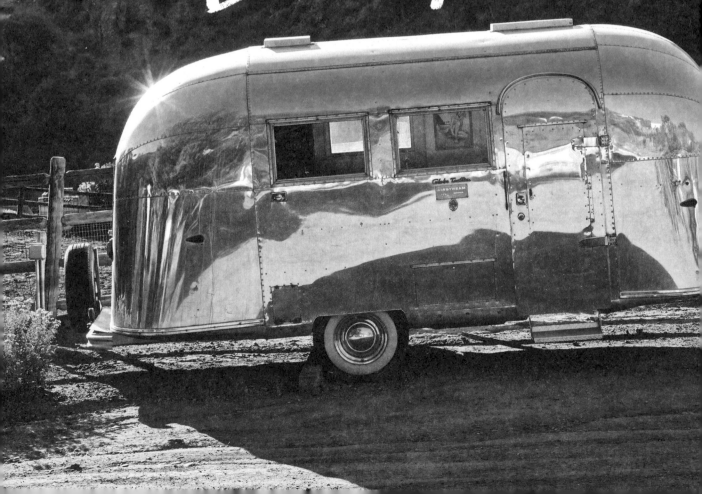

A HOLISTIC AND HARMONIOUS LIFESTYLE is at the heart of One Gun Ranch, our home in the Malibu hills, and we believe we are part of a growing movement. After so many years of moving away from an agrarian society, people have a deep need to reconnect with nature. This shared desire to feel a connection with the earth is elemental, and is currently being expressed more and more all the time in developments, such as the demand for farm-to-table foods, an explosion in urban farming, and a renewed enthusiasm for camping and hiking.

At the Ranch, we feel more in harmony with ourselves, having rediscovered the rhythms of nature and integrated them into our lifestyle. When we eat a just-picked, biodynamically grown salad or sip a homemade bowl of soup, we don't just feel physically nourished, we feel mentally and spiritually nourished. And our daily outdoor exercise, surrounded by nature, invigorates our bodies as well as our minds and souls. It makes us feel grounded . . . rooted.

In our society, there is an overwhelming need to nurture and connect with one another, to be more compassionate, to be genuine social beings, and, actually, to do more to nurture ourselves. But our world is increasingly atomized, polarized, over-digitalized, rootless, and artificial, and it is increasingly difficult for people to realize their authentic selves, to grow and blossom as nature intended.

At One Gun Ranch, our mission is to educate and help people reach their true, natural potential. In these pages, we've harnessed our experience and gathered our knowledge and the knowledge of our biodynamic heroes to help you bring powerful organic-growing methods, effective workout routines, and simple, deliciously nourishing recipes into your life. We hope you benefit from and embrace, as we have, the Malibu Biodynamic Diet.

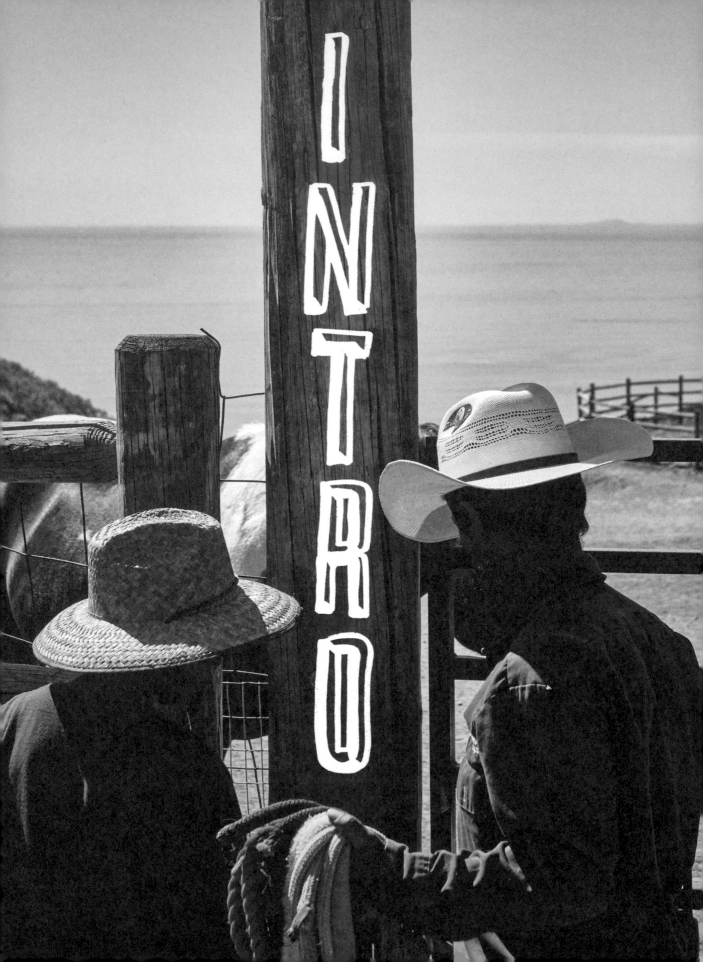

AT One Gun Ranch, our MISSION is to EDUCATE and help people reach their true, NATURAL POTENTIAL

MALIBU:
A place most often ASSOCIATED WITH THE PACIFIC OCEAN

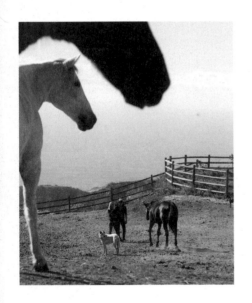

TOURISTS CRUISE UP AND DOWN the Pacific Coast Highway year round to visit such landmarks as the legendary break at Surfrider Beach overlooked by Malibu Pier and the iconic lifeguard towers on Zuma Beach. Or they come to sample the clam chowder at Neptune's Net. On any given day, you might see pods of dolphins or gray whales breaching as they migrate from their Arctic feeding grounds in the north to Baja California, sea lions jostling for space on the rocks off Point Dume—even the odd movie star or two. But turn away from the ocean and you will find another side of Malibu: the majestic Santa Monica Mountains, full of dramatic rock formations, waterfalls, and a profusion of native wildlife and plants. It is a beautiful wilderness that we are lucky to call home.

Long before Malibu became a beach community or a tourist destination, it was home to the Native American Chumash, a tribe of hunters, gatherers, and fishermen. The Chumash believed in balance and sustainability, understood that their lives depended on their environment, and found a use for every part of every plant and animal, wasting nothing and living closely attuned to the seasons. Today, high above Malibu's famous shoreline on twenty acres of land sits One Gun Ranch, home to our biodynamic farm, which we share with an ever-growing number of rescue dogs, retired racehorses, goats, alpacas, pigs, Zebu cows, and Waffle the donkey. We live by nature's time, waking up when the sun rises and going to bed when it sets. We eat, work out, and entertain seasonally, and find a use for everything on the farm so that nothing is wasted—as the Chumash did, as in nature.

Initially in my search for land where I wanted to establish an organic farm, I was looking much farther north. But then, during a weekend visit with friends, I fell in love with Malibu's vast, humbling landscapes. Like many people, I knew Malibu mainly for its beaches and proximity to Los Angeles; but once I turned off the Pacific Coast Highway, I found myself in a magical world, utterly surrounded by nature. I was excited to see how long the growing season was there; the possibilities seemed endless.

When Annie and I first met in Malibu, we immediately connected over a shared passion for an organic, sustainable lifestyle. We had both grown up in an agricultural setting—Annie in nearby Camarillo, known for its walnut and citrus groves; me on a working farm in Staffordshire, England—but the experiences

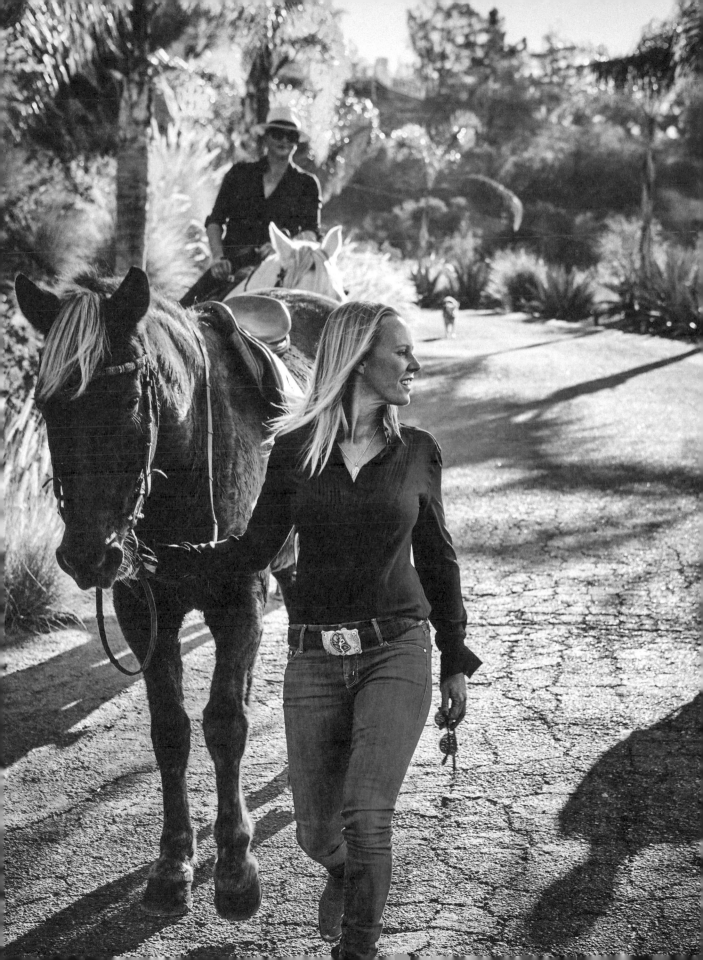

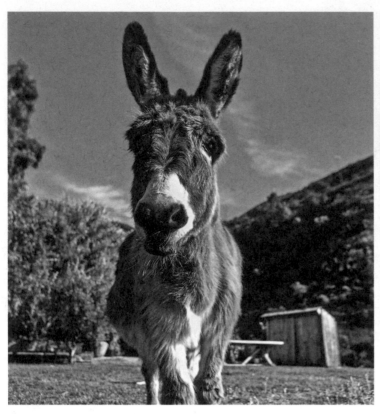
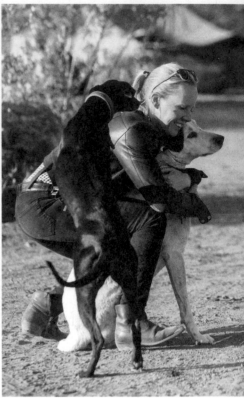

that led us to our current path were very different. Annie had lived in the midst of large, commercial farms that used chemicals and pesticide-spraying crop dusters. After her mother was diagnosed with thyroid cancer, an illness that has been linked to pesticide exposure, she began to search out organic produce and seek out a healthy, chemical-free diet. I, on the other hand, had grown up on my family's organic farm, learning to grow and harvest my own pesticide-free food. I had an awareness of the impact of chemicals on farms from a very early age, as my mother had turned our farm over to organic methods when I was just a baby—after seeing the horrific effects that Roundup herbicide was having on our rose garden. Out of these very

different circumstances, we had both been committed to eating organically, locally, and seasonally for years; next, we became intent on growing food organically and sustainably for the local community as well as for ourselves.

NOT LONG BEFORE MEETING Annie, I had come across a listing for One Gun Ranch, soon to become our slice of heaven—the name came courtesy of its former owner, Guns N' Roses drummer Matt Sorum. After a few years of negotiating, in 2009 we became the proud, and blessed, new caretakers of the twenty acres that we like to call "a cathedral of nature."

Seven years on, we have succeeded in converting the land into a biodynamic,

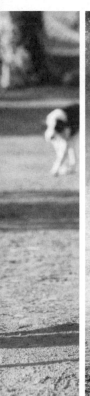

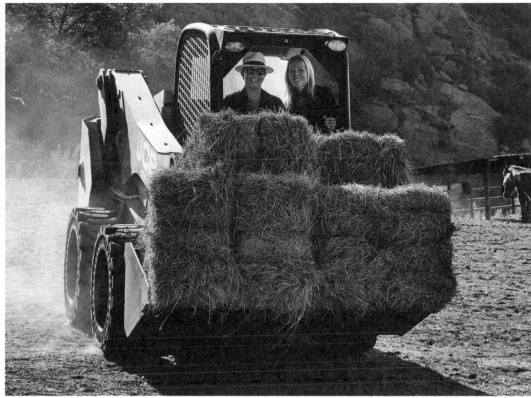

sustainable farm. We grow our own food; we use food waste and manure for our compost; and any unsold produce comes back to the ranch and is fed to the goats and pigs. We use natural methods to provide shade and control pests, including growing passion fruit vines over our raised beds to protect our lettuces from the hot sun and also to deter butterflies from laying eggs on the leafy greens, which otherwise would be eaten by the hatched larvae. This closed-loop process has created a self-sustainable ecosystem on the farm—a sort of halo that provides protection for the animals and plants alike.

Although we can't grow everything here at the Ranch—we buy some fruits and vegetables and meat from local farmers—we find it most joyous to eat our own food. As a child, I always looked forward to the first new crop of fruits and vegetables at our farm, and today I still experience that excitement each season. We want to help people feel the happiness that comes from growing their own food, whether it be a window box of herbs, a fire escape's worth of tomatoes and kale, or a garden full of vegetables.

We all have a choice as consumers: we can eat mindfully, nourishing ourselves and the earth; or we can eat cheap, processed, antibiotic- and hormone-laden foods that hurt our bodies and the planet. Making delicious, nutritious decisions means reconnecting with our food: growing and sourcing it, preparing it, sharing it, and celebrating it.

BIODYNAMIC HERO:

Lady Bamford

MY MAMA WAS MY hero as I was growing up and remains my one true inspiration. She is incredibly passionate about what she does and the way that she lives. From a very young age, she taught me about good food and how to eat it, and my whole attitude and approach to food is a result of her influence.

Her interest in organic farming began at an agricultural show almost forty years ago, where the emerging organic farming movement and its approach to sustainable farming inspired her. She immediately set about converting our family's farm in Staffordshire to organic, responsible farming based on traditional methods, and when we moved to Daylesford Farm in the Cotswolds in Gloucestershire, in the late eighties, she implemented the same methods there. By 1992 the farm was fully organic.

In the move to Gloucestershire, we also inherited a Friesian Herd. Mama wanted to produce something using the milk and found an artisan cheese maker with whom she collaborated to create an organic cheddar cheese, which, within the first year of being available, won a prize at the World Cheese Awards. The Daylesford brand was born out of this first product and Mama went on to open the Daylesford café in the creamery at the farm in 2002, showcasing farm to table, seasonal produce. Today there are four stand-alone Daylesford Farmshops with cafés.

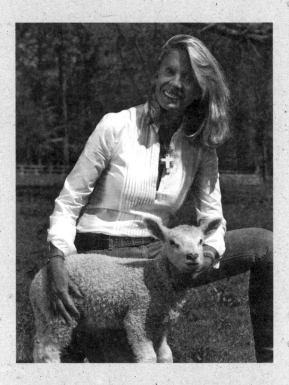

My mother believes that preserving the heritage breeds of both fruits, vegetables, and animals is of great import, and so on the farm, we have Kerry Hill and Ryeland sheep and both Devon and rare Gloucester cattle. The dairy herd of Gloucester cattle in particular is my mother's favorite. She bought the small herd some years ago when there were very few remaining and it has now flourished to about 120 head of cattle, with the cows continuing to milk well into their late teens. These cows are responsible for a true heritage product in the form of a Gloucester cheese made with their milk and this is now one of our best-selling products.

The Daylesford Foundation was launched in 2007 and supports projects in the UK that protect sustainability (most notably saving bees) and educate children and young people in the core areas of organic food growing and the countryside.

Was there a defining moment that set you on this path?

It was a life-changing moment shortly after Alice was born while I was pushing her round the garden of our home—which was in Staffordshire back then. My interest in gardening had just begun; and I looked at the roses and saw them wilting. When I returned to the house, I asked the farmers what they were spraying in the fields and they said, "Roundup." I thought, "Well, those roses don't like it," and I was worried about the effects it might have on Alice.

A couple of weeks later, at an agricultural show, I became inspired by the emerging organic farming movement after spending a couple of hours talking to a man who was there promoting organic food and farming. I came away thinking that we must look after our soil.

The hardest part was persuading my husband. He looked at me as if I was completely barmy; it would be expensive and would mean the crops would be less productive. It took three years to begin farming organically, but thirty years later, we are still going strong.

Why is the health of the soil so relevant in the age of modern farming?

It all starts with the soil. If we have healthy soil, we can grow and produce food that is naturally full of goodness. We must also look after the soil for the wellbeing of our future generations.

Why is eating mindfully so important?

To me, eating mindfully means slowing down and being thankful for the food we are eating. If we take time to think about what we are eating, where the ingredients are from, and how the food has been prepared, we are more likely to enjoy each mouthful and reap the nutritional benefits. If we care about the production and provenance of food, we also nurture the soil, our animals, the environment, and ourselves.

What is your approach to growing or buying and eating food and/or wine?

I have been passionate about organic and sustainable farming for over thirty-five years, and this has been the greatest influence on the way we grow and produce food on our certified organic farms in the UK and the organic and biodynamic wines at our vineyard in the South of France. When I am buying food, I really enjoy shopping at farmers' markets and independent butchers, fishmongers, and grocers. The ingredients I choose will always be in season, because this is when they will be at their best naturally, and whenever possible I buy from local producers.

WHAT IS
Biodynamics?

Biodynamics is a spiritual-ethical-ecological approach to agriculture, food, and nutrition that goes beyond organic.

THE WORD "BIODYNAMIC" REFERS to "life force"—the force that stimulates change and progress, the very energy of life. Proponents of biodynamics view the Earth as a living, self-sustaining organism that is inextricably linked to the Moon, Sun, and planets. Living parallel to the cycles of the Moon and planets is neither a novel idea nor a New-Age fad, but a belief that has existed for centuries. Farmers throughout history have used the Moon and planets as their guides for when to plant and harvest; since its first publication, the *Farmer's Almanac* has included a moon-phase calendar; a guide to the rising and setting of the Moon, Sun, and planets; and a tide predictor.

Biodynamic farming is considered "beyond organic" because no artificial or synthetic chemicals, pesticides, or fertilizers are ever used on the soil or the crops. Instead, nutrient- and bacteria-rich compost is used to revive the soil; biodynamic herbal preparations are used treat specific problems; and pests are managed naturally through peppering, apple cider vinegar, tobacco plants, rotational planting, and companion planting. Biodynamic methods are designed to stimulate and sustain the fertility and health of the soil. These homeopathic remedies have been formulated to treat impoverishments or diseases plaguing the soil (often poor health is caused by the overuse of chemicals) instead of just alleviating the symptoms (weak plants that produce unappetizing fruits and vegetables). Healthy, vital soil provides an environment for plants to thrive, display good root structure and increased vitality, become resistant to disease and pests, and burst with color and flavor.

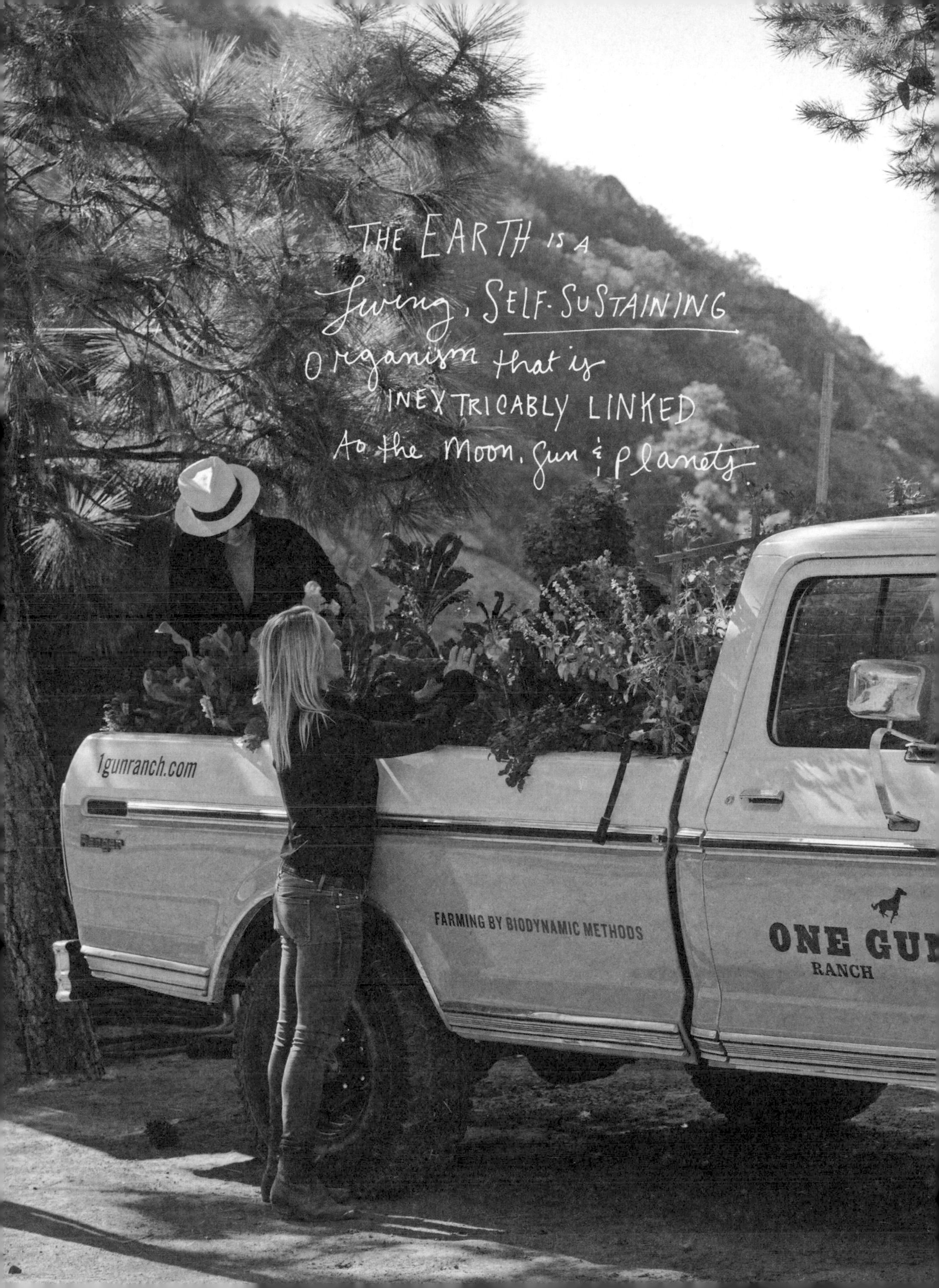

THE EARTH IS A
Living, SELF-SUSTAINING
organism that is
INEXTRICABLY LINKED
to the Moon, gun & planets.

BRINGING
Biodynamics
TO ONE GUN RANCH

I HAD HEARD OF BIODYNAMICS over the years, but worried that its concepts were a bit too esoteric. In an age when religion and spirituality were a much more integral part of everyday life, Rudolf Steiner's philosophy was presumably not as problematic as we might find it today.

In fact, throughout the ages, farming and spirituality have been intertwined in cultures around the world. Harvest festivals in the Americas are believed to date back to 10,000 BC or earlier. In Ancient Egypt, Greece, and Rome, the deltas, fields, orchards, vineyards, springs, and woods all had deities for whom ceremonies were held in every season; and in Great Britain, harvest festivals have been performed since pagan times, when farmers believed that their crops were inhabited by spirits who were released during harvest season.

Then, one night at a dinner party, I met a winegrower called Peter Sisseck. He told me the story of how he successfully used biodynamic viticulture to resuscitate the old vines on his Spanish estate. By tending to the roots of the vines with a nourishing soil preparation, within a few years he was able to produce some of the best wine in the world. I mulled over his methodology while I was having my own problems with the seeds I had brought over to the US from my family's farm in Gloucestershire, England, Daylesford Farm—the tomatoes, cucumbers, and broccoli were growing very poorly, and I soon learned it was because the soil was too acidic. Since I had no idea what kind of chemicals had been used on the property in the past, I started looking into growing in raised beds to maintain the soil integrity. I went to a meeting of the Malibu Agricultural Society to learn more about the region, and the name Farmer Jack came up. Upon learning that he was a local biodynamic compost guru, I realized I had to give it a try.

We started doing some trials at One Gun Ranch using compost that Farmer Jack had made. We planted tomatoes, radishes, jalapeño chiles, and onions side by side in raised beds that had exactly the same conditions—except that some were filled with biodynamic soil and some with conventional soil. The results of the experiment were shocking: The onions in the conventional soil grew to about two to three inches, but the onions in the biodynamic soil were two to three feet high.

Once we were sold on the idea, the next big step was to make our first compost pile. Under the guidance of Farmer Jack, and with the help of a group of volunteers from the Malibu Agricultural Society, we began by mixing together the ingredients of the biodynamic preparation. The process of making the compost was incredible in itself. As we layered all of the elements inside the tepee—vast amounts of dairy cow manure, special herbs like stinging nettles, alfalfa, oak bark, yarrow, and chamomile—you could almost feel the alchemy taking place. Preparing the compost pile felt like a reawakening for the ranch.

Today we are proud to be part of the biodynamic movement that has spread to thousands of successful gardens, farms, and vineyards all over the world. We are part of a giant ecosystem, and if we respect the Earth, we will all benefit: connecting with our food source, reveling in the preparation, making eating a celebration, complete with friends and a real sense of occasion. Taking time to cook and spoil oneself while at the same time being economical by using everything and wasting nothing—this is the essence of Malibu Biodynamics.

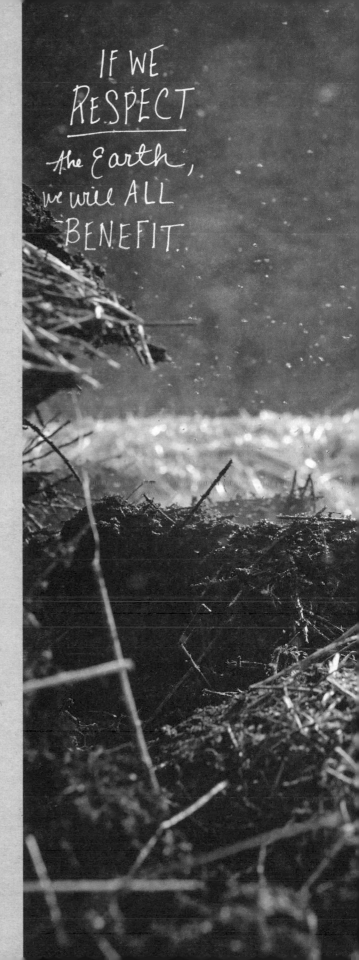

IF WE RESPECT the Earth, we will ALL BENEFIT

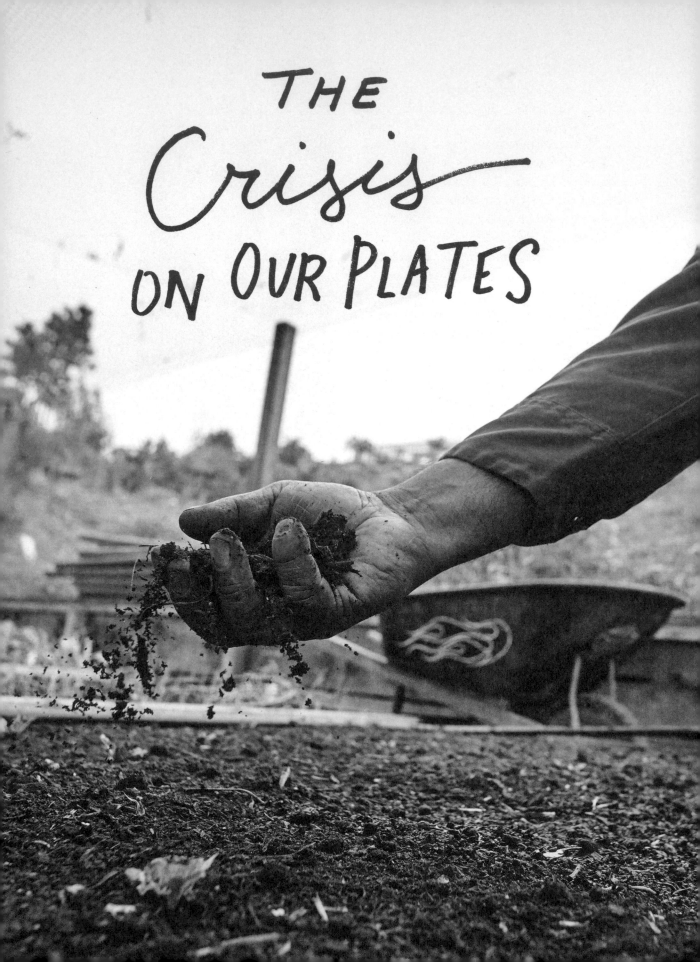

THE Crisis ON OUR PLATES

Spirituality is the essence of biodynamics,
and biodynamic agriculture is an organic extension
of this philosophy of anthroposophy.

IT SEEKS TO RECONNECT the spiritual part of planting, growing, and harvesting with the larger spirit of the universe, as well as remind the farmers of how we are connected to the earth and the universe at a time when large-scale commercial farming seems to be undermining everything we knew. Over the past few years, this lack of connection between the farmer, the consumer, and the food on their plates has once again become a hot topic. Food activist and writer Michael Pollan, one of our modern-day food heroes, is among the growing number of voices warning us that eating is the most direct connection we have with the natural world and that the industrial processing of food is breaking that connection.

Although the intensification of agriculture has vastly increased productivity, there is mounting evidence of the destruction that modern industrial agricultural practices are wreaking, not just on our environment but also on our health. Examples include the rapid decline of the bee population and erosion of fertile top soils; the contamination of drinking water with chemicals such as nitrates; the increase of obesity levels and diabetes diagnoses in urban areas; and pesticide-related illnesses and allergies in rural areas.

When we understand where our food comes from, we are moved to care about the conditions from which it came and how it was produced, which in turn can motivate us to change the way we eat. There is a hunger for truth when it comes to food, and the food we grow here at the ranch *is* truth: It's authentic, sustainable, organic food. Understanding where your food comes from also teaches you to enjoy it more and to eat more mindfully and more responsibly. At One Gun Ranch, we feel the spirituality in the planting, growing, harvesting, preparing, and sharing of food is imperative. We believe in synchronicity and everything having its place in the rhythms of nature and the cycle of life. Our interpretation of this philosophy is simply that nature is a higher power and our greatest teacher.

Many people have lost touch with nature in its truest form in significant ways. They have lost touch with the earth, they have lost touch with themselves, have forgotten how to connect with one another, and have disconnected from too many of the realities underpinning the physical, natural, and manufactured world. There is a real need for us to rediscover and reconnect with our core values, our natural values—values such as integrity, kindness, openness, thoughtfulness, and acceptance.

At One Gun Ranch, we've discovered that the most powerful way to heal and connect is to follow the philosophy behind the Malibu Biodynamic Diet: growing, cooking, eating, and exercising with one another in harmony with nature.

CHAPTER 1

Grow Well

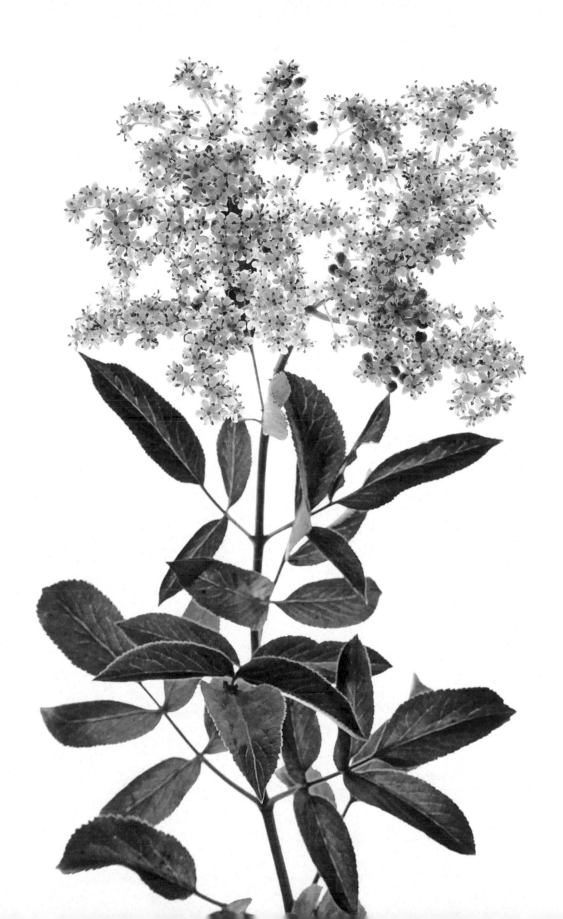

EVERYTHING HAS ITS PLACE
THE
Closed-Loop System
AT ONE GUN RANCH

The synchronicity of farm life is something
I have been aware of since childhood.

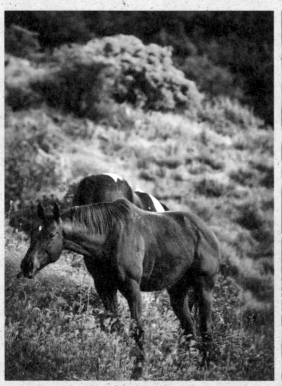
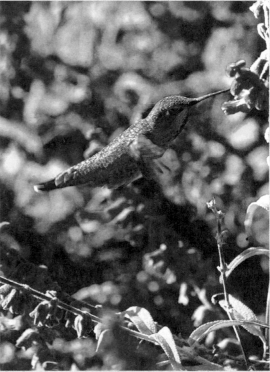

G ROWING UP ON A FARM, you learn that everything has its place and serves a purpose, creating a marvelous closed-loop system where nothing is wasted.

Our horses love their home and are free to roam in wide-open spaces. We use their manure to fertilize crops and exercise them regularly on trail rides throughout the property. Waffle the donkey is a bit of a local celebrity and a regular at our market stall in Malibu—he is a source of great joy to many children, who love to sit on his back and have their photo taken with him.

Lady Gaga the goat is also a superstar, formerly appearing in one of the singer's music videos. She has retired from show business and settled for a quiet life at the Ranch. Along with the other goats, the sheep, and the pigs, she is a big help with our waste-management program, eating unsold vegetables and wilted salads. All of the animals' manure can then be used around the property as fertilizer, which allows us to return everything back into the soil.

The chickens are invaluable when we are making compost, as they control the fly population by eating larvae from the heap before the flies can hatch while also providing us with fresh eggs.

Meanwhile our dogs Ossian, Boo, Snoopy, Dr. Watson, Whiskey Bravo, and Woodstock, to name a few, protect the land and other animals and accompany us on hikes along the beautiful trails that surround us.

This closed-loop ecosystem is a cornerstone of biodynamics, and at One Gun Ranch we are striving to decrease our dependency on external inputs and instead find a use for everything that grows here—either as food, pest control, or fertilizer—and we love that our animals get to be part of the process.

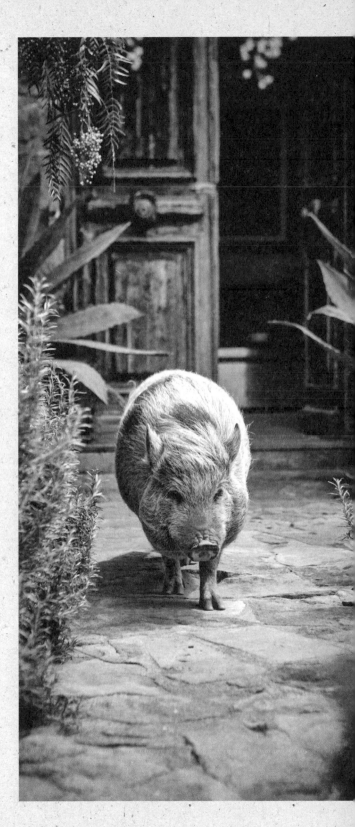

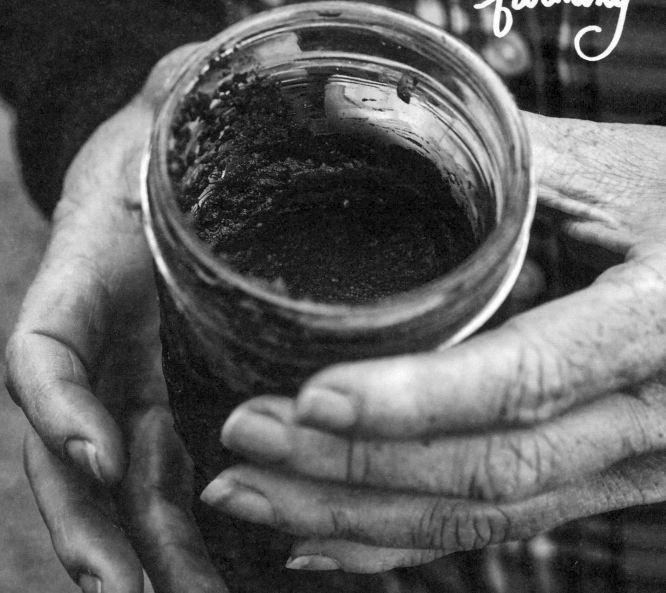

Supersoil
BIODYNAMIC COMPOST,
the CORNERSTONE of
Biodynamic *farming*

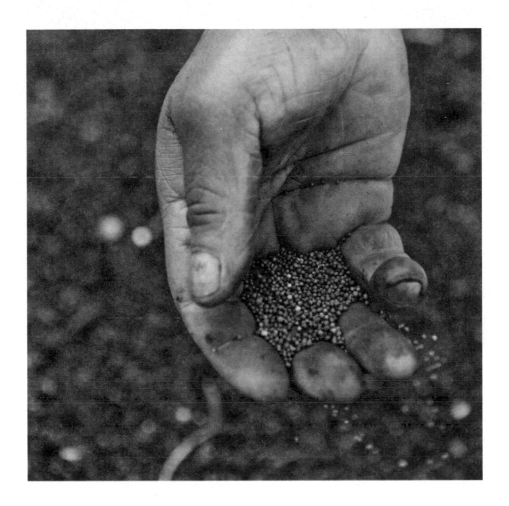

IN ORDER TO BE TRULY SUSTAINABLE, agriculture has to work in harmony with the natural environment. Crops should be rotated throughout the farm to keep the levels of nutrients in the soil stable. Food waste should be fed to animals that graze on the land, and their manure used to fertilize the soil. In turn, this healthy soil holds water and nutrients and supports healthy plant roots, which produce strong crops that are more resistant to pests and disease. As farmers take from the land in this closed-loop system, they also give back and a happy balance is achieved.

I grew up understanding that we farmed in a closed-loop system and that every animal and crop had its place, which instilled in me a great wonder of my surroundings. On our farm, we grew fields of kale next to where the cattle grazed; we then fed the kale to both the dairy herd and the beef cows, all of whose manure was then put back into the land to fertilize it. The following season, we would rotate and plant blue linseed for cattle feed, followed by red clover to lock in the nitrogen, which would produce a nutrient-rich grass the next year.

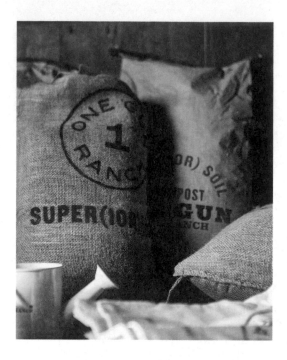

I clearly remember the fields turning from green to blue to red each year. We grew without using any pesticides, which resulted in our food being incredibly delicious and nutritious, and also meant that we were rarely ill. Meanwhile, many of our cattle lived for up to fifteen years (twice or even three times the lifespan of those on industrial farms) and continued to calf and produce milk for most of those years.

Industrial farms do not respect this symbiotic relationship. To keep crops growing out of season, in unnatural locations, and in vast numbers, commercial producers must use a host of toxic pesticides, fertilizers, and genetically modified seeds. These practices have a devastating effect on the soil because the land is used continuously, without rest, and the minerals needed for plant growth (especially nitrogen and phosphorus) diminish more quickly than they can be replaced.

Crops are not rotated in a way that replenishes the soil, intensive plowing eliminates the protective ground cover from the soil surface and destroys root systems that limit soil erosion, and mono-cropping leads to vulnerability to fungi, weeds, insects, and other pests. All of this creates a cycle where yet more fertilizers, pesticides, and genetically engineered crops need to be developed and used, while crop yield declines, soil erosion increases, and pests become more resistant.

The damage does not stop at the boundaries of the farms, as the inorganic fertilizer leaches into underlying groundwater from agricultural fields and runs off into rivers, streams, lakes, and oceans, degrading water quality. Increased pesticide use leads to a loss of biodiversity and the elimination of key species like bees. GMO crops have also had negative effects on beneficial insects like butterflies and bees. Pesticide-related illnesses are endemic among agricultural workers and the rise in allergies is being linked to genetically engineered food. For all of these reasons and more, modern methods of industrial crop production are ultimately unsustainable.

Looking after the soil is essential to our future, and to making delicious, sustainable, and safe food. At One Gun Ranch, we are putting this into practice by farming biodynamically without the use of any harmful chemicals, fertilizers, or pesticides, along with many other farmers across the globe, both large and small scale, and you can, too. No matter how small your space or how little you grow—from a couple of pots of herbs on a windowsill to a kitchen garden—you can use biodynamic methods and participate in this movement. In order to be well, you must eat well. But first, we must grow well.

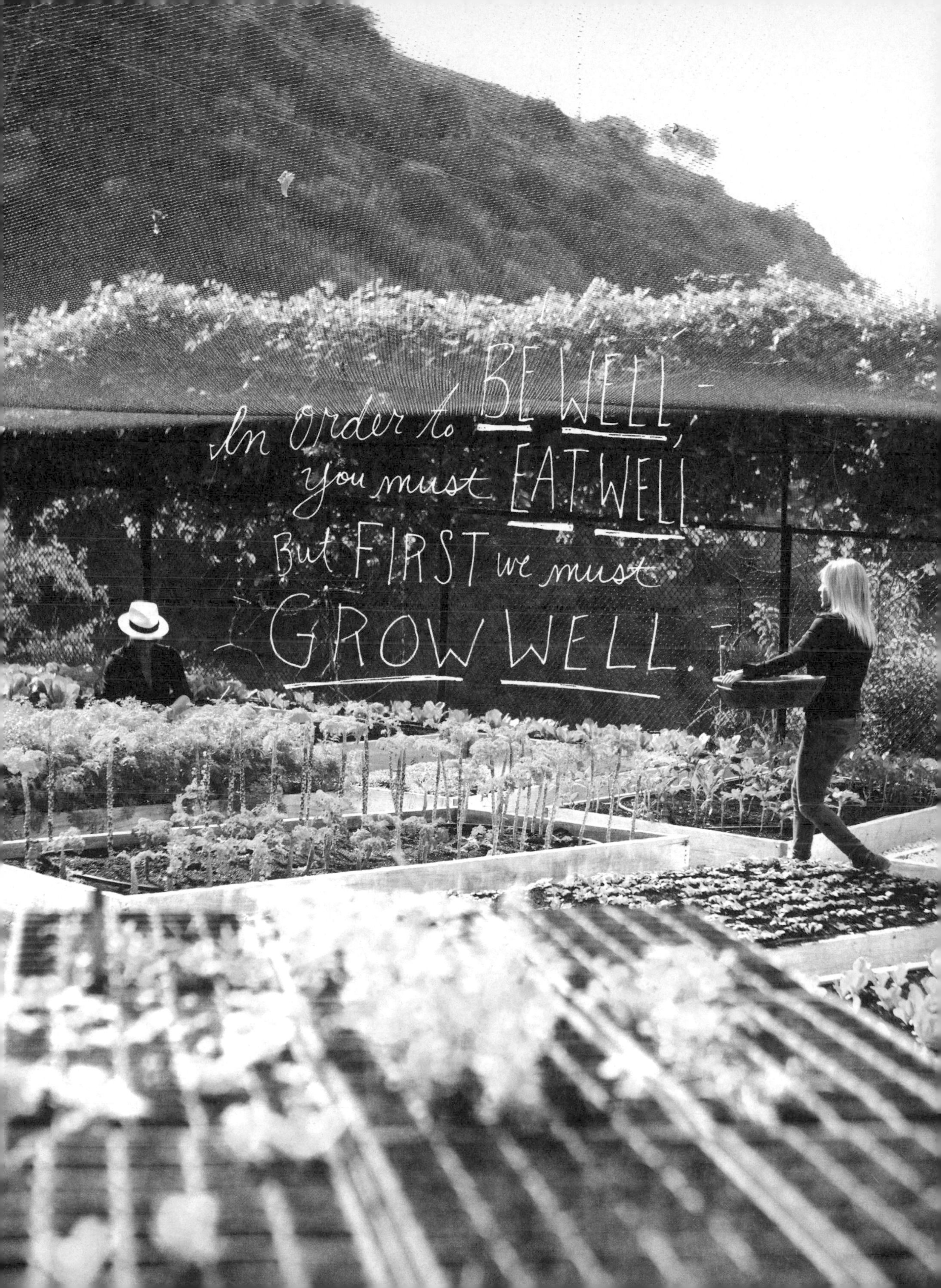

In order to **BE WELL,**
you must **EAT WELL**
But **FIRST** we must
GROW WELL.

Agriculture has to work in HARMONY with the natural Environment.

Organic Farmers DO IT BETTER

A 2014 STUDY IN NEWCASTLE, ENGLAND showed that the organic crops contained amounts of a number of key antioxidants up to 60 percent higher than crops that were conventionally grown. Analyzing 343 studies into the compositional differences between organic and conventional crops, the team found that switching to eating organic fruit, vegetables, and cereals and the foods made from them provided additional antioxidants equivalent to eating between one and two extra portions of fruit and vegetables a day. The study, published in the *British Journal of Nutrition*, also showed significantly lower levels of toxic heavy metals in organic crops.

Furthermore, traces of cadmium, a toxic metal, were found to be almost 50 percent lower in organic crops than in those that were conventionally grown, while nitrogen concentrations were also found to be significantly lower in organic crops (an excess of nitrogen in plants can cause reductions in the levels of other mineral nutrients, such as potassium, calcium, and magnesium). Concentrations of healthy antioxidants, such as polyphenols, were 18 to 69 percent higher in organic crops, and pesticide residues were four times more likely to be found in conventional crops than organic ones. The findings contradicted those of a study commissioned in 2009 by the UK Food Standards Agency (FSA), which found there were no substantial differences or significant nutritional benefits from organic food. The FSA-commissioned study based its conclusions on only 46 publications covering crops, meat, and dairy, while the Newcastle-led meta-analysis was based on data from 343 peer-reviewed publications on composition difference between organic and conventional crops now available.

Put simply, this study shows that organic food is higher in antioxidants and lower in toxic metals and pesticides than conventional crops. Modern industrial growing practices have changed the very composition of our food and while we do not yet know the effects this will have on our health, there is little to recommend conventionally grown produce over organic produce . . . apart from the price. Data from the USDA shows that organically grown produce can be anywhere from 12 to 300 percent the price of conventionally grown fruits and vegetables (www.ers.usda.gov/data-products/organic-prices .aspx). That might be a hard pill to swallow when you are doing your weekly shopping—but, then again, what will be the cost to your health in the long run?

Biodynamic Hero: Patrick Holden

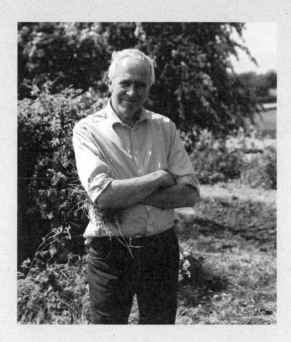

PATRICK HOLDEN IS A true biodynamic hero. He has studied biodynamic agriculture exhaustively and is a champion of organic and biodynamic farming. Patrick was the founding chairman of the British Organic Farmers in 1982; later he joined the Soil Association, where he worked for nearly twenty years leading the development of organic standards and the market for organic foods in Britain. He is currently Patron of the UK Biodynamic Association, is the founding director of the Sustainable Food Trust, and was awarded the CBE for services to organic farming in 2005.

Why is the health of our soil so relevant in the age of modern farming?

Soil is essentially a living biological entity, comprising a vast community of bacteria, fungi, invertebrates, and other higher life forms, many of which species have not yet been named and which coexist in an amazing, complex equilibrium akin to the diversity that exists in a rainforest.

I recently read a book called *Dirt*, by David Montgomery, which shows us that throughout history, the most important single influence on the prosperity and longevity of civilizations lies in their capacity to maintain and build the fertility of their soils. Unfortunately, due to a lack of understanding of these principles, modern intensive farmers have regarded the soil as an inert medium and a recipient for chemical fertilizers and pesticides, the use of which has had a devastating impact on soil health. Half a century of intensive farming has massively reduced soil organic matter, which is the key building block of healthy soil, namely stable carbon in the form of soil organic matter.

Fertilizers and pesticides also act as a biocide, killing off soil bacteria and fungi and thus robbing plants of their capacity to nourish themselves through a remarkable symbiotic relationship wherein sugary saps exude from their roots and nourish the soil organisms upon which the plants depend for their own nutrition—as plants cannot break down soil organic matter, but bacteria and fungi can.

This "mass extinction" of the biology of the soil constitutes an unfolding ecological catastrophe, the impact of which will ultimately threaten the future of mankind if urgent action is not taken to reverse the destructive momentum of modern industrial farming.

Of course it doesn't have to be like that, as I am now finding on my farm in West Wales, where after more than forty years of avoiding the use of any chemical fertilizers or pesticides, our fertility and yields are increasing year on year. I have recently come to a more personal understanding of the earth beneath my feet by imagining the soil of my farm as if it was, as it actually is, the digestive organ of all the plants that are growing there. Without healthy soil, meaning a soil full of the bacteria and fungi upon which plants depend for their nutrition, they cannot thrive. This idea, imagining the soil as the stomach of the plant, gives us a means of understanding its function in an entirely new way—it makes it personal and allows us to apply insights derived from our own digestion of food to that of the soil under our stewardship, whether it be a window box, a garden, or a farm.

What is your approach to growing, buying, and eating and drinking food and wine?

In relation to food growing, our aim has been to move progressively toward self-sufficiency, treating the farm as a self-sustaining ecosystem as described by Rudolf Steiner in his agricultural lectures of 1924, which led to the emergence of biodynamic agriculture. In practice, this means obeying the "law of return": recycling nutrients in the form of animal manures and crop wastes, minimizing the use of non-renewable inputs such as fossil fuels, fertilizers, etc., and moving toward self-sufficiency in animal feeds—in our case for our dairy cows—and recognizing that all plants and animals adapt to the place in which they live over time through extraordinary interactions at a cellular level, now understood through the emerging science of epigenetics.

As an expression of this remarkable principle of adaptation, our herd of Ayrshire dairy cows has been largely homebred since the original introduction of the foundation herd of cows in 1973. It is my direct observation that over time, the descendants of these original animals have adapted in a number of subtle ways to the unique environment of our farm—its weather, its soils, the biodiversity of its vegetation, and even the landscape itself. The arising of scientific understanding of these processes, of continuous co-evolution between all living organisms and the environment in which they live, is one of the great unfolding revelations of our time. For the farmer and grower, it demands a new sensitivity—firstly, to observe the subtle changes of health responses to the farm environment, and secondly, to respond in ways that support the plants or animals in coexisting healthily with their external environment. This is the real meaning of what plant or animal husbandry, farming, and food production is actually about. It is about managing ecosystems, with the person involved being part of the process.

As a general rule, I try to buy food with as sustainable and local a story as I can manage. Like so many areas of modern life, the degree to which I'm able to achieve this varies considerably depending on whether I'm on the farm, the time of year, how busy I am, etc. But my ideal diet would be food that I've grown myself on land near to me, with beautiful fertile soils producing a wide range of in-season vegetables and fruit, as well as fresh eggs, dairy products, and meat.

Of course, most of the time I get nowhere near to this, but just recently, we've had several family meals that actually conform to that prescription! For instance, this week we sat down to Sunday lunch and the menu was whey- and oat-fed slow-roasted shoulder of pork from an Oxford Sandy and Black pig reared on our farm, with *cavolo nero*, and mashed potatoes on the side, all grown in our vegetable patch on the edge of one of our oat fields. This was followed by blackberry-and-apple crumble, again with fruits from the farm, washed down with an elderflower cordial made every June by my wife, Becky.

There is something about eating meals where you know that every ingredient is connected with soil under your care that is not only deeply satisfying but actually more delicious, even more than the wonderful meals I have eaten in well-known restaurants prepared by celebrity chefs (something I have been lucky enough to experience a few times). In saying this, I'm mindful I might be upsetting one or two chefs, but I'm sure they would agree that this is the ultimate eating experience. The reason why meals like this are so satisfying is not just because the ingredients are so fresh, seasonal, and properly grown but also because they are connected to our relationship with place, in the same sense that evidence now emerging shows that the digestion systems of animals, plants, and people are all intimately linked to the unique populations of bacteria and other organisms that form the signature mark of specific ecosystems all over the world. This means that when I eat a meal grown in my own soil, it is actually more digestible and compatible with the ecology of my stomach than something that is shipped from the other side of the world, however well it was grown.

Needless to say, in the twenty-first century, very few of us can rigidly stick to this prescription, and would probably become boring and obsessive if we did, but as a direction of travel for a way of eating, it is surely a good place from which to start. When I go shopping, I try to buy foods which conform to a similar prescription: namely, sustainably produced, local where possible, and ideally from a producer whose identity and particular production system is known to me or described on the packaging. This is increasingly hard to do in supermarkets, since nowadays they are mostly buying "commodity" crops from very large-scale producers whose systems, even if they are based on organic production methods, are not the kind of places that you would want to read about in a children's storybook. So because of this, my priority places to purchase food are box schemes, farmers' markets and CSAs, small retail outlets whose proprietors are dedicated to this philosophy, mail order—including the growing number of online innovative virtual distribution hubs made possible through the Internet—or direct from the farm.

What are you working toward?

Since leaving the Soil Association, I've set up a new organization, the Sustainable Food Trust, with a mission to accelerate the transition towards more sustainable food systems. Although more and more of us are becoming aware that there is a real urgency about the need for fundamental changes to our farming, food systems, and practices, it is often difficult to know how citizens can respond—that is, in which ways can individual action make a difference, both on a personal and societal level. Consequently, the work of the SFT is to promote an improved understanding about these issues. We work in three areas: building collaborative partnerships with individuals and organizations, influencing the research and policy and economic environment for sustainable production, and building public awareness, both about the problems and potential solutions.

What is something you tell people they can do to make a difference?

The most important action is to start with ourselves, based on the understanding that exactly the same laws and principles that manifest in the universe as a whole can be experienced in microcosm in ourselves. This means that any positive action we take, however small, can be amplified through parallel responses from millions of other individuals, thus creating an impact that is potentially more than the sum of the individual parts, and yet at the same time is truly a collective reflection of the action of the individual. This understanding—that everything is connected, that the world is in a state of constant evolution and development, and that each individual has it within their own capacity to understand the beauty of the whole, the disharmony resulting from the industrial age, and the corrective action necessary through one's own personal actions—is a profound truth that is potentially available to all of us if we start with ourselves.

In practice, that means acting as a consumer and a citizen. As a consumer, use your buying power by making sure that all the staple foods you buy have a story behind them that you actually know, including, ideally, the identity of the producers themselves. But make your voice heard as a citizen, too, because right now making our food systems sustainable is not yet on the political agenda. Even President Obama and his family grow and eat organic food at the White House. I should know, because I visited the garden and actually picked spinach for the president's supper, although he might not know that.

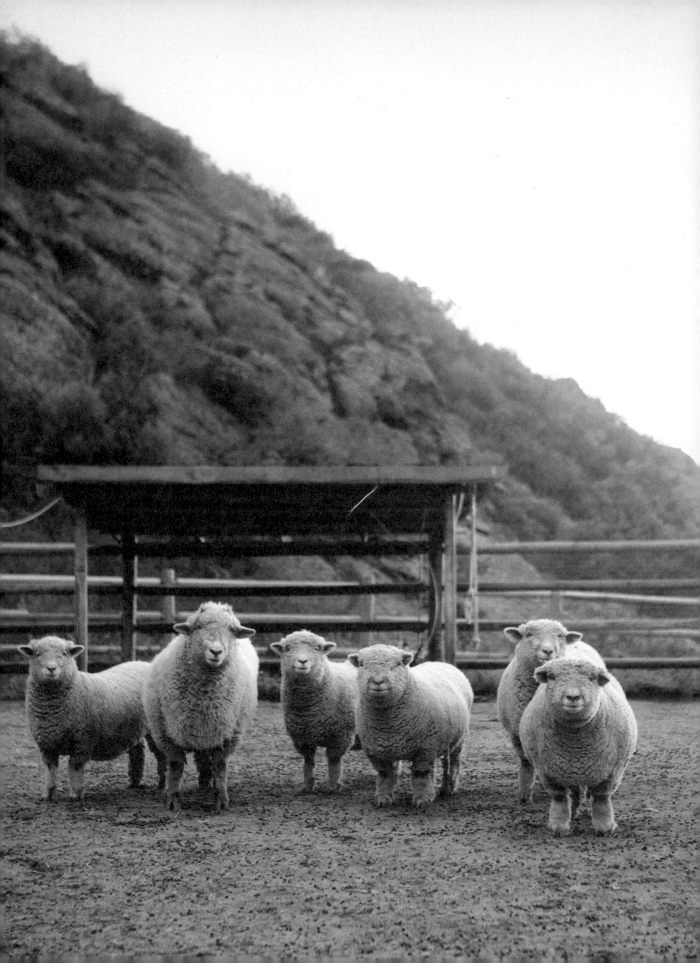

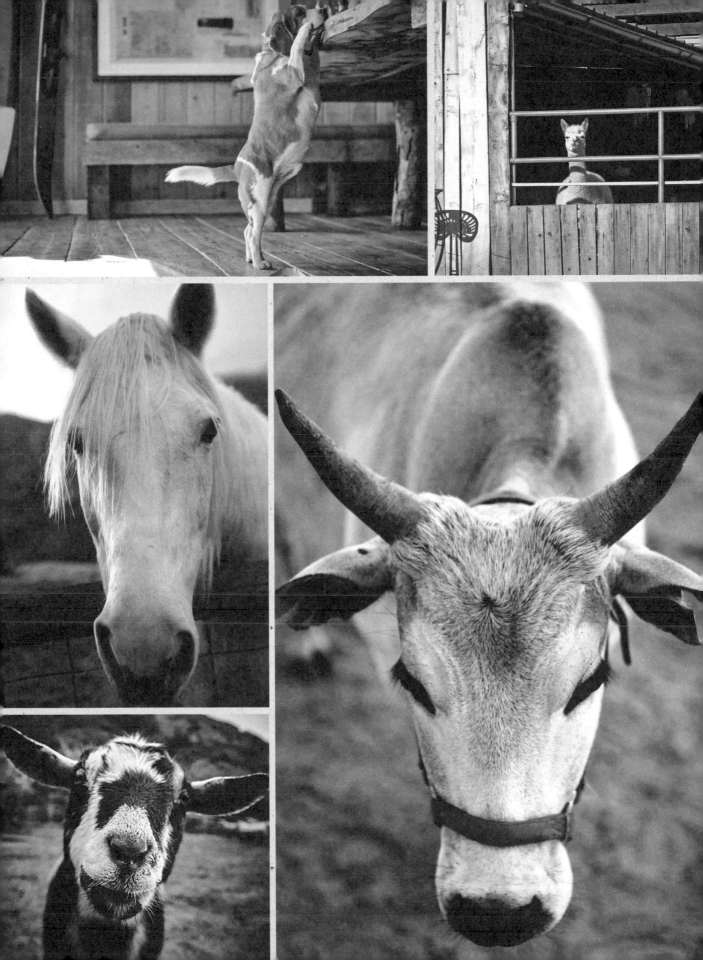

THE TRUE COSTS
OF EATING
Cheap food

THE TRUE COSTS OF cheap foods are hidden. This is the message of the Sustainable Food Trust in the UK, which is carrying out extensive research on the subject under Patrick Holden's leadership. The question he puts to us is: How is it possible that a vegetable grown halfway around the world—which then must be packaged, stored, transported, marketed, and distributed—can cost less than a vegetable grown and sold close to home? The answer is that it doesn't. We must look beyond the cost of our grocery bill to see the bigger picture. The food that lines the supermarket shelves today may be cheap, but tomorrow the enormous cost of the damage the production of that food has wreaked on our environment and our health will prove it to be a false economy.

Today, food prices are on the rise, and the UN predicts a further 40 percent increase over the next decade as the global population increases, resources are depleted, and the effects of climate change become greater. Now is the time when we should be looking toward increasing the diversity and capacity of national production, implementing climate-resilient systems, and building food security.

We are not saying that food has to be expensive to be good. On the contrary, fruit and vegetables found at your local farmers' market are often comparable to those at the supermarket, but stay fresh for longer since they have just been picked.

We encourage the use of every part of the plant. Make a pesto out of those carrot tops or sauté beet greens instead of throwing them out (these delicious parts of the vegetable barely ever make it to the supermarket, as they wilt and rot quickly). And leftovers can always be used to make another meal. Traditional dishes like pot pies are a wonderful way of using up the remains of a Sunday roast; vegetable soups and even green juices or smoothies can be made up of whatever odds and ends you have on hand, like a few pieces of kale, a stalk of celery, an apple, and a sprig of mint.

Organic, locally produced, and seasonal foods are not exclusive or a luxury—they are simply food as it should be. As the bumper sticker reads: "Organic food . . . or as your grandparents called it, 'food.'"

BENEFITS OF A
BIODYNAMIC TOMATO
VERSUS A
COMMERCIALLY PRODUCED TOMATO

BIODYNAMICALLY GROWN TOMATO

Is grown seasonally, and crops are rotated to ALLOW THE SOIL TO MAINTAIN NUTRIENTS. No chemical fertilizers, which damage soil health, are used.

———

Biodynamic compost and companion planting REDUCE THE SUSCEPTIBILITY TO PESTS AND DISEASE, so no chemical pesticides are needed.

———

The tomato is picked when it's ripe and most nutritious and delicious. It's distributed and sold locally, so it is FARM-TO-TABLE FRESH AND HAS A MINIMAL CARBON FOOTPRINT.

———

Organically grown food has been shown to be have HIGHER LEVELS OF ANTIOXIDANTS than commercially produced food.

COMMERCIALLY PRODUCED TOMATO

Is grown in a greenhouse out of season, which requires heating and therefore produces GAS EMISSIONS THAT CAUSE ENVIRONMENTAL DAMAGE.

———

Toxic pesticides are used, causing environmental damage and PESTICIDE-RELATED ILLNESSES, including asthma, cancer, diabetes, and Alzheimer's and Parkinson's disease.

———

The tomato has been genetically modified to have a thicker skin so that mechanical pickers will not damage it. It is picked while still green, so it LACKS THE FLAVOR OF A BEAUTIFUL RIPE TOMATO.

———

The tomato must be transported a great distance, running up "food miles" and creating HIGHER POLLUTION LEVELS THAT DEGRADE AIR QUALITY.

The dirt on
HEALTHY SOIL and
HAPPY BODIES

BEFORE THE Second World War and the advent of widespread intensive, industrial farming, people either grew their own food or bought produce from small, local farms. Before chemical pesticides and synthetic fertilizers were commonplace, one would simply brush the dirt off of fruits and vegetables prior to eating them. As a result, we had much healthier guts and immune systems, thanks to the proliferation of the soil-based organisms and bacteria we ingested. When I was growing up, dirty, funny-looking carrots were a sign of them being honestly farmed and truly delicious vegetables, and we were rarely ill.

Today, most of our pesticide-covered food no longer carries probiotic strains. Instead, we are sold a profusion of lactobacilli and bifidobacterium probiotic products in the form of yogurt, drinks, and supplements, which, while beneficial, actually represent less than 1.5 percent of the range of bacteria found in the human gut; are sensitive to heat, light, and pressure; and don't fare well

in our stomachs. The bacterial strains found in healthy soil, on the other hand, can survive heat, pressure, and stomach acid, and thrive in the human gut, helping to regulate the immune system, reduce inflammation, break down food, and assist with detoxification.

Geophagia, or the deliberate consumption of earth, soil, or clay, was common in Europe until the nineteenth century—the simple explanation for the practice being that soil contains minerals such as calcium, sodium, and iron, which support energy production and other vital human biological processes. There is a Danish saying: "To stay healthy, you have to eat seven pounds of dirt a year." While we are not suggesting you eat dirt, there is no denying that with all of the carbon, nitrogen, minerals, and vitamins in our body derived from soil through the food that we eat, we are not just nourished by the soil, our health is intrinsically linked to its health.

Natural microbial substances from soil bacteria are also at the root of most antibiotic drugs developed during the past century, including lifesaving medicines such as

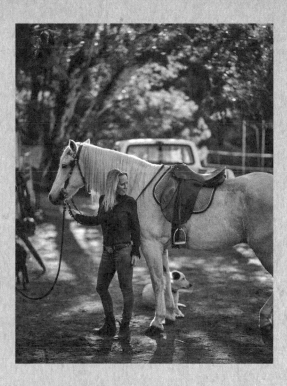

penicillin. But only about 1 percent of these organisms can be grown in a lab—they only thrive in healthy soil. Furthermore, widespread use of antibiotics in the twentieth century has led to pathogens that have developed a resistance to these drugs.

Healthy soil also contains fulvic acid, a natural compound found in humus—the dark, organic material that forms in soil when plant matter decays, created by the process of microbes breaking down the organic matter. A powerful, natural electrolyte, fulvic acid aids the absorption of minerals and vitamins into the soil by enriching it and encouraging healthy plant growth. Containing seventy-two trace minerals, fulvic acid has the ability to balance cells within the body by either giving or taking electrons as needed and destroying free radicals, protecting cells from oxidative damage; it enhances the absorption of vitamins and minerals and aids in the production of enzymes. It can also help regulate the thyroid, thymus glands, and immune system and increase the ability of cells to discharge toxic metals. Fertilizers, pesticides, herbicides, and fungicides all hinder fulvic acid from forming in the soil, leaving it void of this vital mineral, and therefore the natural ingestion of plant-based fulvic acid in the human diet has decreased in the last century.

New research is also showing that soil can affect our mood. While many people find gardening therapeutic and love getting elbow-deep in dirt, a recent study carried out at Bristol University found that a strain of bacterium in soil called *Mycobacterium vaccae* can actually trigger the release of serotonin, a neurotransmitter that elevates mood and decreases anxiety. The bacterium has also been found to improve cognitive function. A further study at Sage Colleges in New York found that just inhaling *M. vaccae* when out taking a walk in the wild or rooting around in the garden, or ingesting it through eating vegetables had a similar effect on mood.

Mounting scientific evidence is backing up what we have already learned through our experiments with biodynamic compost at One Gun Ranch: Healthy soil is the key to our health. As American nature writer Michael Pollan recently noted, "Some researchers believe that the alarming increase in autoimmune diseases in the West may owe to a disruption in the ancient relationship between our bodies and their 'old friends'—the [bacteria] with whom we coevolved." Putting these microbes back into the soil and back into our bodies can be achieved through adopting a biodynamic lifestyle.

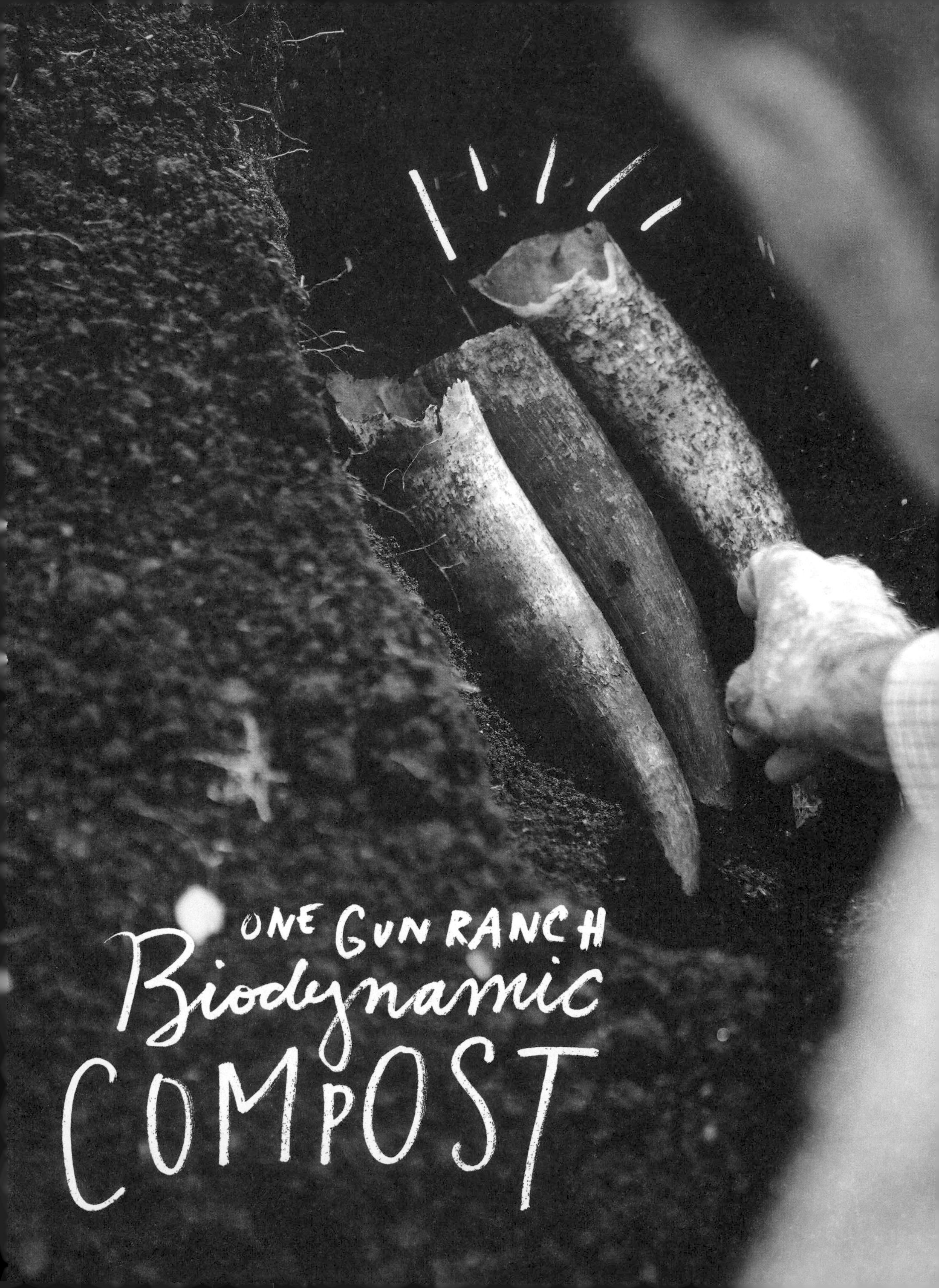

ONE GUN RANCH
Biodynamic
COMPOST

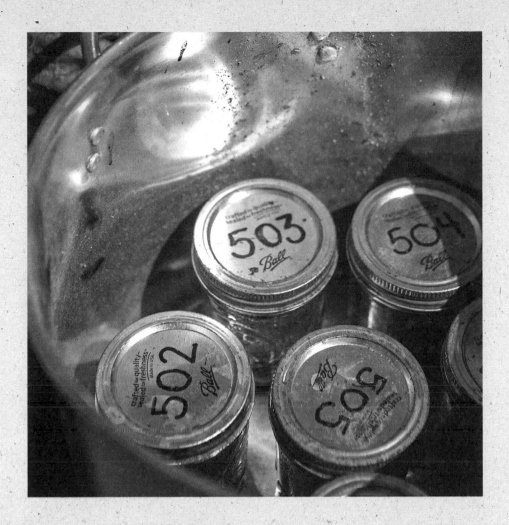

BECAUSE BIODYNAMIC AGRICULTURE TREATS the soil as a living organism rather than just a support system for crops, at One Gun Ranch we seek to feed the soil and revitalize it using biodynamic compost that we make according to a technique devised by Rudolf Steiner, the father of biodynamics himself, with the help of our resident biodynamic expert Jack McAndrew.

After we met Jack at a Malibu Agricultural Society meeting, he introduced us to his rich, nutrient-loaded, black gold that is recognized in agricultural circles—whether fans of biodynamic methods or not—as the finest quality compost available, capable of growing the most vibrant, nutritious food on Earth. He has been overseeing our compost-making process ever since, and we know that our produce looks, feels, and tastes different from anything else grown nearby. The colors are brighter, sharper, and crisper, and the taste is exciting, full of vitality, moisture, and clarity of flavor. It's also so full of nutrients it tastes alive!

MAKE YOUR OWN
COMPOST

THE AVERAGE HOUSEHOLD throws away around two pounds of organic waste each day—and if you're eating a healthy diet full of fresh produce, you might be throwing out even more. So, if you have a garden or backyard and would like to start growing some of your own food, you should think about starting your own compost pile to make the most of that waste and to start your own mini closed-loop system within your household. You may not grow all of the food you eat, but any foods leftover from your meal preparations can be put to work in the compost pile, and then back into the soil.

A compost pile needs to be outside, and you need room for a three-foot-square structure to house it. Apart from that, it's a pretty simple process.

WHAT YOU WILL NEED

Compost bin or tumbler for the garden

Bags of organic soil or compost

Pitchfork or shovel

Compost crock or pail to keep by the kitchen sink

While there are many types of compost bins and tumblers available to buy online and in garden stores, you can also build one quite easily using chicken wire, hardware cloth, and a simple wooden frame (a slatted box about three feet in every dimension is a good small starter bin). This is the best way to compost. Tuck the bin away somewhere at the bottom of the garden, out of view of the neighbors, and make sure to cover it with wire or a plastic tarp so as to avoid any problems with scavenging animals.

To start your pile, line the bottom of your compost bin with a one-inch layer of soil or compost, then cover it with an inch of green or brown organic material, such as garden cuttings, mown grass, or raked leaves. You are ready to start adding your kitchen scraps.

FEED YOUR COMPOST PAIL

KEEP YOUR COMPOST PAIL in the kitchen in a convenient place so that you can throw in any scraps or peelings that come from food preparation instead of throwing them in the trash or down the garbage disposal.

WHAT GOES IN

- A wide range of vegetable or fruit peelings and general scraps are appropriate for the compost pile.

- Salad leaves that have wilted or have started to rot, bad fruit, limp carrots, moldy berries, eggshells, coffee grounds, tea leaves, dead flowers.

- Bread, rice, and even pasta.

- To provide a good nitrogen balance, shredded paper, newspapers, and wood chips should also be added to the mix.

WHAT DOES NOT GO IN

- Do not add meat or dairy products to your compost.

Periodically dump your compost pail into your pile, then cover the food scraps with a layer of soil and then a layer of garden

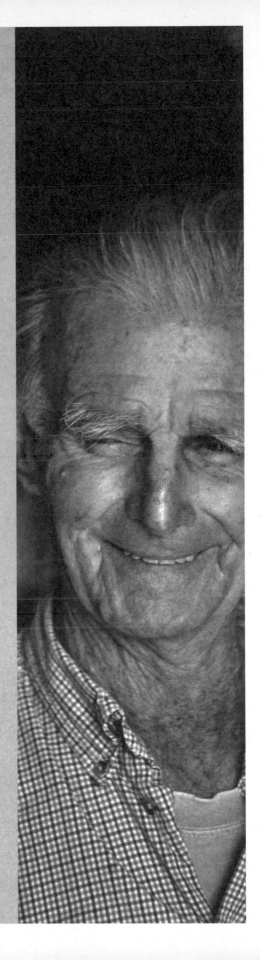

Jack McAndrew's
BIODYNAMIC COMPOST

A NEW MOON OR a full moon or your birthday or your husband or wife's birthday . . . there is never a bad time to make compost. Making this compost is very simple: All one needs to begin is one ton of organic milk cow manure and two bales of alfalfa. The ratio of carbon to nitrogen must be twenty to one. For the breakdown process to happen between the manure and the alfalfa, an herbal bacterial starter must be added, just like the starter in a loaf of bread. We have to have a critical mass of ten tons, and it has to reach a temperature of 130°F (54°Celsius). This is not something you can do in your backyard!

First, we put down a layer of manure and then an equal layer of alfalfa and manure—carbon and nitrogen, carbon and nitrogen—and so on. The moisture content is very important: if it's too dry, the pile will get too hot and burn up; if it's too wet, it becomes anaerobic and can't breathe. The right balance is achieved by fine-tuning with additions of either manure or the grass. Finally, the pile is sprayed with a biodynamic herbal bacteria mixture made of chamomile, oak bark, valerian, stinging nettle, yarrow, and dandelion to call forth elements from the cosmos into the compost pile. After about six months, it will be nicely dark and crumbly with a forest-like aroma.

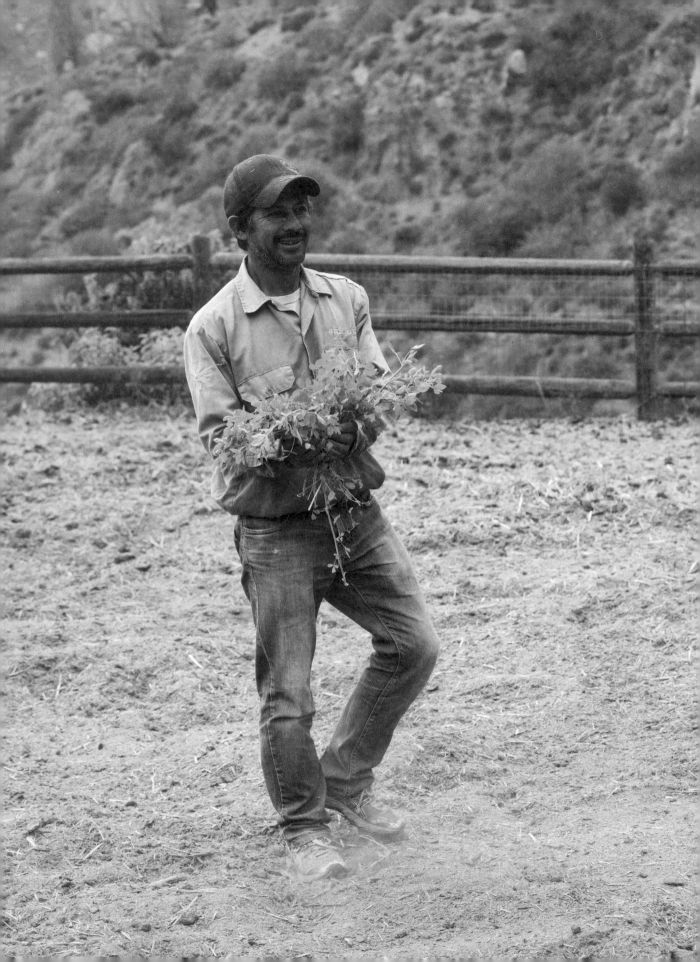

cuttings or leaves again. Ask your neighbors if they have any food scraps or garden waste they would like to throw in, too.

After several weeks, the scraps will begin to break down and you can give the pile a quick turn with a pitchfork or shovel in order to aerate it. You should continue to add to the pile and aerate it every couple of weeks. If you want to, and have some at hand, you can add organic manure into the mix to activate the composting process. Adding hay is also a great way to aerate the pile if you are not going to be able to turn it manually for a while. Once your compost pile is established, you can just start mixing your scraps in. When the bin is full, leave it for another few months to allow the entire pile to fully decompose and turn into a rich, dark, crumbly homemade compost.

Use this biodynamic compost for everything from houseplants (just a handful in a potted houseplant will rejuvenate it) to your window boxes, raised beds, and kitchen garden for the most nutritious, delicious biodynamic produce.

HOW WE KEEP THE SOIL HEALTHY
BIODYNAMIC PREPARATIONS

WHILE CROP ROTATION and companion planting are excellent ways to nurture, nourish, and keep the soil alive and healthy, biodynamic farmers also use a variety of "preparations," developed by Steiner, to help regulate biological processes and enhance and strengthen the life forces on the farm.

Steiner concocted nine different preparations to enhance soil quality and stimulate plant life using a combination of mineral, plant, and animal extracts. These include quartz, cow manure, cow horns, yarrow flowers, chamomile blossoms, stinging nettle, oak bark, dandelion blossoms, and valerian flowers that are aged or fermented and then applied in small amounts to the compost piles, the soil, or even directly onto the plants.

Perhaps of all the unusual aspects of biodynamics, these preparations are met with the most skepticism, as the process of making them is very alchemical, even mystical. Some preparations are packed into cows' horns and buried for six months, others are stitched into a stag's bladder and hung in the branches of a tree facing the sun before being buried. A lot of animal organs are used in the making of the preparations, but we must remember that in Steiner's day, offal was an everyday part of country life, and cooking and using it would not have been thought of as bizarre or "gross." It's primal stuff, but there is also real chemistry at work here: Some of the preparations moderate the temperature curve of the thermophilic stage in the compost pile, slowing the temperature's ascent, keeping the peak temperature slightly lower, and holding the warmth in the pile longer; others act as a homeopathic remedy for fungal diseases.

Preparations are an integral part of what makes biodynamic compost unique. At the Ranch we have preparations 500 and 501 (see next page) buried around the property, and we have also created our own Compost Tea. Biodynamic preparations can be bought online from trusted biodynamic sources, such as the Josephine Porter Institute, and used in the garden; or you can try some of these DIY preps at home.

BIODYNAMIC
COMPOST PREPARATIONS

Nettle (stems from *Urtica dioica*): stimulates soil health

Yarrow (flowers from *Achillea millefolium*): encourages trace element uptake for nutrition

Chamomile (flowers from *Matricaria chamomilla*): stabilizes nitrogen and stimulates plant growth

Oak Bark (bark from *Quercus robur*): provides healing forces to combat plant disease

Dandelion (flowers from *Taraxacum officinale*): stimulates relationship between silica and potassium to attract cosmic forces into the soil

BIODYNAMIC PREP 500

PREP 500 IS THE CORNERSTONE of biodynamic farming, made each fall by packing cow manure into cow horns and then burying them for six months until the manure has fermented. Earthy, sweet-smelling, and bursting with rich, soil-enhancing nutrients, the prep is then stirred into pure rainwater for an hour to simulate the Earth's rotation and add energy to the prep. This solution is then sprayed onto the soil directly to improve the soil structure and microbiological activity of the earth by stimulating the soil's own bacteria and life source, promoting the richness of the soil and enabling nutrients to permeate the plant roots for healthy plant growth.

BIODYNAMIC PREP 501—QUARTZ

IN THIS PREP, FINELY ground quartz is crushed into a paste, packed inside a cow horn, and buried over the summer to ferment. When the horns are dug up in the fall, within is a paste that has fermented, matured, and intensified to the extent that only half a teaspoon is needed per acre. As with Prep 500, the paste is stirred into pure rainwater for an hour to simulate the earth's rotation and add energy to the prep. This radiating liquid is sprayed on the leaves of the plants to stimulate, regulate, and promote healthy growth.

BIODYNAMIC PREP 502—YARROW

THIS PREP IS MADE from yarrow flowers harvested at peak bloom, then dried and sewn into a stag's bladder. The bladder is hung in the branches of a tree for the summer, with direct exposure to the sun. In the fall, the bladder is buried in the soil for the winter, and then the yarrow is removed from the bladder and immediately inserted into the compost pile the following spring. Yarrow influences plant reproduction and growth by stimulating sulfur intake. The whole yarrow plant can also be used to make a liquid manure for areas where potassium and selenium are needed in the soil. The plant is also useful as a border plant for garden beds, aiding general fertility, and is excellent as a nourishing tea.

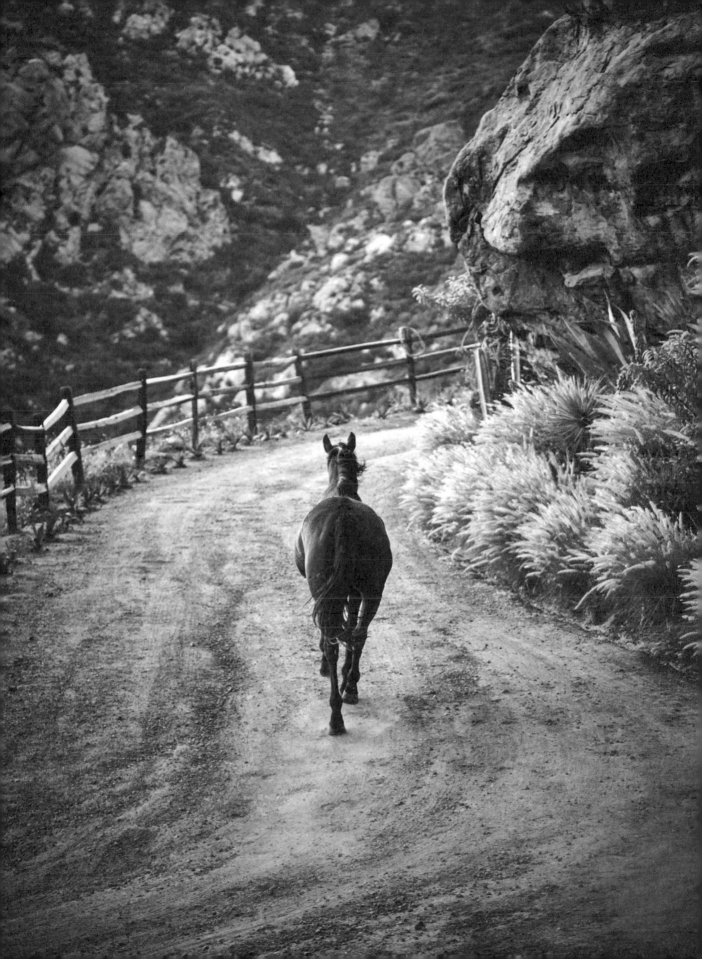

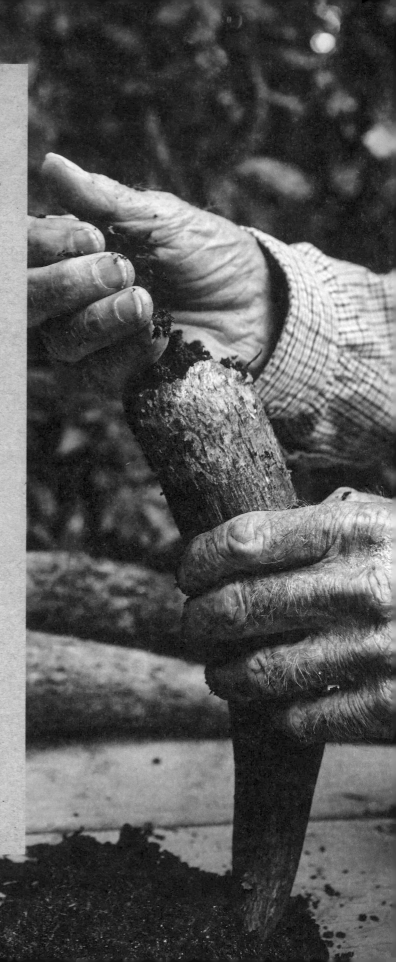

DIY

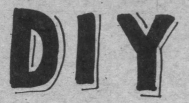

Nutritious
NETTLE TEA
FOR HEALTHY SOIL

WILD NETTLES THRIVE IN moist woodlands and thickets, along rivers, and along partially shaded trails. Next time you are out on a walk or hike, bring along a pair of shears, gardening gloves (nettles are covered with tiny hairs that sting the skin and cause redness and irritation), and a bag to collect the nettles.

To make a tea for your soil, simply add water to the leaves—about 2 cups of water to 1 cup of leaves—and heat to a near boil, then reduce the heat and simmer for a couple of minutes.

Remove from the heat, leave the tea to cool unstrained, then pour through a strainer and into a spray bottle. Spray directly onto the soil before planting seeds or seedlings. Spray regularly to enliven the soil, as well.

ONE GUN RANCH
COMPOST TEA

MAXIMIZE YOUR PRECIOUS biodynamic compost by making this simple tea.

Fill a 5-gallon bucket with water. Add a scoop of compost to the bucket, stir, and then allow it to stand for at least an hour to really homeopathically infuse the water. Distribute evenly over your pots and garden beds.

BIODYNAMIC PREP 503—CHAMOMILE

THIS PREP IS MADE from chamomile flowers harvested at peak bloom, dried, and then stuffed into cow intestines, which are buried in the soil over the winter and then inserted into the compost pile the following spring. Chamomile contributes to plant reproduction and growth by stabilizing nitrogen within the compost, simultaneously influencing the calcium and potassium content. It also promotes a good breakdown of proteins in the compost to humic substances, which are the major organic constituents of soil.

BIODYNAMIC PREP 504—STINGING NETTLE

THIS PREP IS MADE from whole stinging nettle leaves that are harvested in early summer, dried, and then buried in the soil in an unglazed earthenware pot until the following spring, when they are removed and inserted into the compost pile. Stinging nettle is thought to "enliven" the soil by influencing sulfur, potassium, calcium, and iron content.

BIODYNAMIC PREP 505—OAK BARK

MADE FROM THE BARK of the English oak tree (*Ouercus robur*), this prep encourages calcium and phosphorus absorption into the earth. It also helps prevent fungal disease and, when used over time, will raise the pH levels in the soil. The oak bark is grated into a fine powder, then packed tightly into a clean, washed animal skull, preferably that of a cow or sheep. The oak-filled skull is then submerged in a barrel of water, which is filled with plenty of rotting vegetation, such as leaves and grass clippings. The barrel should be placed under a downspout where rainwater can refresh it.

BIODYNAMIC PREP 506—DANDELION

TO MAKE THIS PREP, dandelion flowers must be cut first thing in the morning during early to midsummer and then dried. In the autumn, the flowers are stuffed into a cow's mesentery, the sac that holds its digestive organs, and buried in an unglazed earthenware jar until spring. This preparation stimulates the potassium and silica bacteria in the soil and aids in the flowering and fruiting processes of plants.

BIODYNAMIC PREP 507—VALERIAN

FOR THIS PREP, ONE PART fresh Valerian flowers is ground up in a mortar with a pestle and then placed in a jar with four parts pure water. The mixture is allowed to ferment on a windowsill for seven days. Filter the extracted valerian and use 1 teaspoon per 2 gallons of pure water to spray all over the compost heap, stimulating the phosphorus process and aiding the phosphorus-activating bacteria in the soil. If sprayed onto fruit blossoms in spring, it will also provide protection from a late frost. Experiment making it yourself!

PLANTING, HARVESTING & EATING
ACCORDING TO THE
Cycles of the Moon

The Moon replenishes the Earth; when she approaches it, she fills all bodies, while when she recedes, she empties them. —PLINY THE ELDER

BIODYNAMIC FARMERS PLANT and harvest their crops according to the cycles of the Moon. Every month, as the Moon ascends, descends, and orbits around the Earth, passing through the constellations of the zodiac, its magnetic pull affects not only our tides, but also the Earth's water table and moisture levels into the soil.

Moon-planting recognizes that different plants benefit from being sown during different phases of the Moon, as the moisture levels in the ground change. This is a practice that has existed for centuries and has been traced back to ancient Babylon, Egypt, China, India, and Greece, when early civilizations were working on establishing accurate calendars with which to organize the planting and harvesting of their crops.

Biodynamic methods also use a combination of lunar and astrological calendars to determine the best times to sow, cultivate, and harvest various plants. Crops are organized according to four key lunar variables: Moon phase, Moon path, Moon constellation, and plant aspect—and four categories of days defined both by specific, dominant parts of the plant—root, flower, leaf, and fruit. Each plant category also has a corresponding element—earth, air, water, and fire—and associated zodiac signs. Roots are ruled by earth, flowers by air, leaves by water, and fruit by fire. Additionally, Taurus, Virgo, and Capricorn are earth signs; Gemini, Libra, and Aquarius are air signs; Cancer, Scorpio, and Pisces are water signs; and Aries, Leo, and Sagittarius are fire signs. According to biodynamics, plants should be sown according to the corresponding element of the zodiac through which the Moon is passing. We take all of this information and create a biodynamic planting calendar to show us the ideal days to sow, harvest, and eat our roots, flowers, leaves, and fruits.

CROP
CATEGORIES

ROOT DAYS

ASSOCIATED WITH THE EARTH SIGNS (Capricorn, Taurus, and Virgo), these days are best for cultivating potatoes and other root crops including carrots, beets, parsnips, onions, garlic, and radishes. Root crops harvested during Root Days produce good yields and storage quality.

LEAF DAYS

ASSOCIATED WITH THE WATER SIGNS (Pisces, Scorpio, and Cancer), these days are best for sowing salads, spinach, leaf herbs like mint and basil, leeks, cabbages, cauliflower, fennel, and grasses. But note, while these leafy plants should be sown and tended to on Leaf Days, they are best harvested and stored during Fruit and Flower Days.

FLOWER DAYS

ASSOCIATED WITH THE AIR SIGNS (Gemini, Libra, and Aquarius), these days are best for cultivating flowers, flowering herbs like lavender and chamomile, flowering hedges, and flowering trees. All flowering plants should be sown and tended to on Flower Days—and cut then, too, so they remain fresh and retain their color for longer.

FRUIT DAYS

ASSOCIATED WITH THE FIRE SIGNS (Aries, Sagittarius, and Leo), these days are best for sowing all fruits, like strawberries, raspberries, apples, and plums, as well as fruiting vegetables like tomatoes, cucumbers, zucchini, beans, peas, bell peppers, pumpkins, and broccoli. Fruit plants are best harvested on Fruit Days.

Each month we sow, harvest, and eat our root, leaf, flower, and fruit foods on the days when they are enhanced by the Moon and the planets.

CROP
VARIABLES

MOON PHASE

DURING A WAXING MOON, the Earth is exhaling. This is the time to sow non-root plants. During a waning Moon, the Earth is inhaling. This is the time to water and fertilize crops.

MOON PATH

DURING AN ASCENDING MOON, sap is drawn up. This is the time to graft, and to harvest non-root plants. During a descending Moon, sap is drawn down. This is the time to plant or prune crops.

MOON CONSTELLATION

THE PASSAGE OF THE Moon in front of the constellations emphasizes the effects of the Moon phase and Moon path on different parts of the plant, giving rise to the root, flower, leaf, and fruit days explained below.

PLANT ASPECT

BIODYNAMIC FARMING TAKES INTO account what aspect of the plant needs to be stimulated.

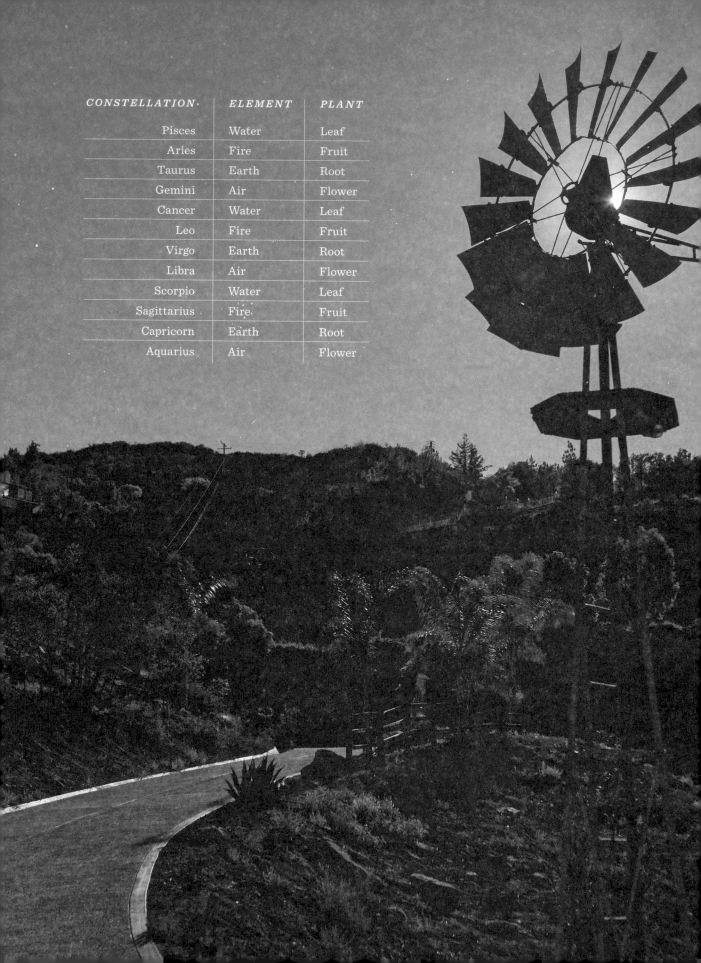

CONSTELLATION	ELEMENT	PLANT
Pisces	Water	Leaf
Aries	Fire	Fruit
Taurus	Earth	Root
Gemini	Air	Flower
Cancer	Water	Leaf
Leo	Fire	Fruit
Virgo	Earth	Root
Libra	Air	Flower
Scorpio	Water	Leaf
Sagittarius	Fire	Fruit
Capricorn	Earth	Root
Aquarius	Air	Flower

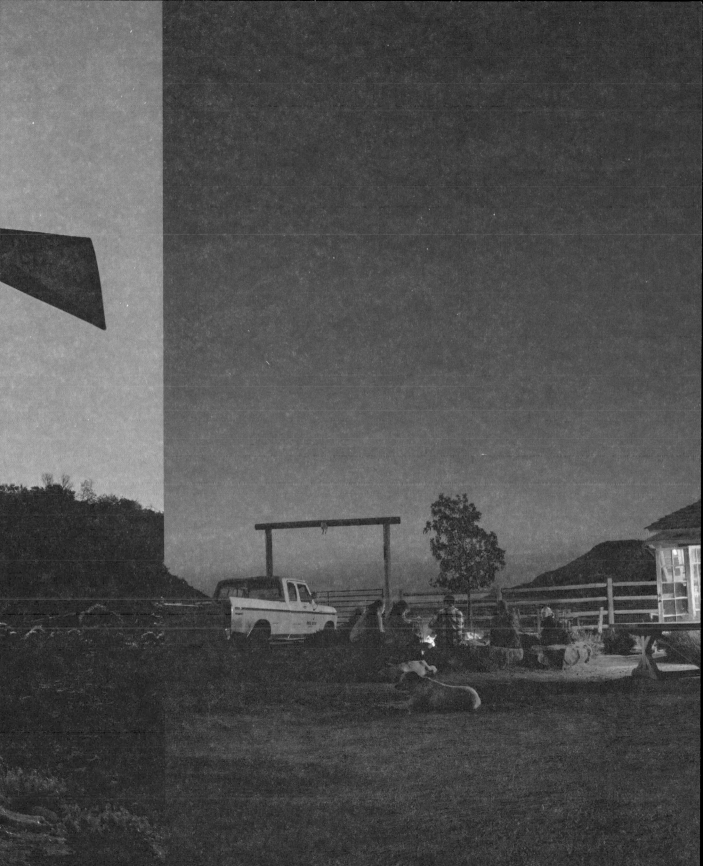

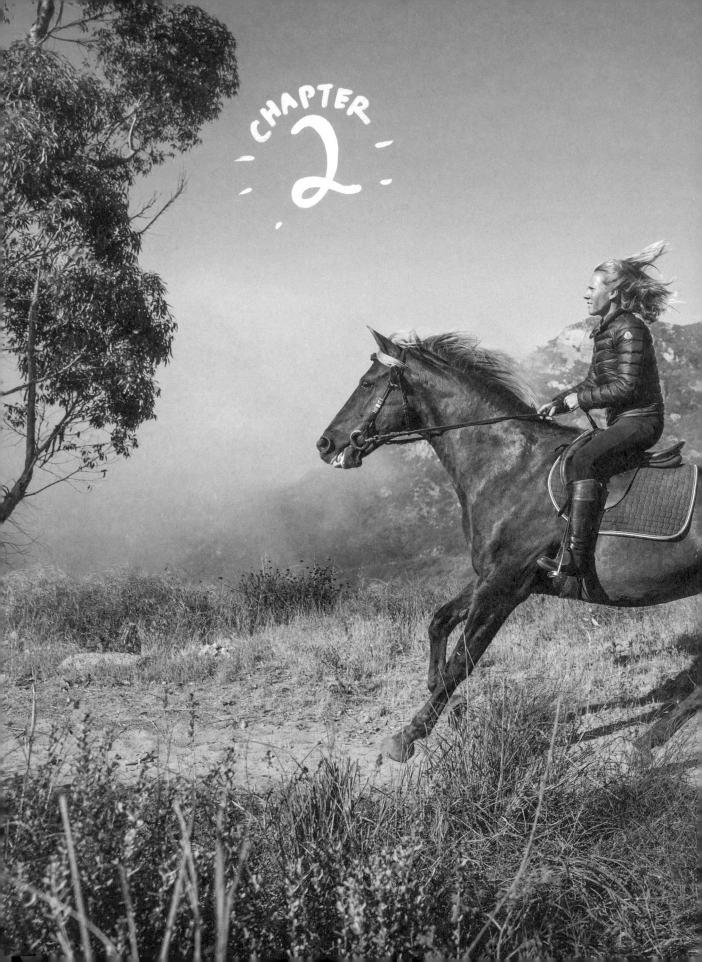

CHAPTER

2

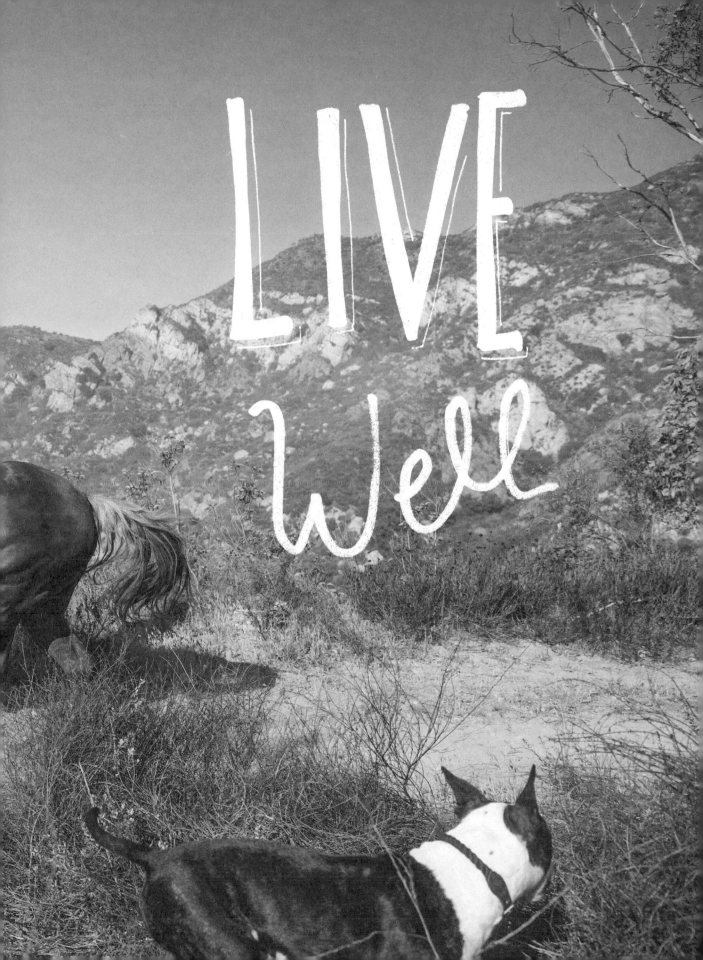

RISING with the SUN

All humans, animals, microbes, and even plants have a built-in circadian rhythm. Circadian rhythms are physical, mental, and behavioral changes responding to external cues—mainly daylight and darkness.

THE HUMAN BRAIN'S INTERNAL circadian clock, which we often call our body clock, is in effect using sunlight to naturally synchronize itself each day to within just a few minutes of the Earth's twenty-four-hour rotation cycle. This is the reason that traveling across time zones causes "jet lag," as any disruption to the cycle throws your body clock off and leaves you feeling disoriented. Eventually, using daylight, your body is then able to adjust its circadian rhythms to the new environment and synchronize itself again. In modern life, the majority of the disruptions to our internal body clocks are related to our environment and lifestyle habits. Artificial light, televisions, computer screens, and mobile devices all keep us stimulated much later and/or longer than in a more natural setting and disrupt our circadian rhythms.

Humans are diurnal animals, which means we are naturally active during the daytime, and our natural circadian rhythms reflect this. Various studies have shown that after melatonin production stops, around 7 a.m., our energy increases, hitting a peak between 10 a.m. and noon every day, followed by a low at around 3 p.m. Alertness then tends to increase again, hitting a second peak around 6 p.m., and then declines for the rest of the evening until melatonin production kicks in around 9 p.m. Alertness hits the very lowest point between 2 a.m. and 3:30 a.m. before increasing again, and the cycle repeats itself. A number of studies have also shown that a short period of sleep during the day, a "power nap" or *siesta*, around 3 p.m., when energy is at its lowest, can decrease stress and improve productivity.

But circadian rhythms are about more than knowing when it's time to wake up or go to sleep. This internal clock also regulates our appetite, alertness, core body temperature, brain wave activity, hormone production, glucose and insulin levels, cell regeneration, and many other vital biological activities. The most important hormones affected by our circadian clock are melatonin (which is produced in the pineal gland in the brain, and causes drowsiness and a lowering of our body temperature, helping us to sleep) and cortisol (which is produced in the adrenal gland, and is used to form glucose or blood sugar, and helps to enable anti-stress and anti-inflammatory functions in the body). Abnormal circadian rhythms are therefore often associated with obesity, diabetes, depression, bipolar disorder, and seasonal affective disorder.

At One Gun Ranch, as on most farms, we get up when the cock crows, just as the sun starts to rise, and often find ourselves turning in by 10 p.m. We have a routine that is defined by the Sun and the Moon, and it makes us feel at our best. In Ayurvedic medicine, it is believed that a daily routine, or *dincharya,* merging one's daily cycle with the natural cycle of the Sun, Moon, Earth, and other planets in the solar system, is the key to a balanced, healthy life. The Ayurvedic rishis honor *dincharya* as the healing force, stronger than any other curative medicines. Traditional Chinese medicine also believes that the flow of the vital energy, or *qi*, through the various organ systems (called meridians) in the body is governed by circadian rhythm, and that observing and respecting this rhythm allows our body to function more efficiently and defend against illness.

An EDIBLE Education

A CORNERSTONE OF STEINER'S PHILOSOPHY is that we must act as stewards of the land. But in order to do this, one must first learn about the land; and another crucial part of the biodynamic movement is to share that knowledge. So since day one, we've opened the Ranch to education and charities. Alice Waters is the inspiration behind our educational program, because we believe, as she does, that how we eat can change the world. Alice gave me the seeds to start this project, and her Edible Schoolyard in Berkeley is the model for our learning initiatives in Malibu.

At the Ranch, we like to provide a haven for children and adults to learn about layering compost, planting flats, and transplanting and harvesting the corn, beans, squash, peppers, herbs, vegetables, pumpkins, and wide variety of leafy greens and micro greens that we grow here. Student groups visit the Ranch regularly for a morning in our outdoor classroom, learning biodynamic gardening principles, the importance of fresh and healthy food, and composting and recycling methods. All visitors have the opportunity to try their hand at planting, or experience a healthy-cooking demonstration in our campfire kitchen. Each time we start a new compost pile, we invite groups up to watch the process. Hundreds have come through our Secret Garden and planted lettuces, kale, and edible flowers. Many of these children have never done any kind of gardening or planting before, and it's a joy to witness their openness to the experience.

We have also been very community driven when it comes to education, with our goal of building sustainable, "farm to fork" collaborations both in Malibu and around the city. We have been working with Jane Semel and Wendy Slusser, two of our biodynamic heroes, at UCLA to create a "living amphitheater" on the campus in Los Angeles, part of their Healthy Campus Initiative. We started by installing garden beds among the existing seating, which are planted with produce for the on-campus restaurants, and we designed a living sort of padded seat-back of hanging rosemary and thyme on the terraces that provides a sensory experience for the audience as they rest against it. Going forward, the student garden will provide seedlings for the amphitheater, and a composting program is in development.

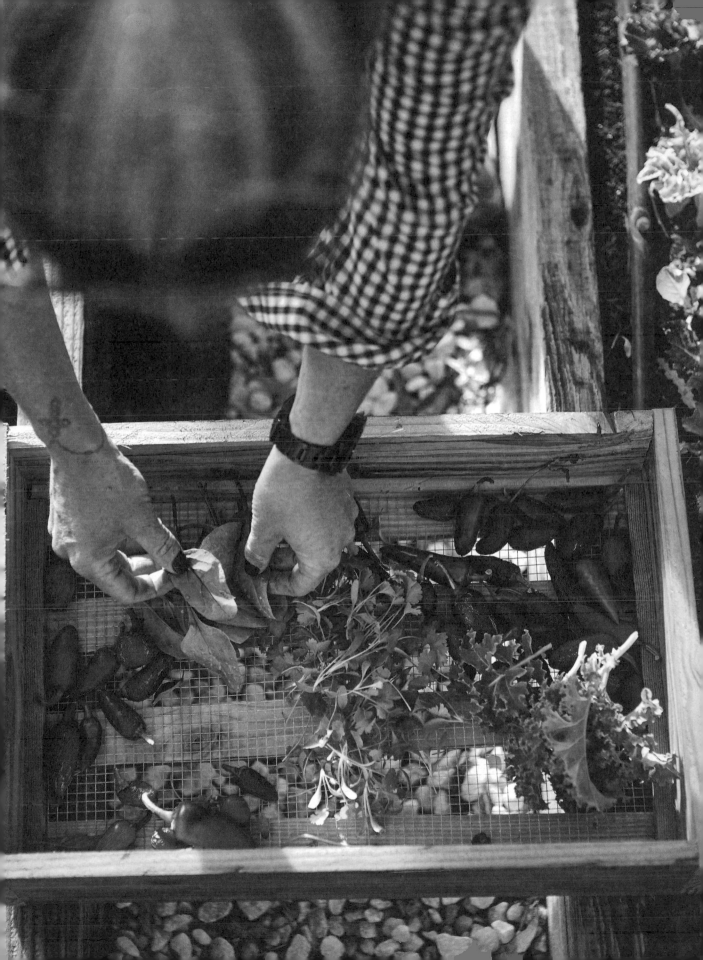

BIODYNAMIC HERO:
Dr. Wendelin Slusser

I FIRST MET WENDY SLUSSER, the associate vice provost for the UCLA Healthy Campus Initiative, at an environmental event here in Malibu. We were instantly drawn to each other. She's very grounded, incredibly warm, and truly practices what she preaches, which is really all about healthy eating and movement.

It was Wendy's work promoting fruit and vegetable consumption among low-income elementary schoolchildren in the Los Angeles Unified School District that triggered national legislation and led to First Lady Michelle Obama's Let's Move Salad Bars to Schools (LMSB2S) program. She is currently the lead on the UCLA Healthy Campus Initiative and heads the nutrition pod for the Initiative.

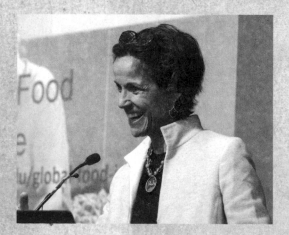

What is your approach to growing, buying, and eating food and wine?

I strive to walk the talk. I buy from farmers' markets, grow my food when and where I can, and direct my purchases to organic products. I am an omnivore but minimize my meat intake and mostly eat nuts, legumes, fruits, vegetables, and eggs. I recognize that it is a process and I admit to not always eating organically—and I love to bake.

What are you working toward?

I strive to work with others to impact each level of the health pyramid, exploring how we can promote the health of others and a healthy food system and, in turn, our own health.

What is something you tell people they can do to make a difference?

Let your passion be your vocation, and along the way, observe, reflect, study, and take action. I usually end my "advice" talks with this quote from His Holiness the Dalai Lama: "With realization of one's own potential and self-confidence in one's ability, one can build a better world."

BIODYNAMIC HERO:
JANE SEMEL

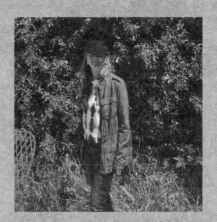

JANE SEMEL IS A FORCE of nature. Annie has known her for fifteen years and has worked with her often. I met her on the same night I met Wendy, and I was immediately blown away. She's truly someone who makes things happen. Her spirit is incredibly courageous and wonderfully fierce. She just says it like it is, and has the ability to simplify and really see the big picture with issues. The issue she is most passionate about is mental and physical health and how they relate to nutrition.

Jane and her husband, Terry Semel, are the founders of the Institute for Neuroscience and Human Behavior at UCLA, an interdisciplinary research and education institute devoted to the understanding of complex human behavior, including the genetic, biological, behavioral, and sociocultural underpinnings of normal behavior, and the causes and consequences of neuropsychiatric disorders. In addition to conducting fundamental research, the institute faculty seeks to develop effective strategies for the prevention and treatment of neurological, psychiatric, and behavioral disorders, including improvement in access to mental health services and the shaping of national health policy. With abundant energy, Jane is tireless in her mission.

Was there a defining moment that set you on this path?

When I was hospitalized with colitis at twenty-three, a doctor said, "There must be something in your life that is making you unhappy and you will not heal until you address it." I did so, and in addition went on a very strict diet of no red meat and only soup for six months, introducing solid food gradually over the subsequent six months. This healed my colitis. Stress and bad food are toxic.

Why is the health of the soil so relevant in the age of modern farming?

If the nutrients are not in the soil, they will not be in the food.

What is your approach to growing, buying, and eating and drinking food and wine?

I grow my own vegetables in biodynamic soil and I scrutinize all product labels. I buy only organic.

What are you working toward?

Gradually teaching the population to learn about food and also focus on their mental well-being.

3

EAT
well

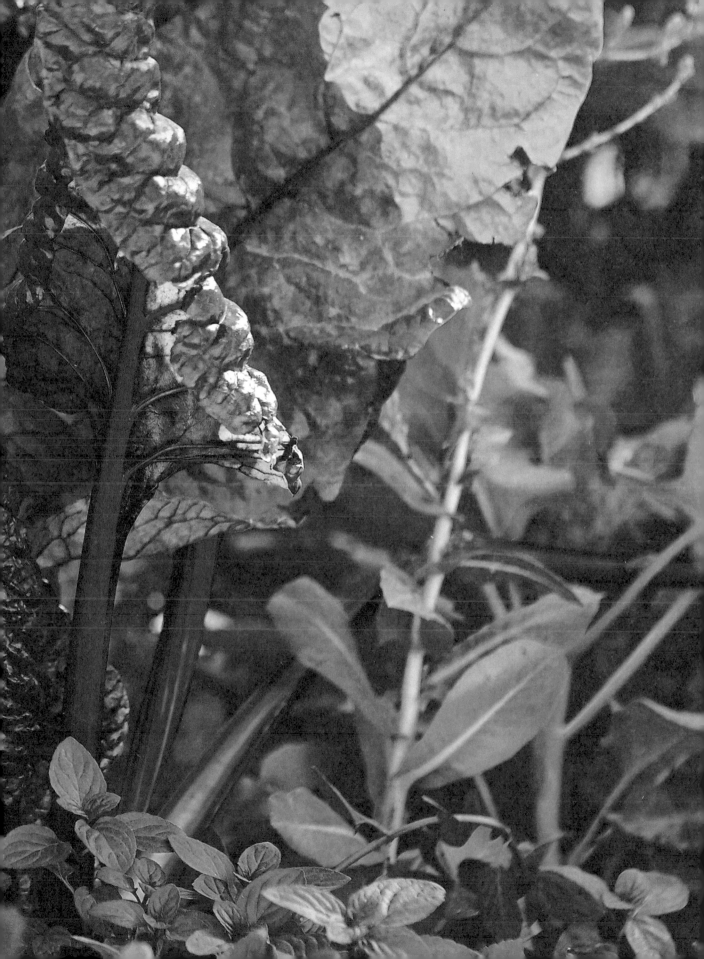

THE IMPORTANCE OF

Growing your Own

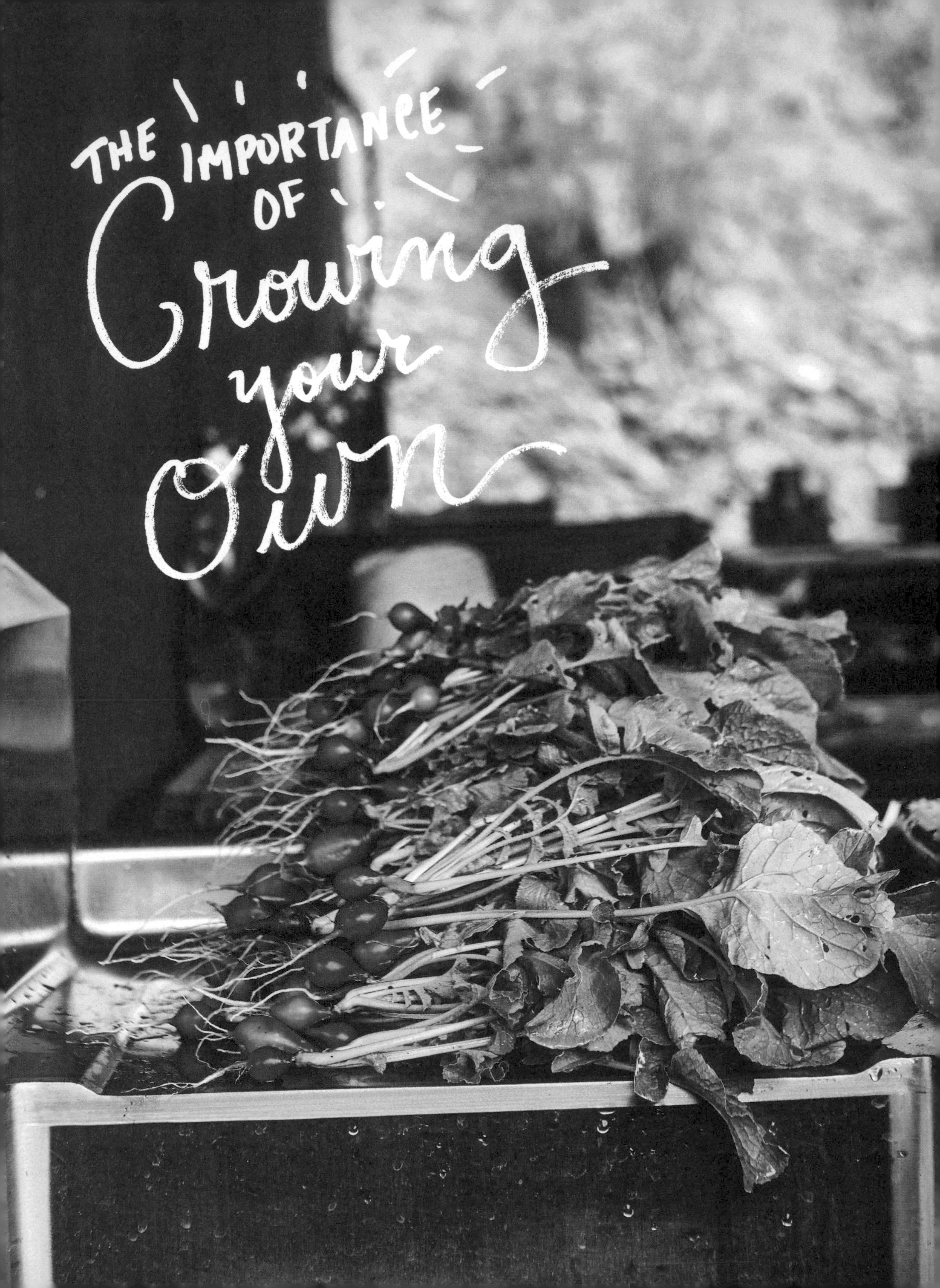

IN ENGLISH nursery schools, sprouting cress and mustard seeds in empty eggshells stuffed with cotton balls to grow "hair" of sorts (we would also draw a face on the shell to make an egg head) is part of the national curriculum. This kind of simple project was my introduction to "growing your own." I went on to grow my own plants in pots, and fruits and vegetables in a little vegetable patch in the garden with my brothers, before becoming a farmer myself. This is what we teach the children who visit the Ranch: Everyone can have a green finger and learn to grow plants. You can start small and then learn your way up, experimenting with different plants in different spaces. Whether it's a few pots of arugula on a windowsill in a city apartment or a bed full of carrots, onions, and tomatoes in a proper kitchen garden, everybody can grow something using biodynamic methods and experience the joy that comes with eating what you've grown from scratch. At the same time you're learning to appreciate healthy foods and cultivating a deep understanding of harvesting, cooking, and consuming clean, energy-enhancing food.

Experimenting with growing and harvesting plants and food—whether you do it yourself or occasionally help a friend or relative in their garden or just go to a pick-your-own farm on a weekend in the country—is an invaluable and deeply rewarding experience. When you see firsthand food being planted, grown, and harvested, you gain a deeper and wider knowledge of fruits, herbs, and vegetables than you get from a trip to the supermarket; you may also be inspired to try, and appreciate, new foods that you never would have otherwise. A recent study conducted by Cornell University showed that if children grow vegetables themselves, they are more likely to eat them. The study, conducted at a local high school, found that when the salad bar in the cafeteria contained produce grown by students, the percentage of those who selected salads with their meals increased from 2 to 10 percent, and overall salad consumption for the entire student body increased from approximately five to twelve servings per day.

Similarly, research has shown that the more knowledgeable you are about food, the more likely you are to feel comfortable purchasing, preparing, and cooking your own food. Moreover, a dislike of cooking has been associated with lower fruit and vegetable intake. When cooked from fresh or raw ingredients, food prepared at home also tends to be more nutritious and healthier, as it makes you more aware of the fat, salt, and sugar that goes into a dish. A breakfast blueberry muffin from your local coffee chain may seem like a virtuous and healthy start to the day until you make a batch of your own muffins and see that many recipes use over a cup of sugar and a stick of butter. The salt content in store-bought soup, meanwhile, can often exceed the recommended daily intake by three or four times.

Many studies have also shown that having family meals or eating dinner with others is significantly associated with a more nutritionally adequate diet that includes higher intake of fruits, vegetables, grains, and calcium-rich foods, while conversely, eating food prepared away from home and eating on the run is linked to a poorer diet, with higher intakes of saturated and total fats. The takeaway? The key to eating healthfully is to reconnect with the earth and with your food. It's never too late to begin educating yourself, experimenting, and getting your hands dirty!

How To
PLANT YOUR
Garden
OF ANY SIZE

I F YOU ARE NEW to growing your own or are short on space and looking to grow a few things in pots or window boxes, don't fear! You can grow in pretty much anything. First, look around the house for empty coffee cans, old wooden crates, old buckets or watering cans. Seeds can be started in old egg boxes, halved tennis balls, or paper cups.

WHAT YOU WILL NEED

A tape measure. Measure the space you have before you go shopping for pots, window boxes, and planters.

Landscaping cloth

Kitchen scissors

Hand trowel

Dredge shaker

Trigger spray bottle

Watering can

A biodynamic lunar calendar to help you plan when to sow and harvest. You should plant two days before the full Moon, as this is when the Moon's energy is being pulled down into the earth.

FOR THE BIGGER GARDEN

Garden hose with a spray attachment

Rake

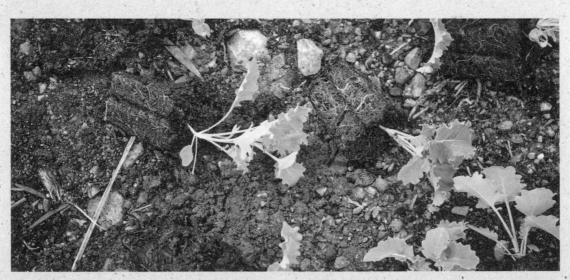

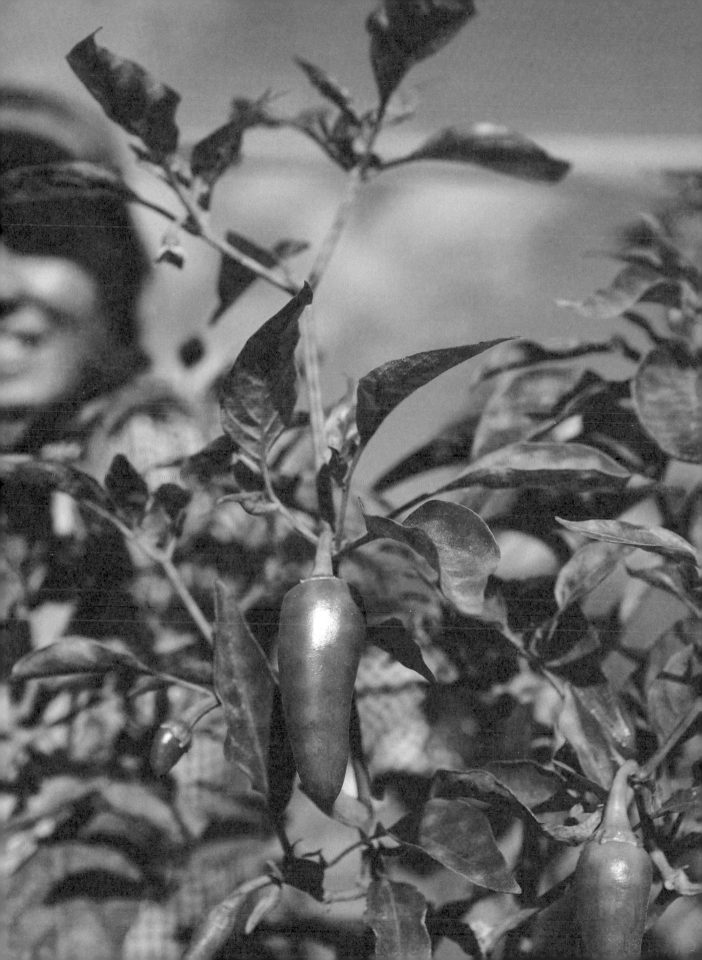

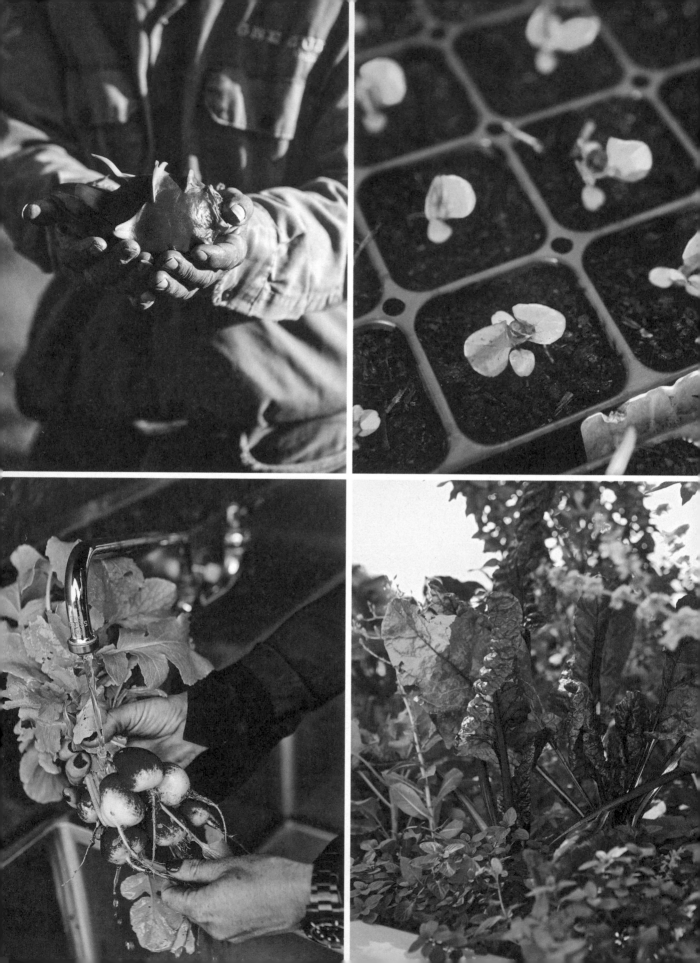

BUYING & SAVING
SEEDS

THERE ARE MANY PLACES to buy organic, biodynamic, and heirloom seeds today, all of which conserve biodiversity and soil health. Technically, a variety is an "heirloom" once it has been cultivated for over fifty years and is open-pollinated (meaning the pollination has occurred by insect, bird, wind, or other natural means). You may ask, why not just buy what is for sale at the local supermarket or hardware store? Buyer beware: The majority of seeds sold today are hybrids or genetically modified, so read the fine print.

Hybrid seeds are the result of two varieties being cross-pollinated to produce a vigorous hybrid with the best traits of each, such as resistance to disease and a higher yield. The seeds from these plants, however, are often sterile and therefore cannot be saved and replanted. This is bad for farmers and for sustainable farming, as new seeds have to be bought every year.

Genetically modified seeds (GMOs) have been created in a laboratory. These seeds have had changes made to their DNA by scientists to allow for the introduction of new traits such as the ability to act as a pesticide or to be resistant to weed killer. These seeds are largely only available to farmers.

The seeds you choose are important because it is the combination of the best seeds grown in the best soil that produces the best-tasting and most nutritious vegetables, fruits, and herbs.

PLANTS YOU CAN GROW
FROM SEED

MOST PLANTS grow from seed; it is more economical than buying grown plants. It is a great way to guarantee the integrity of the soil.

IN POTS, BOXES, OR BASKETS:	IN BIGGER CONTAINERS AND RAISED BEDS:
Arugula	Beets
Basil	Carrots
Chard	Cucumber
Cilantro	Onions and green onions
Cucumbers	Radishes
Green beans	Tomatoes
Kale	Zucchini and other squashes
Lettuces	
Mesclun	
Mint	
Mustard greens	
Nasturtium	
Parsley	
Peppers (bell and chiles)	
Sage	
Spinach	
Sweet peas	

PLANTING
IN POTS, HANGING BASKETS, OR WINDOW BOXES

YOU CAN GROW IN pretty much anything. From window boxes, pots, hanging boxes to old wooden crates and watering cans. Make sure the bottom has a few small holes, evenly placed to allow drainage. To stop spillage on your windowsill or tabletop, place a tray or large plate underneath the growing container to catch the excess water. This in turn can be put back on the growing produce acting as a compost tea.

PLANTING YOUR FIRST LETTUCE MIX

THE EASIEST THING to start edible gardening with is a lettuce mix. At the Ranch, we have mixtures of arugula, tatsoi and mustard greens, different butter and romaine lettuces, and a micro green blend.

1. Fill your containers with biodynamic or organic compost. Containers should hold at least a gallon; window or other boxes should be at least 12 inches deep and wide.

2. Dampen the soil a little before sprinkling the seeds evenly on top. A gallon pot requires about ⅛ teaspoon of seeds, or a small pinch. For larger containers, put your lettuce mix in a dredge shaker and sprinkle evenly. Salad seeds can be very close together, so don't worry too much.

3. Cover the seeds with a very light layer of compost—the motto here is "over-sow, under-cover."

4. Mist the soil with water using a spray bottle after planting, and then once or twice a day thereafter.

5. When you are ready to harvest, cut off the leaves about an inch above the soil and they will regrow.

Nasturtium are also easy to grow and colorful, and the edible flowers can be added to your salad mix. Plant seeds 10 inches apart and ½ inch deep, then cover lightly with compost and mist with water. Plants should appear within 2 weeks.

Kale and chard can be grown fairly close together in pots—about 3 inches apart and ½ inch deep.

Peas, peppers, and green beans are all also easy to grow in pots, but they require a trellis to grow up. You can construct one easily using some bamboo sticks tied together, or some chicken wire. Plant green beans 4 inches apart and 1 inch deep. Plant peas 3 inches apart and 1 inch deep. Peppers should be kept to one plant per pot, planted ½ inch deep. As with all seedings, cover lightly with compost and mist the soil with water.

Strawberries are delicious but also notorious for being among the most pesticide-laden fruits at the market, so growing them at home is a wonderful idea. You will have to buy plants from your local nursery and plant them either in narrow planter boxes 8 inches apart or individually in hanging baskets. Make sure the roots are well covered but that the central crown is exposed to light and air. Place your strawberries in a sunny spot for the sweetest fruit.

Lemon and lime trees can be planted in large pots on a terrace or patio, and moved inside during the winter months if your climate requires.

PLANTING
IN BIGGER CONTAINERS & RAISED BEDS

WHAT YOU WILL NEED:

Garden hose with a spray attachment

Rake

MOST VEGETABLES NEED to grow at least 2-inch roots, so you will need deep containers for beets and radishes and beds for carrots, onions, squash, and tomatoes.

Raised beds and deep containers allow you to start experimenting more fully with

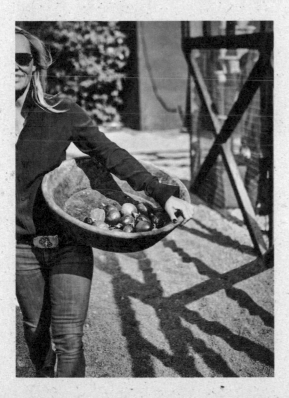

companion planting and using compost tea to enrich the soil.

The best times of year to plant your seeds vary by region, but a biodynamic calendar will tell you the most favorable days to sow your salads, spinach, and leafy herbs and to harvest your carrots, beets, and radishes.

COMPANION PLANTING

COMPANION PLANTING IS the practice of planting two or more plant species together for their mutual benefit. No matter what size biodynamic food container you start with, from a window box to a full-sized raised garden bed, understanding this principle is an invaluable tool. A diverse mix of plants makes for a beautiful and healthy garden with nutritious soil, but the benefits go beyond that.

A wonderful example of companion planting is the "Three Sisters" system used by Native American tribes. Corn, beans, and squash are planted together to provide the nourishment needed for a balanced diet all within a single plot of land. Each of these crops also benefits the others in some way. The tall corn stalks provide a support structure for the climbing beans; the beans do not compete with the corn for nutrients, as they supply their own nitrogen; and the squash provides a dense ground cover that shades out weeds, which otherwise would compete with the corn and beans.

In the wild, the companion effect occurs naturally as the flora and fauna of fields, meadows, forests, swamps, and deserts evolve to create the perfect balance. At the Ranch, we strive to re-create this by planting crops alongside good companions.

SOME EXAMPLES OF THE BENEFITS OF COMPANION PLANTING

- **Companion Plants Support Each Other:** Taller plants provide shade for sun-sensitive plants or protection from the wind for more delicate ones; members of the legume family and alfalfa have the ability to capture nitrogen from the atmosphere and add it to the soil, benefitting plants growing in proximity.

- **Companion Plants Prevent Pests:** Tomatoes exude a chemical that repels the asparagus beetle; sage and carrots drive away each other's pests; likewise, leeks repel the carrot fly and in lovely synchronicity, carrots repel onion flies and leek moths.

- **Companion Plants Attract Beneficial Insects:** Garlic chives, rosemary, and lavender all attract the pollinators crucial to seed and fruit production.

- **Companion Planting Makes the Most of the Available Space:** Planting vining plants, which cover the ground, next to upright plants, which grow upward, allows you to maximize the number of plants you can grow in one patch.

FRIENDS WITH BENEFITS

- **Artichokes:** tarragon

- **Asparagus:** basil, cilantro, dill, parsley, tomato

- **Beans:** beets, cabbage, carrots, cauliflower, cucumbers, celery, corn, eggplant, lettuces, radishes, rosemary, strawberries

- **Beets:** beans, broccoli, carrots, celery, corn, kohlrabi, lettuces, onions, potatoes

- **Cabbage Family:** beets, celery, chard, cucumbers, dill, garlic, lettuces, mint, onions, oregano, peas, potatoes, rosemary, sage, spinach, thyme

- **Carrots:** beans, chives, garlic, lettuces, onions, peas, peppers, radishes, tomatoes

- **Celery:** beans, cabbage, cauliflower, leeks, onions, spinach, tomatoes

- **Corn:** beans, cucumbers, melon, parsley, peas, potatoes, radishes, squash

- **Cucumbers:** beans, cabbage, celery, corn, lettuces, onions, peas, radishes, tomatoes

- **Eggplant:** beans, mint, peppers, potatoes, spinach, thyme

- **Lettuces:** beets, cabbage, carrots, chives, cucumbers, dill, garlic, onions, radishes

- **Melons:** corn, oregano, radishes, squash

- **Onion Family:** beets, broccoli, cabbage, carrots, celery, lettuces, squash, strawberries, tomatoes

- **Peas:** beans, carrots, chives, corn, cucumbers, mint, potatoes, radishes, spinach, turnips

- **Peppers:** basil, carrots, eggplant, onions

- **Potatoes:** beans, corn, cabbage, eggplant, peas

- **Radishes:** beans, carrots, chervil, cucumbers, garlic, lettuces, melons, peas, spinach, sqaush

- **Squash Family:** corn, melon, onions, peas, radishes

- **Tomatoes:** asparagus, basil, celery, cucumbers, garlic, onions, parsley

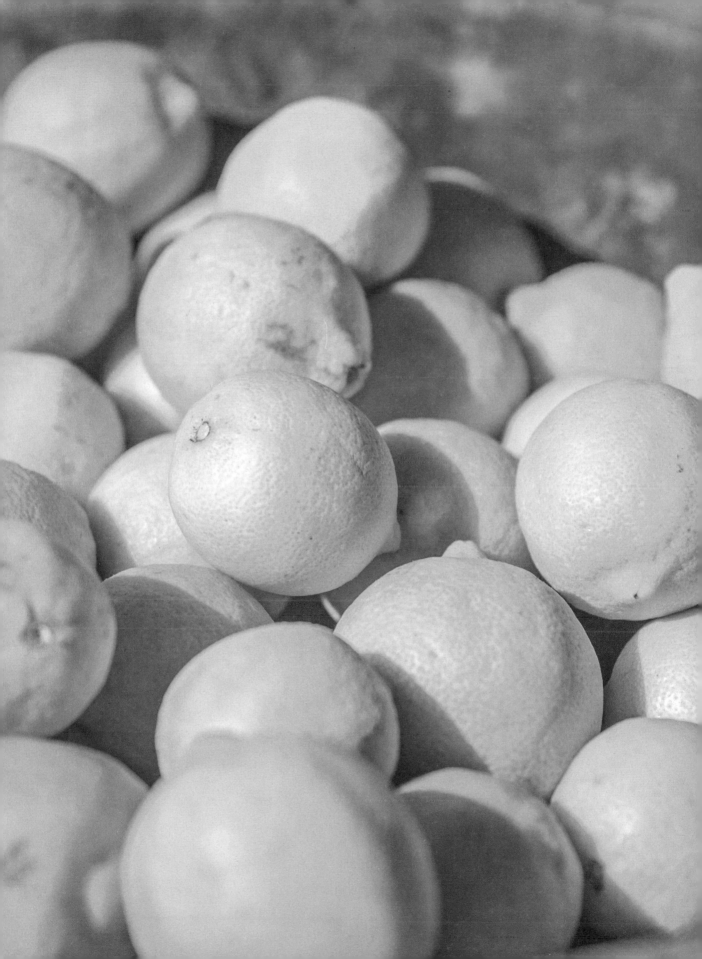

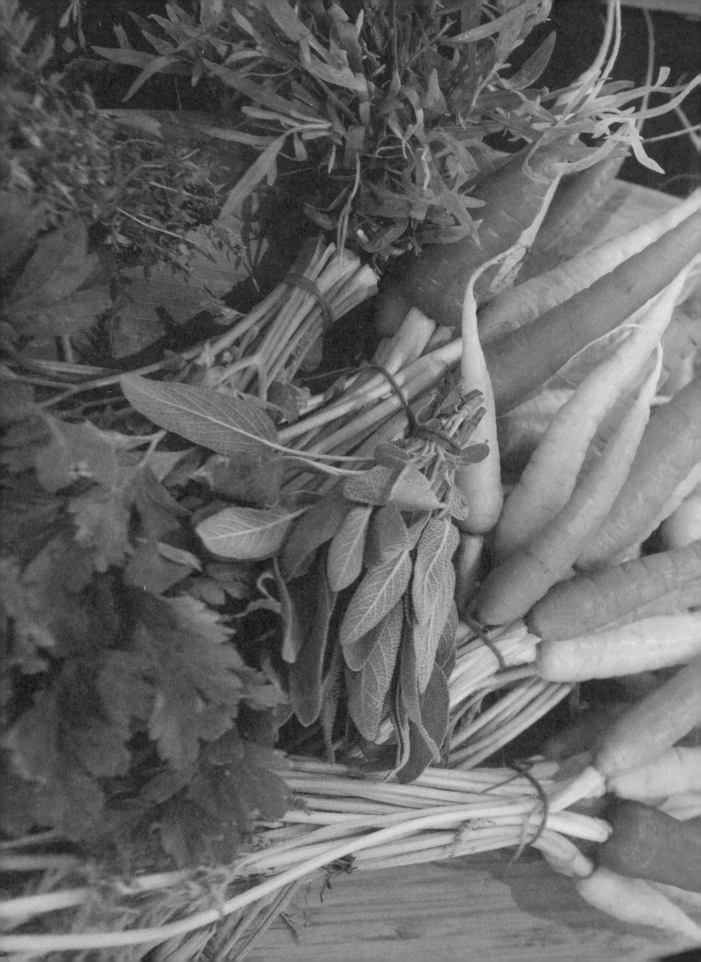

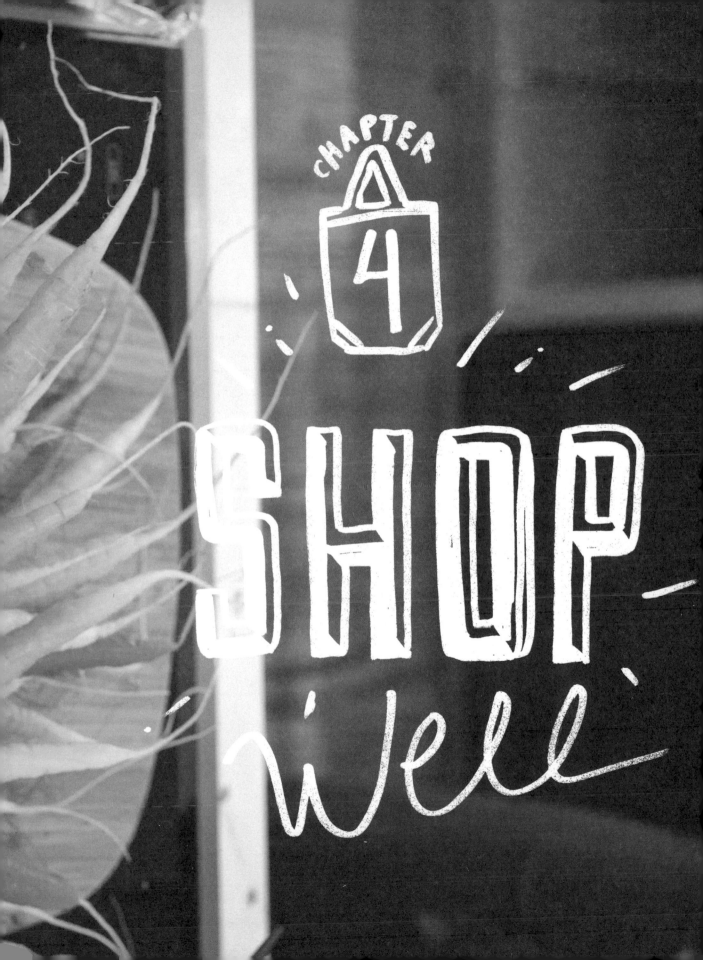

CHAPTER

4

SHOP
well

Your Local
FARMERS' MARKET

W E GROW a lot of fruits, vegetables, herbs, and spices at the Ranch, and our chickens provide us with eggs. We do not grow everything, however, so we like to shop at local farmers' markets for the rest of our needs. In the process, we are supporting other small organic growers and producers from the surrounding area.

In many countries, farmers' markets are the only places that people buy their food, but in the Western world, for far too many years, there has been a glorification of the supermarket in their stead. Shelves piled high with out-of-season produce flown thousands of miles across the world, perfectly formed and shiny, washed in chlorine and peracetic acid, over-packaged in layers of plastic has long been seen as the height of luxury. Now that we know that much of this produce is tainted with toxic fertilizers and pesticides and is often lacking in both flavor and nutrients, there has been a swing back to recognizing the value of locally, responsibly grown food. And as we have become more aware of the negative effects this type of food marketing is having on both the environment and our health, farmers' markets have been experiencing a great resurgence in towns and cities everywhere.

Going to the farmers' market is a completely different affair than going shopping for food at a supermarket. While going to the supermarket is a chore, a mindless task that often entails walking around with a list that you never veer from (subconsciously limiting yourself to the same foods), going to a farmers' market is an inspirational experience that can lead you to buy and experiment with all kinds of new foods you may never have tried before. That said, shopping among the stalls can also be an intimidating experience for first-timers, who may not recognize much of what is being sold, much less know if it's ripe or how to prepare it. Well, another wonderful thing about farmers' markets is that, unlike a supermarket, the stalls are usually staffed by people who grew the produce themselves and are eager to explain what is what and how best to use it.

FARMERS' MARKET CHECKLIST

1. BRING YOUR OWN BAGS.
Many stalls provide plastic baggies for
individual items, but you will need bags with
handles to carry all of your groceries.

———————

2. If you plan on doing your weekly shopping
at the market, you may also want to **INVEST
IN A FOLDING SHOPPING CART,** and bring
a cooler in your car for meat, fish, and dairy
purchases. Some vendors will give you a bag
of ice to tide you over during the drive home,
but on a hot day, a cooler is the safest bet.

———————

3. BRING CASH. Smartphone technology
has led to an increase in vendors
accepting credit cards, but cash is still king
at the farmers' market.

———————

4. KEEP THE TOPS ON. When a vendor
asks if you want the tops torn off your
carrots or beets, say "No!" Carrot tops make
great pesto, and beet tops are delicious
sautéed with olive oil and garlic. Save other
sometimes overlooked parts like celery and
fennel leaves for salads, soups, and stocks.

———————

5. Remember to **TALK TO THE VENDORS**
while shopping. Unlike the supermarket,
the farmers' market is a place where you can
learn about the provenance of the produce,
the best ways to prepare it, what it goes well
with, and many other great details.

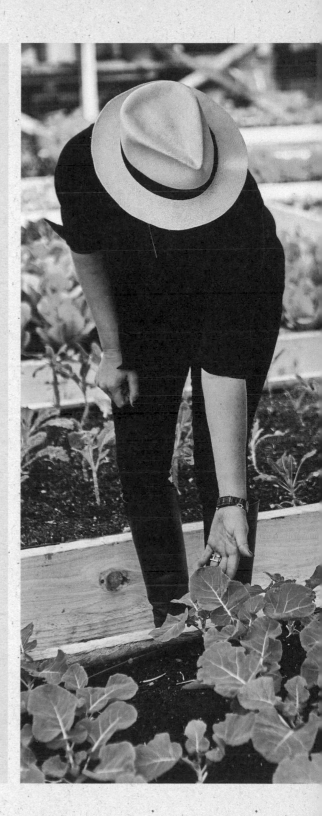

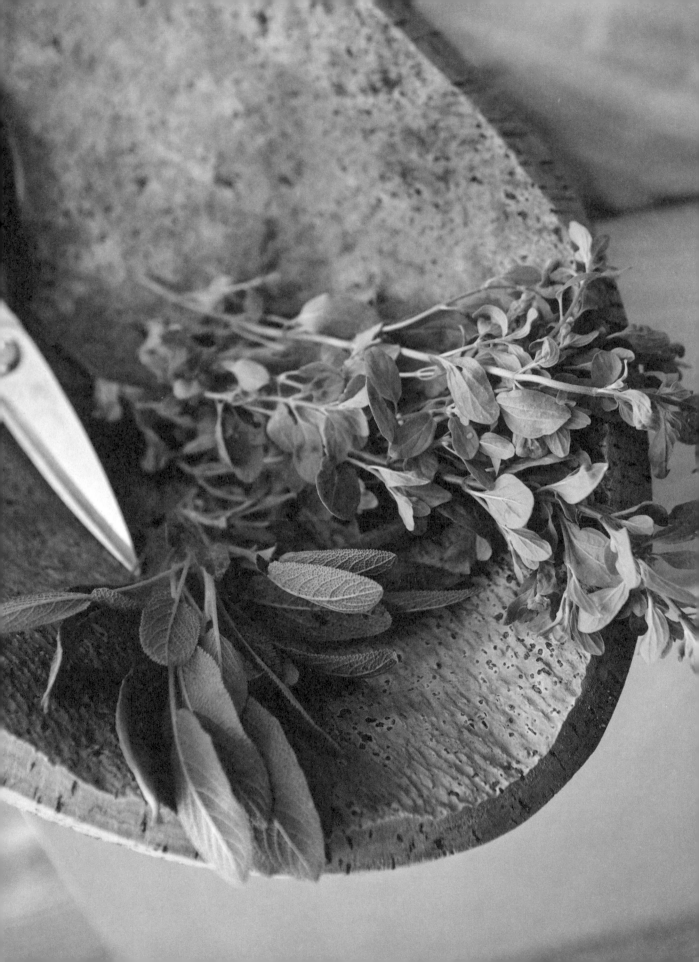

The Internet is a great place to find your local farmers' market. Sites like localharvest .org and farmersmarketonline.com have comprehensive listings of every market nationwide, along with CSAs and farms that sell to the public. Once you have identified your local market, take a look at our tips below for making the most of your shopping trip.

QUESTIONS TO ASK
AT THE FARMERS' MARKET

WHAT IS IN SEASON RIGHT NOW?

There may be strawberries at the market all year round, but that doesn't mean they are in season (strawberries are at peak from April through June in many places, but almost year round in warmer climates). Seasonal produce tastes the best, is higher in nutrients because it's picked at its prime, and is usually cheaper, as it's in abundance and needs to be sold quickly. Eating seasonally also provides an opportunity to broaden your palate as you get to experiment with foods not commonly on your shopping list.

HOW SHOULD I PREPARE THIS?

Ask the vendor for tips on how to prepare or feature a vegetable, fruit, or herb you've never used before. They should know what goes best with what. At One Gun Ranch, our rule of thumb is: what grows together goes together on a plate. So for example, combine eggplant, onions, and peppers; tomatoes and basil; lettuces and kale; beets and carrots; strawberries and mint; and so on.

DID YOU GROW THIS FOOD? IF NOT, WHO DID?

It may seem hard to believe, but not all farmers' markets are producer-only markets. Some of the "farmers" at your local market may in fact be reselling produce they bought wholesale from out of state or out of the country that has been harvested by an exploited workforce or sprayed with toxic pesticides banned in the US. The vendor should know a good amount about the provenance of the food they are selling. If they do not, move on.

DID ALL OF THE PRODUCE COME FROM ONE FARM, OR MULTIPLE FARMS?

The vendor may be a farmer selling his or her produce directly, or they may be acting as an agent for a local cooperative. Either way, again, they should be able to tell you about the provenance of the food they are selling.

HOW LONG HAS THE FARM BEEN ESTABLISHED? WHAT WAS IT BEFORE?

It is always nice to know if a farm has been growing organically or biodynamically from the start, or if at some point they were conventional and then switched over, as this will give you more insight into the producers.

DO YOU HAVE ANY CERTIFICATIONS?

Organic products in the US have strict production and labeling requirements overseen by the USDA. Farms that are not certified cannot make any organic claim—unless they make $5,000 or less a year. So if your local farmers' market is made up of these smaller businesses, ask the following two questions:

WHERE IS YOUR FARM AND CAN I VISIT?

Vendors should not have anything to hide, and ideally the farm should be close enough to the market for customers to travel to it. By the same token, your food should travel as few miles as possible before reaching your table. That is truly local food.

DO YOU USE ANY TYPE OF SPRAYS ON YOUR PRODUCE? HOW DO YOU CONTROL PESTS?

"No spray" is a common sign at farmers' markets these days, but some organic farmers still use a host of organic pesticides, such as seaweed-based sprays, while biodynamic farmers aim to optimize soil health in order to strengthen plants against pest infestations. There is usually some method of pest control being undertaken, so find out what it is.

TOP FARMERS' MARKET
PICKS

IF WE WERE TO buy only five things from the local farmers' market this is what we would choose and why:

EGGS

The nutrient content in eggs from farm-fresh, free-range, grain-fed, hormone-free naturally raised chickens is higher than in commercially raised eggs. And unlike supermarket eggs, which can be over thirty days old, eggs sold at your local farmers' markets are usually gathered shortly before bringing them to market. These eggs are also less likely to contain salmonella, as the waxy layer (called the cuticle, or "bloom") that seals the pores of the shell and helps keep out bacteria has not been removed by commercial egg washing, which uses chlorine, hydrogen peroxide, lye, and peracetic acid.

GREENS

The selection of leafy greens at the farmers' market is always stunning, often covering the full range from mizuna, bok choy, mesclun, micro greens and sprouts, kales, chards, spinach, collard greens, and lettuces to beet tops and carrot tops and edible flowers. The variety is endless—and they have not been sprayed with pesticides or washed with chlorine, as is so often the case with supermarket greens.

HERBS AND SPICES

The farmers' market is a great place to find herbs and spices not commonly sold in supermarkets. Sorrel, fenugreek, lavender, Thai basil, lemon verbena, chocolate mint, fresh garlic, and a rainbow of mild to fiery-hot chiles are just some of the more hard-to-find items we have picked up over the years.

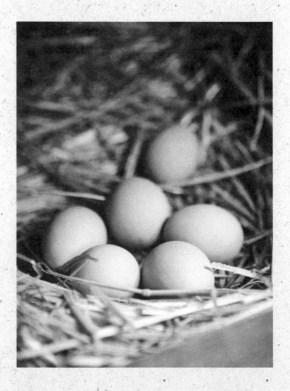

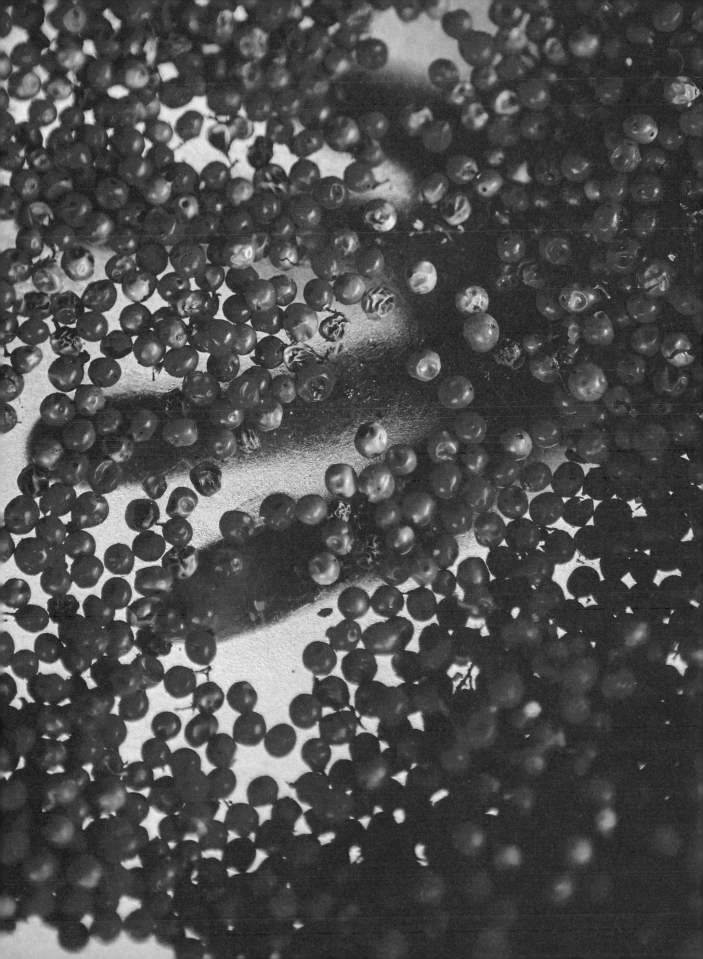

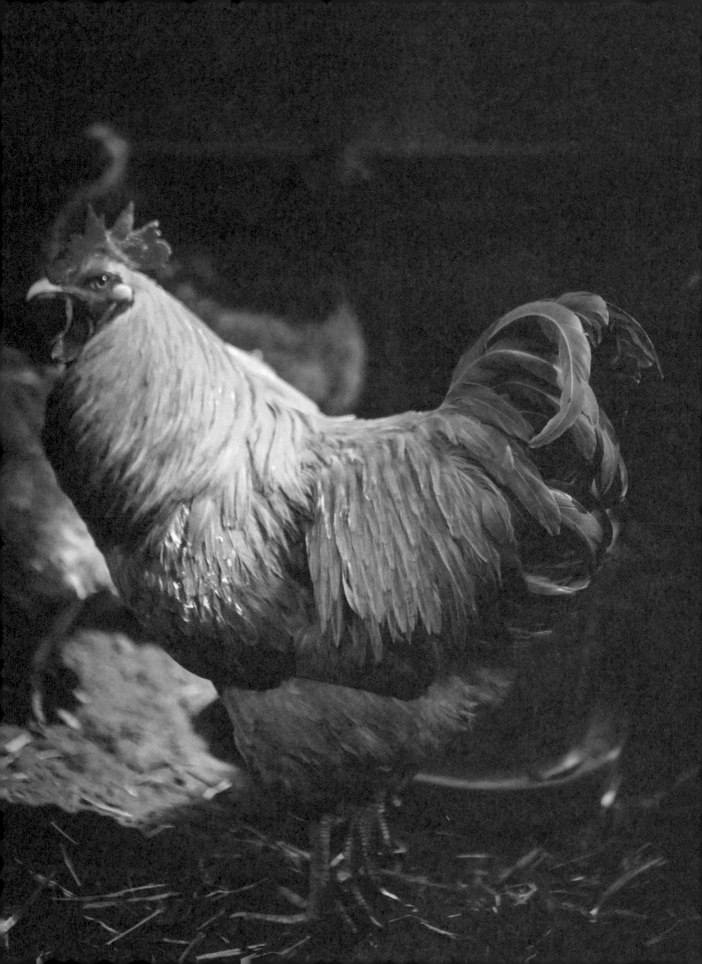

STONE FRUITS

Peaches, nectarines, apricots, plums, and cherries really don't hold up well during transport, which is why supermarket stone fruits are picked while green and then put in cold storage, creating a mealy texture. Buy cherries anywhere from early to mid-June; apricots from late June to early July; and peaches, nectarines, and plums from July through August. These all taste best ripe, at the height of their season, and should be eaten on the day of purchase.

TOMATOES

A supermarket tomato will never come close to the taste and texture of a ripe, just-picked organic tomato. Why? Because, as explained by a study published in *Science* magazine, commercially farmed tomatoes have been bred for uniform color, and as a result, they are actually missing a gene. Supermarket tomatoes have also been picked long before they were ripe as they need an extended shelf life, and so the starches in them never fully convert to sugar either. The result? A tasteless or sour tomato with a dry, cottony texture.

Once you get home, make sure you wash all your fruits and vegetables. Cut off any leafy green tops, wash and dry them in a salad spinner, and store in the high-humidity drawer of your refrigerator along with all your leafy greens like arugula, spinach, and herbs. By holding water vapor in the drawer, the moisture will keep your greens crisper and fresher for longer.

We like to keep fruit in bowls on the counter. A bowl of ripe fruit looks and smells fantastic, and keeping it out where you can see it means you are more likely to eat it! If you are worried about it spoiling, keep fruit in the low-humidity drawer of the fridge to allow naturally produced ethylene gas to escape.

MEAT
AT THE FARMERS' MARKET

THE FARMERS' MARKET IS also an excellent place to buy meat. That said, meat can be more expensive at the farmers' market because it is more expensive to raise fresh, nutritious meat using sustainable agricultural practices (which are more beneficial to the local economy and less damaging to the environment) than it is to factory farm. Most markets will only have a couple of stalls selling chicken, lamb, beef, and pork from small, local, sustainable farms, which means you can really learn about how the animals were raised, fed, and slaughtered.

QUESTIONS
FOR YOUR FARMERS' MARKET MEAT VENDOR

1. Did you raise the animals yourself? If not, do you know the farmer who did?

———————

2. How confident are you that your meats are hormone and antibiotic free?

———————

3. FOR BEEF: Is this 100 percent grass-fed and finished or were the cattle fed grain?

———————

4. FOR CHICKEN: Was this chicken pastured (meaning left to forage on grass, seeds, and insects during the day) and air-chilled after slaughter? (Factory-farmed chickens are water-chilled in chlorinated pools after slaughter.)

EAT with THE Seasons:

A MONTHLY CALENDAR OF SEASONAL FOODS

FRUITS and vegetables taste best when eaten in season, but these days it can be hard to tell what is and is not in season, as so much of our food is flown in from thousands of miles away. California is blessed with an incredibly long growing season and a huge variety of produce is available year round. That said, as a general rule of thumb, most fruit is in season during the summer months; root vegetables during winter, spring, and fall; and leafy greens early summer to late fall.

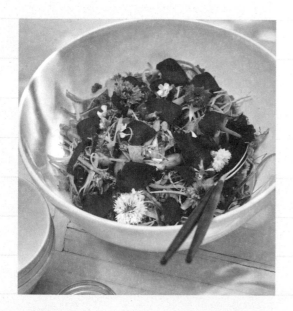

THE MANY BENEFITS OF EATING SEASONALLY

• **When produce is in season locally,** the abundance of the crop and the fact that it needs to be sold fast means it is usually less expensive.

• **Produce that is in season** is more flavorful and nutritious.

• **The natural cycle of produce is perfectly designed to support our health.** As the seasons change, our bodies need different kinds of food. In the winter, squashes and root vegetables provide sustained energy, while ginger and garlic generate warmth and promote circulation. In the spring, leafy greens give us a boost of much-needed vitamin D. In the summer, water-heavy tomatoes, cucumbers, and watermelon keep the body hydrated.

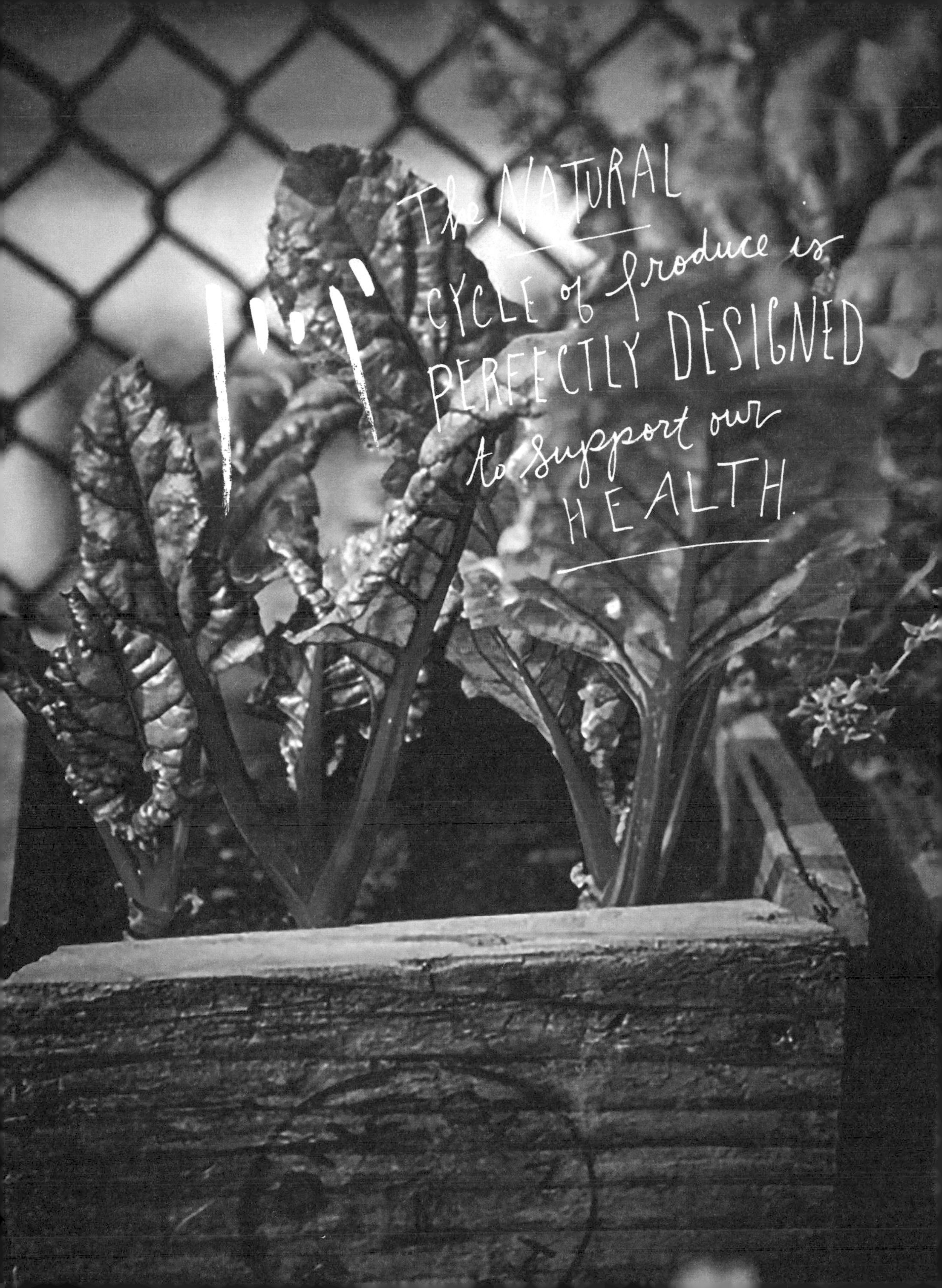

The NATURAL
CYCLE of produce is
PERFECTLY DESIGNED
to support our
HEALTH.

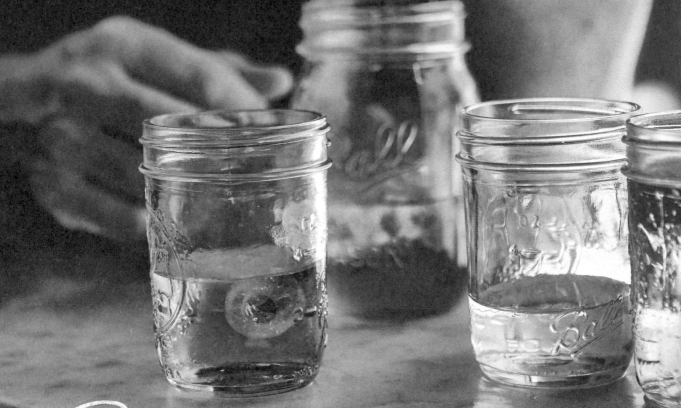

Biodynamic
WINE -
A success STORY

A T THE CORE OF biodynamics is the tenet that the farm is a holistic entity, and there is no crop in which the final product is a truer expression of its *"terroir,"* or environment, than the grapes grown to produce wine. Many of the world's most well-known wine regions, however, have seen the soil that they have grown their grapevines in for centuries deteriorate because of the destructive effects of monoculture agriculture. As a result, many have turned to organic and biodynamic farming to revive the ailing vines.

The "bio" wine movement, as it's known in Europe, is already well established with famous names such as France's Zind-Humbrecht, Domaine Leroy, Nicholas Joly, Château Latour, Château Figeac, Domaine Huët, and Chapoutier, and the trend is catching on in the US, too. There are currently estimated to be over five hundred biodynamic wineries among producers in France, Italy, Australia, New Zealand, South Africa, Chile, Argentina, Portugal, Spain, Austria, and Germany, with about one hundred American winemakers among them, including influential wine writer Robert Parker and his brother-in-law Mike Etzel, who use biodynamic methods at their Beaux Frères vineyard in Oregon.

Why are winemakers embracing biodynamics in such large numbers? Because biodynamic's holistic practices truly take into account the terroir—a word that attempts to capture the concept of all the combined characteristics of a vineyard, including the soil, topography, and climate, that help shape a wine. Traditionally, wine lovers across the world have waited anxiously for each new vintage to see how the wine has expressed the conditions of the past year. But with the widespread use of sulfites and chemicals on vineyards, much of that has been lost, completely stripping the industry of what made it so special.

Biodynamic practices, on the other hand, take care of the soil and promote cover cropping in between the vines to replace nutrients and minerals. Biodynamic practices also take into account the water levels in the soil at different times during the lunar cycle, giving growers an insight on how much water content is in the grapes and when to prune the vines or harvest the grapes for wine. Biodynamics reduce the incidence of disease and pests on the farm, allowing the grapes to speak for themselves, once again. It's an easy choice for any winemaker who wants to bring the industry back to its former glory.

BIODYNAMIC HERO:
PETER SISSECK
of DOMINO DE PINGUS WINERY

PETER SISSECK, OR "PINGUS," as he was known growing up in Denmark (it means "penguin" in Danish), and I met through a mutual Danish friend about fifteen years ago. Over the course of many conversations about biodynamics and how he started his vineyard, Pingus truly inspired me to try the biodynamic route. In 1995, he bought a vineyard in the Spanish town of La Horra in the Ribera del Duero wine region of Spain. It had very ancient, gnarled Tempranillo vines that had originally been planted in 1929. Having studied biodynamics at the Rudolf Steiner School in Basel, he knew the soil was the key to making exceptional wine. The first 1995 vintage of Pingus was awarded an unheard of 96-100 point score by Robert Parker—the highest score given to any young wine from Spain. Since 2000, Pingus wines have been fully biodynamic, and they now have a cult following. Peter has a very refined and emotional intelligence, and it's this harmony and alchemy within him and in biodynamics that I find so special and attractive.

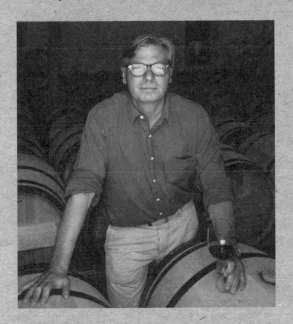

dead from lack of microbiological life. One of the very best ways of getting life back into it is through the biodynamic method. Modern farming relies so much on herbicides and fungicides and kills a great many of the organisms in the soil, especially fungi. The fungi that are a precursor to mycorrhiza are of the utmost importance. Mycorrhizae are fungi that live in symbiotic association with the plant roots, providing nutrients and minerals that are often difficult for the plants to accumulate otherwise. In winemaking this will help the grapes to have more complex taste and, normally, better balance.

Why is eating mindfully so important?

As the saying goes: We are what we eat.

What is your approach to growing, buying, and eating and drinking food and wine?

I try, for the most part, to grow my own, which is why I decided to live in the countryside. We can do full circle out here. What we cannot produce we must buy, but we always try to find local alternatives and to eat in season (no strawberries in December). We also try to buy and support organic and free-range producers as much as possible.

What are you working toward?

I try basically to leave the smallest footprint. I also believe that beauty is important for everybody, so we try to create beautiful landscapes and places. I think it is what gives me the greatest joy.

What is something you tell people they can do to make a difference?

I tell people to try to do everything with love and attention. A beautifully pruned vineyard is a joy for everybody: the people and the plants. It may take more time and work in the short run, but it will keep everybody in good health in the long run.

Was there a defining moment that set you on this path?

My interest in biodynamics comes from way back when I went to agricultural college, where I saw an experiment carried out using carrots. Around Christmastime, three carrots, one normal, one organic, and one biodynamic, were cut in half and left in a tray with water. After two weeks, the conventionally grown carrot had rotted away; the organic carrot lasted about a month or more. But the biodynamic one kept until April, and even sprouted. That was special. Then, in 1995, I tasted some biodynamic wine from Lalou Bize Leroy, a famous biodynamic grower from Burgundy. It was her 1993 vintage and I had never tasted anything like it.

Why is the health of the soil so important in the age of modern farming?

The health of our soils are very important for all agriculture, but even more for viticulture. The best wines are made with natural yeasts that come from the soil, but the soil in old vineyards is often quite

CHAPTER 5

BE well

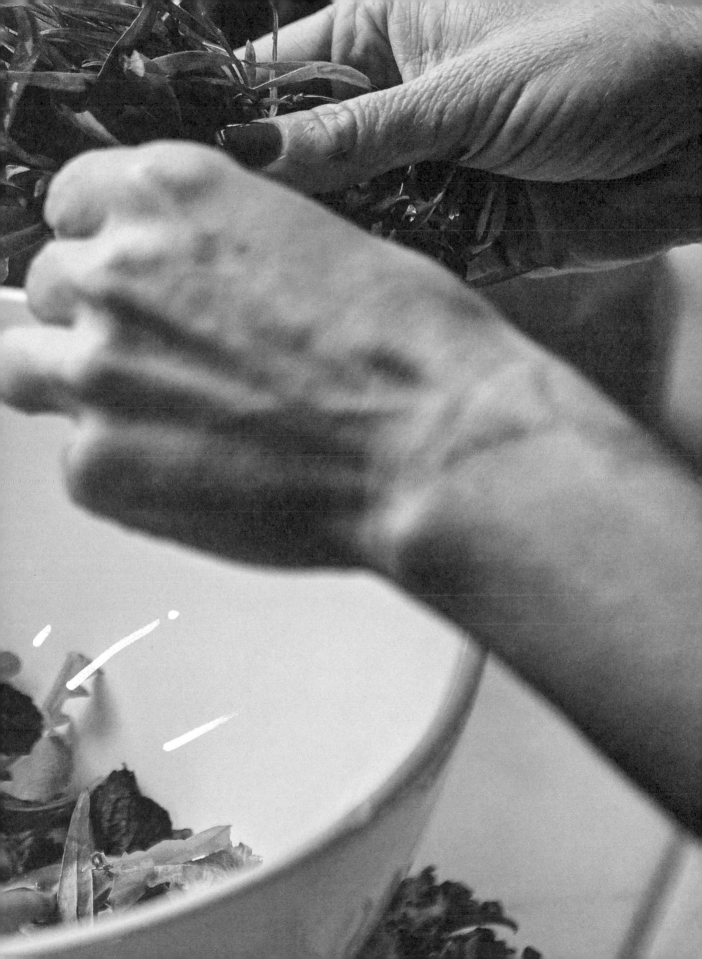

You Are what you Eat

YOU WOULD never guess judging by the walls of vitamin supplements that line the aisles of pharmacies and health-food stores today, but there actually is scant evidence that vitamin supplements make healthy people healthier—and they are certainly no substitute for a healthy diet. Herbal supplements are not regulated or required to be safety tested in the US, and a recent investigation by the New York attorney general's office found that a large number of the herbal supplements on store shelves did not contain the ingredients listed on the label at all.

The best way to take your vitamins and supplements, therefore, is through your food. A balanced diet containing plenty of fruits, vegetables, and whole grains offers a mix of vitamins, minerals, and nutrients that combine perfectly to meet the body's needs, and it is the synergistic interactions of these nutrients that deliver the most benefit.

Of late, research has been done to understand more about so-called "superfoods" and other nutrient-dense foods that contain high levels of micronutrients, vitamins, minerals, phytochemicals, and antioxidants. While there has been a lot of hype in the last few years surrounding exotic foods such as Brazilian acai berries and chia seeds, the most nutrient-dense foods can actually be found a lot closer to home, and there so are many to choose from that it is easy to incorporate them into your diet.

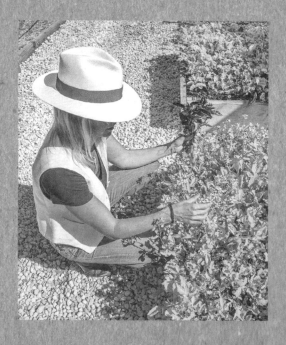

EAT YOUR
VITAMINS

THE BEST WAY TO absorb your daily intake of vitamins is to eat them!

VITAMIN C, VITAMIN K, AND CALCIUM

Bok choy

Brussel sprouts

Collard greens

Kale

Mustard greens

Spinach

Swiss chard

RIBOFLAVIN AND BIOTIN

Mushrooms

VITAMIN A AND POTASSIUM

Potatoes

Sweet potatoes

Yams

VITAMIN C AND LYCOPENE

Blackberries

Blueberries

Raspberries

Red bell peppers

Strawberries

Tomatoes

VITAMIN E, NIACIN, AND MAGNESIUM

Almonds

Avocado

Cashews

Peanuts

Pine nuts

Pistachios

Pumpkin seeds

Sesame seeds

Sunflower seeds

IRON AND LYSINE

Black beans

Chickpeas

Kidney beans

Lentils

Peas

FOLIC ACID

Barley

Brown rice

Oats

Quinoa

OMEGA-3 FATTY ACIDS AND ZINC; VITAMINS D, B12, AND B6

Beef

Chicken

Eggs

Lamb

Salmon

Sardines

Shellfish

Turkey

BIODYNAMIC HERO:
RON FINLEY, the GANGSTA Gardener

RON FINLEY IS A creative phenomenon: an urban horticulturalist with a strong vision for community gardening. Nicknamed "the Gangsta Gardener," Ron started growing food in abandoned city lots after he realized that in his neighborhood of South Central Los Angeles, unhealthy fast-food drive-thru foods were killing more people than drive-by shootings.

South Central was a food desert with a high obesity rate and a population suffering from illnesses due to poor diet. He got tired of his community not having access to healthy food, so he started planting organic vegetables in an abandoned strip of land in front of his home. Unbelievably, the City cited Ron for gardening without a permit. But this slap on the wrist did little to dissuade his green thumb. Instead, he fought back and started a petition with fellow green activists to demand the right to garden and grow food in his neighborhood. They won.

Ron now spends his time turning food deserts across the country into food forests by planting fruits and vegetables in unused parkways and vacant lots. These gardens are community hubs where people learn about nutrition and join together to plant, work, and unwind. We were instantly blown away by Ron's fresh approach to eating and gardening and his "just do it" attitude. Ron has inspired so many people with his incredible energy. He really grasps what needs to be done to empower people: Show them that they can grow their own food and take control of their health. This is exactly the message that we want to put out, and why he is one of our heroes of the contemporary food movement.

Was there a defining moment that set you on this path?

Yes, it was when I walked into a local grocery store for an apple and couldn't find one that wasn't coated with shellac and pesticides I couldn't pronounce. I'd been to grocery stores in other neighborhoods and I saw the difference. There weren't any healthy organic options in my neighborhood and that's when I knew: If I wanted organic, I had to grow organic.

Why is the health of the soil so relevant in the age of modern farming?

Not only have we become disconnected from our food source, we've become disconnected from the soil. We are made of the same stuff that the earth is made of. If it's not healthy, we're not healthy. Plants eat soil, they don't just grow in it; therefore, we need healthy, nutrient rich soil to get the best crops we can get. It's real simple: good in, good out.

What is your approach to growing, buying, and eating and drinking food and wine?

If you can't read that shit, don't eat that shit! Almost nothing natural has sixteen letters in it. Truth is, it's important to know where your food comes from. That's why it's great to have farmers' markets, where farmers are held accountable for their growing techniques and their business practices. But the easiest thing is to have your food growing right outside your door! That way you know where it comes from and what went into it.

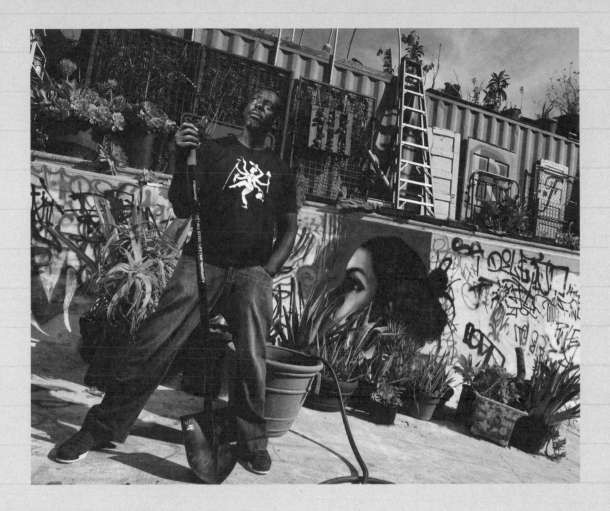

What are you working toward?

A plan to take over the world! (But don't tell anyone.) What we're doing is working toward changing the culture. At this time, we're in the process of securing land for our biggest project yet. It's going to be the poster child for urban renewal and it's going to be right here in South Central LA. On our land, we'll have large garden plots where members of the community will come to learn everything from how to plant, grow, glean, harvest, cook, share, sell, store, and trade the food that they grow. There will be a café made from repurposed shipping containers that will serve the food that has been grown right there by the very members of the community, and a maker space with classes on everything from yoga to painting, weaving, and entrepreneurship. Ultimately, we're changing the culture and showing people that they have the power to design their own lives instead of falling victim to the life that was systematically created for them.

What is something you tell people they can do to make a difference?

Plant some shit! Get gangsta with your food. Grow a garden for you and your family. Growing your own food is like printing your own money. Take back your health and your power. Change your food; change your life! You save your food, you save your life!

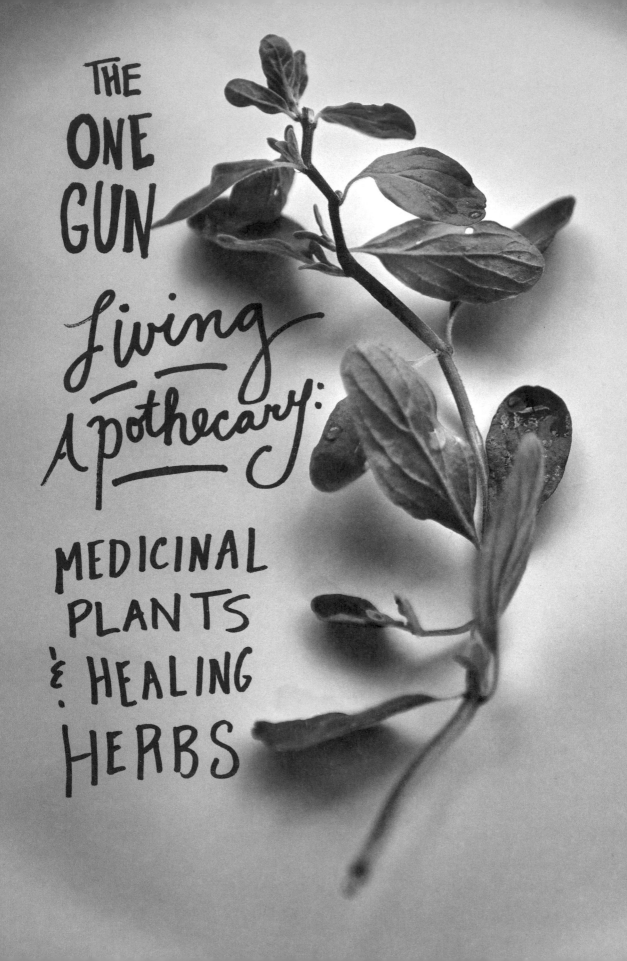

THE ONE GUN

Living Apothecary:

MEDICINAL PLANTS & HEALING HERBS

THERE ARE A LOT OF plants and flowers growing wild at One Gun Ranch, and while we identified many on our foraging hikes and began to use them in the kitchen, it turned out we also had a wild apothecary right under out noses. We discovered this when, through the burgeoning biodynamic community in Malibu, we had the good fortune to meet Marysia Miernowska, a skilled herbalist, biodynamic gardener, and director of the Gaia School of Healing and Earth Education in California.

Originally from Poland, Marysia grew up studying Earth wisdom and ancient healing practices from different cultures around the world. Her knowledge of our indigenous plants' healing properties was truly a revelation. We learned that just as fruits and vegetables are a wonderful way to get all of your daily vitamin requirements, there were a wealth of plants and herbs growing untended at the Ranch that had been used for centuries to treat common ailments such as colds, flu, inflammation, minor cuts and wounds, bacterial infections, sore throats, upset stomachs, muscle pain, anxiety, poor digestion, and insomnia.

We asked Marysia to walk the property with us to help identify the wealth of healing and medicinal herbs growing on the Ranch, and then to create a living apothecary for us in the form of both a medicinal garden and a wilderness area that would not only prevent soil erosion and reduce the risk of landslides (a common problem in drought-stricken Southern California) but also attract native insects and birds.

Medicinal plants can be included in a daily health regimen to strengthen the body and nourish the nervous system, and are a safe and effective source of vitamins,

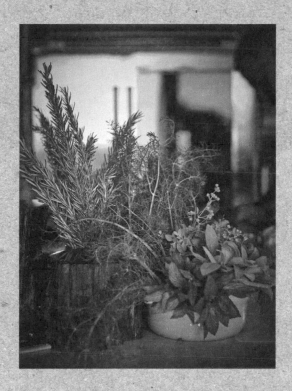

minerals, and enzymes. Just as the food you have grown yourself always tastes better, the simple act of growing and making your medicine is a deeply healing experience.

Here are some of the healing plants we are growing at One Gun Ranch, along with wonderful recipes from Marysia for how to eat, drink, and apply them to our bodies for whatever ails us.

CALENDULA

CALENDULA (*CALENDULA OFFICINALIS*) has beautiful golden flowers that are easy to grow from seed and will continuously reseed themselves in the garden. The flowers are edible and make a beautiful addition sprinkled on a salad, but they can also be dried or tinctured for medicinal use. A strong antifungal and antiviral, calendula can be taken internally to combat the flu or any other infection, while a wash of calendula, an infused calendula oil, or a calendula salve heals wounds, dry skin, and fungal skin conditions.

COCONUT CALENDULA
ANTIFUNGAL SALVE

1 cup virgin unrefined coconut oil

⅓ cup dried calendula flowers

2 tablespoons beeswax pastilles

¼ teaspoon concentrated vitamin E oil, or up to 1 teaspoon 5,000 IU oil

20 drops lavender essential oil

Using a double boiler over very low heat, melt the coconut oil and add the calendula flowers. Stir occasionally, allowing the warm oil to extract the properties of the calendula flowers over a period of a couple of hours. Replenish the water in the bottom pan of the double boiler as needed. The oil is ready when it has taken on a beautiful orange color. Make sure you keep the water at a very gentle simmer and that it doesn't touch the bottom of the top pan of the double boiler. Do not fry the flower petals—if they start to smell like burned popcorn, you must discard the oil and start over.

Once the oil is orange, strain out the flowers and add the beeswax. Stir until the beeswax and oil melt together. Add the vitamin E oil and stir to mix well.

Prepare a clean, dry salve container; a glass Mason jar will do. Drop the lavender essential oil into the bottom of the container. Pour the wax and oil mixture into the jar, closing it quickly to prevent the essential oils from escaping with the vapor.

Allow to cool. Your salve is ready, and does not need to be refrigerated. It has a shelf life of up to three years.

Borage

BORAGE (*BORAGO OFFICINALIS*) IS EASILY identified by its periwinkle-colored, star-shaped flowers. The flowers are edible and have a mild, cucumber-like taste, making them a great addition to any salad, drink, or dessert. The hairy leaves are characteristic of plants that support the lungs and respiratory system, and tea made from them can be used for dry coughs, while also stimulating the adrenals (which may explain the old saying, "Use borage for courage"). The fresh leaves can be juiced, too, and the juice is wonderful for new mothers, as it encourages the production of breast milk. Borage oil, made from the seeds, can be taken internally or applied externally to help clear up skin conditions such as eczema.

BORAGE FLOWER
ICE CUBES

Fill an ice-cube tray with spring water and submerge a washed borage flower into each cube. Freeze. Serve in a lavender lemonade or iced tea.

STINGING NETTLES

STINGING NETTLES (*URTICA DIOICA*) ARE rich in vitamins, minerals, and enzymes. An infusion of nettles nourishes and revives in a way that no multivitamin can! Tonifying to the blood, nettles carry good amounts iron and vitamins A, B, and C, making this a wonderful herb for those with anemia and blood deficiencies. And nettle has a cumulative effect, so if you begin to take it daily, you will notice an increase in energy and vitality, more stamina, a beautification of the skin, and stronger hair and nails. Nettle helps with digestion as well as absorption of nutrients from our food, nourishes the womb, and rebuilds the blood around the menses, as well as creating more nutritious and abundant breast milk when breastfeeding. Finally, nettle also repairs the adrenals, which can become exhausted from chronic stress, making it a valuable remedy in our modern times.

Nettles are at their most vibrant and green in the spring, so best harvested then. You can bruise or dry the leaves for tea, or use them in soup, quiche, or any other dish that calls for greens. The sting is nullified upon cooking or blending, so I love making this raw nettle pesto that preserves the enzymes that would otherwise be destroyed by cooking.

MARYSIA'S VIBRANTLY ALIVE
RAW NETTLE PESTO

3 large handfuls of fresh nettle leaves (seeds can be included, but avoid the tough stems for this recipe)

½ cup extra-virgin cold-pressed olive oil

½ cup pure spring water

½ cup pine nuts, toasted

½ cup freshly grated Parmesan cheese

2 cloves garlic

Salt and freshly ground black pepper to taste

Use gloves when handling the stinging nettles. Place all of the ingredients in a high-powered blender and blend until you have a smooth pesto.

Olive Trees

OLIVE TREES (*OLEA EUROPAEA*) GROW wonderfully in the Mediterranean climate of Southern California, and we have plenty at the Ranch. Sacred to the ancient Greeks, the olive tree is deeply rooted in legend and lore. Myth says it first appeared when the goddess of wisdom, Athena, planted her spear into the ground. Olives, olive oil, and even olive leaves are high in antioxidants and are full of medicinal properties. Herbalists tincture the leaves in alcohol to make a strong antibacterial and antiviral extraction that can be used in acute conditions; however, a tea of the leaves can be used more regularly, to increase energy, lower blood pressure, calm the nerves, strengthen the heart and circulatory system, and boost immunity. The fruit and oil of the tree are rich in vitamin E, iron, copper, and healthy fats and have anti-aging properties.

OLIVE LEAF
TEA

Put a small handful of leaves in a quart-size Mason jar. Pour in boiling water to cover, close the lid tightly to trap the vapors, and let steep for 15 minutes.

Strain the tea into a mug and sweeten with honey, if desired.

MINT

MINT (*MENTHA*) IS A VERSATILE PLANT, both in the kitchen and medicinally. Mint is wonderful in the garden, but it can spread copiously and even invasively. Consider growing it in containers and clip it regularly to encourage fresh new growth. Iced mint tea is refreshing on a hot summer's day, but drink it hot on a cold day, too, to give your circulation a boost when your hands and feet feel cold. Drinking a cup of mint tea after a heavy meal quickly aids the digestion and relieves any bloating. Mint also sharpens the mind, strengthening the brain and improving concentration, focus, and memory. Inhaling the essential oil will increase your mental alertness, open up your lungs, and relieve headaches and nausea.

MINT MIST
FOR ALERTNESS

Fill a mister bottle with purified water and add 10 drops of mint essential oil. Shake well, then spray it around your face. Inhale deeply.

Keep a bottle near your computer at work, in your car, or in your purse. Use any time you need a pick-me-up.

Rosemary

ROSEMARY (*ROSMARINUS OFFICINALIS*) is both a common culinary and powerful medicinal herb. Known as the herb of remembrance, rosemary is a tonic to the brain and helps to strengthen the mind and uplift and energize the spirit. Rosemary tea increases circulation and strengthens the heart. Hot rosemary tea is wonderful for fatigue and sluggishness, and can be helpful in opening up the respiratory system or fighting infection during a cold or flu. High in essential oils, rosemary aids digestion, so adding it to rich meals helps us to digest the fats and protein. Topically, rosemary essential oil can be mixed with a carrier oil such as almond, jojoba, or even olive oil and massaged onto aching muscles and sprains. As a hair rinse, it will stimulate the scalp and combat hair loss.

ROSEMARY
HAIR MIST

Put some rosemary sprigs in a pot and cover them with water.

Cover the pot with a lid to trap the vapors, bring to a boil, and simmer the rosemary for about 20 minutes, to make a strong tea. Remove from the heat and allow to cool with the lid on.

Massage into your scalp after washing your hair. No need to rinse it out.

NASTURTIUM

NASTURTIUM (*TROPAEOLUM MAJUS*) can be recognized by its bright orange flowers and green leaves that resemble little lily pads. Nasturtium is incredibly easy to grow from seed in the garden and will reseed itself year after year without requiring much care or water. The flowers and leaves are edible and have a peppery, spicy taste, making them a great addition to a salad. Nasturtium has antibiotic properties and is high in vitamin C, which makes it a great go-to when you feel a cold coming on.

FESTIVE SALAD

Make a salad of mixed greens fresh from the garden and sprinkle the top with any combination of petals from the following edible flowers: calendula, rose, and rosemary. Finish by decorating with whole nasturtium flowers.

Yarrow

YARROW (*ACHILLEA MILLEFOLIUM*) IS named after the Greek hero Achilles who, according to legend, was the greatest warrior in Agamemnon's army and used this herb to staunch the wounds of his fellow soldiers. Because of this, yarrow also became known as *herba militaris*, meaning "soldier's herb." Yarrow is, in fact, an incredible wound healer and a plant of protection and strength. It is a key plant for any first-aid kit as it can be used in emergencies to stop bleeding. Simply chew up some of the leaves and apply them to the wound. Yarrow is also a powerful remedy for a cold or fever.

YARROW EMERGENCY POULTICE

If you or a companion is wounded and bleeding, chew up some yarrow leaves and place them on the wound. In case of a nosebleed, insert a fresh leaf in the nostril to stop bleeding.

SAGE

SAGE (*SALVIA OFFICINALIS*) IS, AS THE name suggests, a plant that connects us to the wisdom of the elders. A memory-enhancing herb and a tonic for the brain, sage is also very calming to the mind and helps us feel more centered, peaceful, and quiet. A tea of sage calms the nerves and quiets the inner chatter. Sage tea with honey is wonderful for sore throats and colds and as a digestive. And an infusion of sage can be used as a mouthwash, disinfecting the gums and teeth.

SAGE TEA FOR MEDITATION & PEACE OF MIND

Steep some fresh or dried sage with hot water in a covered pot, so the essential oils do not escape with the vapors.

Sweeten with honey, if desired, but make sure to breathe in the vapors of the tea while sitting in a peaceful place, allowing your breath to deepen and your mind to quiet.

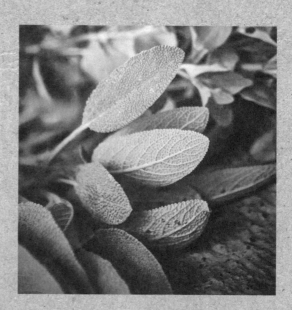

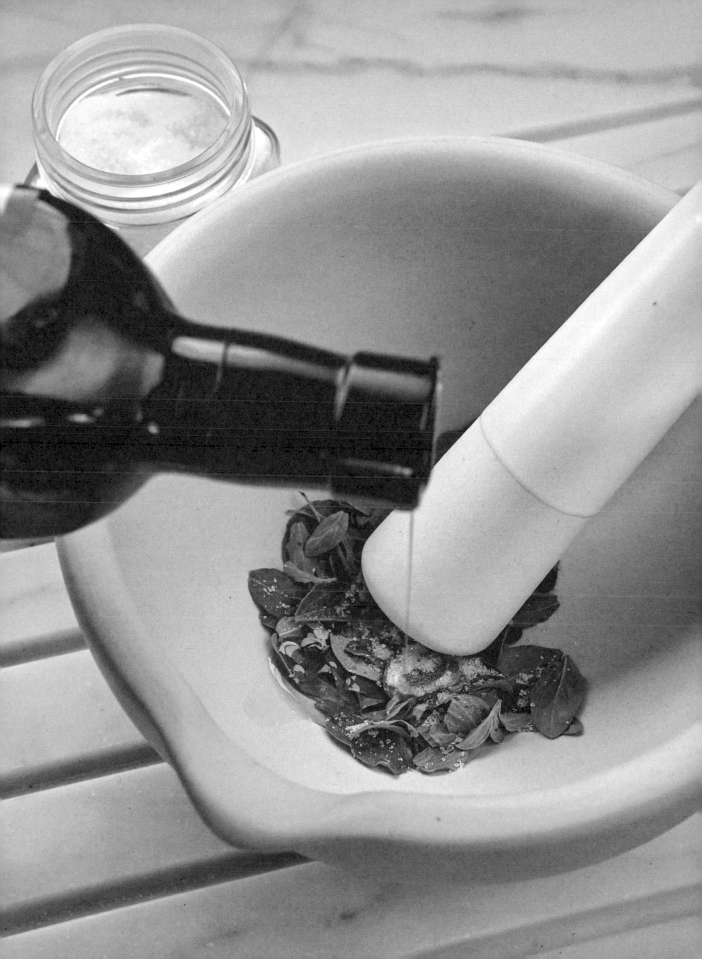

CHAPTER

6

the
Elements

EARTH, Air, AND WATER

Strength & Conditioning Programs

WORKING OUT in Nature

Part of reconnecting with nature means spending as much time surrounded by it as possible.

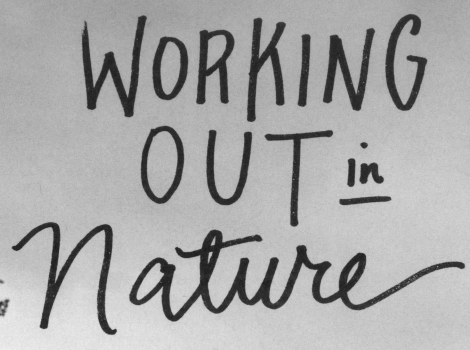

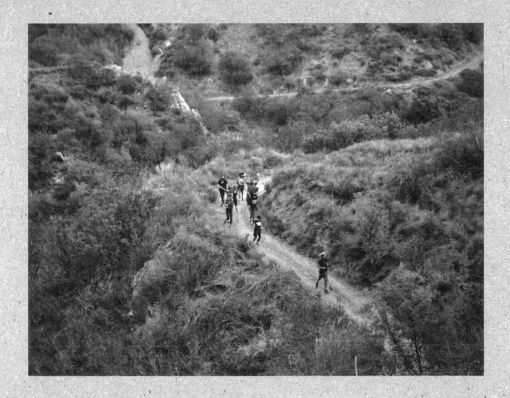

FOR US, WORKING OUT in the open air is not just physically invigo-
rating but also mentally calming, spiritually uplifting, and beneficial
in so many more ways than exercising in a gym could ever be. While
personal trainers strive to create constantly changing workouts for
their clients to keep their muscles and minds engaged, nature gives us a different workout each day. At the Ranch, we ride or hike daily, practice yoga,
invite friends up for a boot camp–style workout, or head down to the beach for
paddle-board sessions when the mercury rises.

All of the exercise we do at One Gun Ranch is meant to be functional. That
means we don't just work out for the sake of it; we want exercises that are useful
to our everyday lives. Yoga connects us to the earth and calms the mind and the
nervous system. Hikes and trail runs connect us to the wildlife and plant life
growing on the property, and we often gather food for lunch or dinner as we go.
The Stable boot-camp workouts we have devised help keep the muscles we use
when we are working on the farm, riding horses, or enjoying a day out on the
water strong, stable, and supple. We switch things up according to the season
and the cycle of the Moon, respecting our bodies and what feels right for us on any
given day. This "functional" approach to fitness gives it purpose and engages not
just the muscles but also the mind and the senses. Finally, there's the feeling of the
sky, the rocks, the ocean, and the elements as you meditate. There's nothing like it.

Earth

YOGA

AT ONE GUN RANCH we start every morning with a yoga session with Jasmina Hdagha, our Ashtanga yoga teacher. Yoga has a special place on the Ranch because, as in biodynamics, the Moon plays an important role and many practices revolve around the Moon's cycle. Just like for the tides and the Earth's water table, yogis believe that our bodies are also affected by the phases of the moon, as we are composed of 50 to 65 percent water.

According to Vedic astrology, the Moon's positions also create different energies that correspond to the breath cycle. The new moon energy corresponds to the end of exhalation when the force of apana—a contracting, downward moving force that makes us feel calm and grounded—is greatest, while the full moon energy corresponds to the end of inhalation when the force of prana—the universal principle of energy or force and the invisible energy behind the breath—is greatest. The new moon is therefore a good time to begin a meditation or yoga practice, while the full moon allows us to reap the rewards of our practice. In Ashtanga yoga, full and new moon days are observed as yoga holidays, as the prana is unbalanced, leaving the body more vulnerable to injury either through lack of energy or through too much energy. For this reason, the new moon and the full moon are often set aside for special meditation sessions.

Yoga is more than just a physical practice. Although it's great for improving flexibility, strength, and balance and the functioning of the respiratory, circulatory, digestive, and hormonal systems, it is also a mental and spiritual practice that can truly bring about emotional stability and clarity of mind. We love being able to do our sessions outside as much as possible to really feel that connection to the earth—in Sanskrit, the word "yoga" means "to unite" or "to join."

THE PRACTICE OF YOGA

THE PRACTICE OF YOGA is dedicated to creating union between body, mind, and spirit. In the ancient sage Patanjali's *Yoga Sutra*, a guidebook of classical yoga, he describes an eightfold path called Ashtanga (meaning eight limbs) that forms the structural framework for a yoga practice. Each limb is part of a holistic focus that together eventually brings completeness to the individual as he or she finds the path to enlightenment.

NEW MOON MEDITATION

A NEW MOON MARKS the beginning of a new cycle, a fresh start, birth and rebirth. Therefore, new moons can also be a time of new beginnings for us. This day, marking the new cycle, when the Moon is receptive and full of potential, is a perfect time to plant seeds of intention for what you wish to manifest in your life going forward. On the day of the new moon, we usually organize a yoga session followed by a New Moon Meditation at the Ranch. This gathering is a fun way to create a circle of connection, gently encourage one another to face our fears, and magnify the

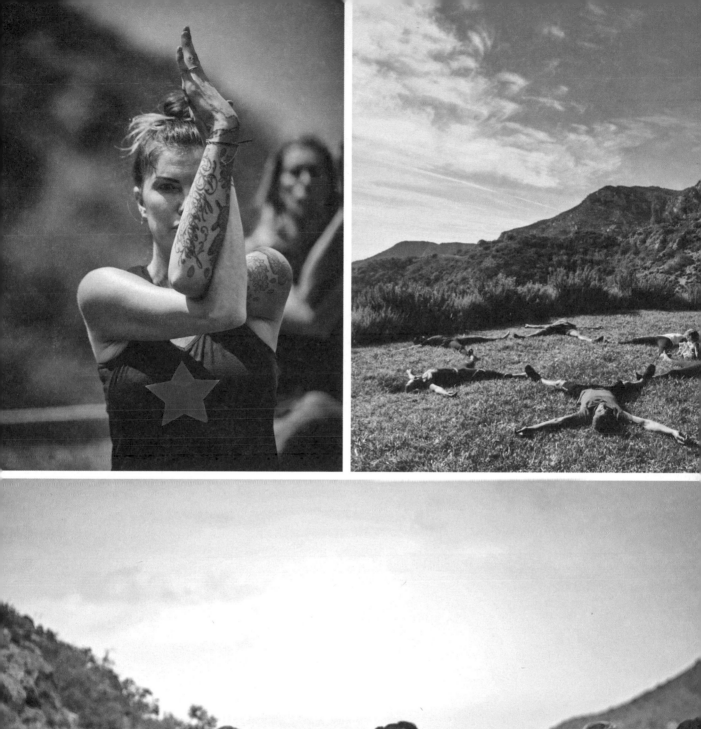
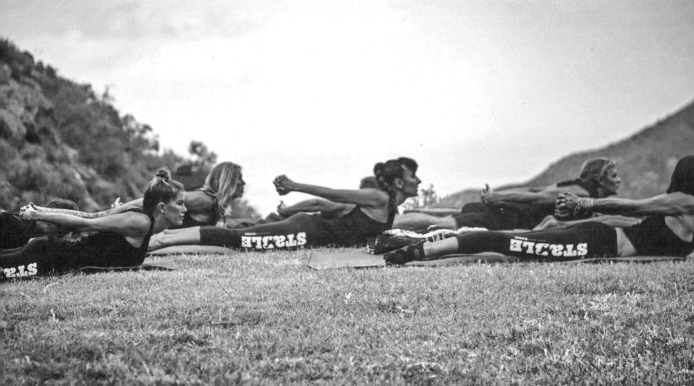

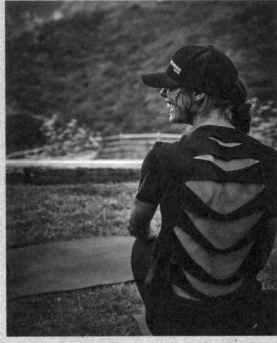
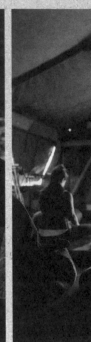

THE
EIGHT
LIMBS

YAMA
ethical disciplines, our attitude
toward the environment

NIYAMA
internal ethical observances, our
attitude toward ourselves

ASANA
poses, the practice of body
exercises, physical practice

PRANAYAMA
breath control, breathing exercises

PRATYAHARA
sensory control and withdrawal or
restraint of our senses

DHARANA
concentration, or the ability to
direct our mind

DHYANA
meditation, or the ability to
develop interactions with what we
seek to understand

SAMADHI
blissful absorption, the ability to
develop interactions with what we
seek to understand

power of our intentions. We hand everyone a piece of paper with an invocation or blessing on it and take turns reading it aloud. Next, everyone writes down their intentions on a piece of paper, and visualizes how they will come about and how it will feel when they manifest. They then read them out to the universe before burning the list.

THE ONE GUN RANCH NEW MOON SALUTATION

ON NEW MOON DAYS, when our energy is lower and a more gentle practice is recommended, we incorporate Chandra Namaskara, or Moon Salutation, which is a series of poses performed in sequence to create a cooling flow of movement that restores and replenishes. Just like Surya Namaskara, the Sun Salutation, each pose in a Moon Salutation is coordinated with your breathing. But unlike Sun Salutations, which are heating and stimulating, Moon Salutations are cooling and quieting and used to calm the mind and draw your awareness inward.

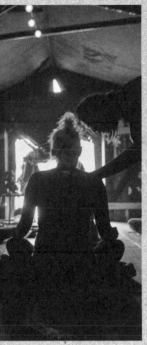
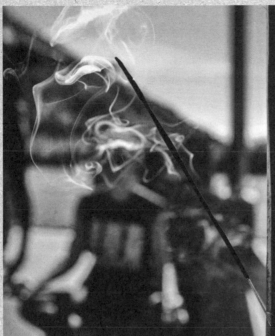
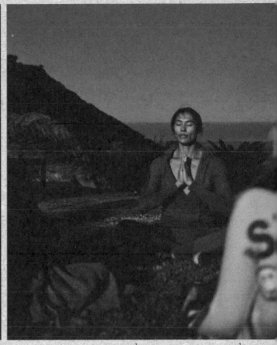

FULL MOON GROUNDING SEQUENCE

TO MARK THE FULL MOON, we often do 108 sun salutes. The full moon illuminates the things that are interfering with our spiritual advancement and is a time for releasing or purging the things in our lives that no longer serve us, breaking down old ways of being, and letting go of bad habits.

The number 108 is sacred in yoga as there are 108 pithas (sacred sites) throughout India, 108 upanishads (sacred texts), and 108 karma points on the body. Malas (garlands of prayer beads used by yogis during meditation to count their mantras) hold 108 beads and one guru bead, around which the other 108 turn like planets turn around the Sun. Vedic mathematicians viewed 108 as a number of the wholeness of existence. And the number 108 also connects the Sun, Moon, and Earth, as the average distance of the Sun and the Moon to Earth is 108 times their respective diameters.

That said, we practice nonattachment in everything we do, so we don't get attached to the final number even as we are working toward it. The moment you lose track of the breath and you can't keep up with one breath per movement, stop. This is intended to be a meditative practice, a moving prayer, and for an advanced student this is truly a wonderful way to stop that internal chatter and direct the mind exclusively towards an object, sustaining that direction without any distractions. If you are dealing with injuries or building up your strength, you can modify: Take child's pose after every ten sun salutes, even *Tadasana* (Mountain Pose). The options are endless and if you listen to your body and heart you will find the right number for you at the given moment.

FULL MOON MEDITATION

THE FULL MOON IS a time to acknowledge what you have accomplished since the last full moon and what you are grateful for. Meditating at the time of a full moon, when there is a lot of energy in the air and emotions can run high, can really help you look within, center yourself, and calm any inner conflict. Full moons are about completion, change, releasing, and cleansing, so we will often practice Pranayamas (yogic breathing practices) to calm and balance our energy.

FULL MOON NADI SHODANA

TO BEGIN, SIT IN A CIRCLE in a comfortable cross-legged position. Place your left hand on your left knee with the palm facing upwards, close your eyes, and start to bring awareness to the breath. Close your right nostril with your right thumb and inhale deeply through your left nostril. At the peak of the inhalation, close your left nostril with your right ring finger and pinkie finger, removing your thumb from the right nostril and exhale fully. Switch back to the left nostril; repeat nine times.

This breathing technique produces optimum function of both the right and left sides of your brain, therefore enhancing creativity and logical verbal activity. What this means for you is it's a quick way to balance out, cleanse, and rejuvenate the vital channels of energy in your body, keeping you refreshed, grounded, and at ease.

ON THE TRAIL:

Trail Running, Hiking, Mountain Biking, Horseback Riding, Running, Cycling, and Other Physical Journeys

IF GETTING OUT ON THE TRAIL is your thing, this workout is for you. Trails can change on a dime, so it's really important to have good lower-body stability, coordination, mobility, power, speed, and endurance.

Inclines, declines, level changes, rocks, trees, loose dirt, creek beds . . . whether you're running, on a bike, or on a horse, the trail can be a total obstacle course, so you'd better be prepared. This program will help all trail athletes improve performance and reduce injury. Cyclists and horseback riders should pay extra attention to posture and lower-body imbalances.

The Warm-up (page 117)

Single-Leg Romanian Dead Lift (page 119)

- Using your body weight and a kettle bell or dumbbell
- 10 to 12 controlled reps on each side

Monster Steps and Side Steps (page 120)

- Using resistance bands
- 2 to 3 sets, 30 to 60 seconds

Squat Jumps (page 120)

- 2 to 3 sets, 8 to 12 controlled reps

Lateral Lunge (page 123)

- 2 to 3 sets, 12 to 20 on each side, then 20 to 30 explosive seconds, alternating

Sprints (page 123)

- 2 to 3 sets, 20 to 30 seconds

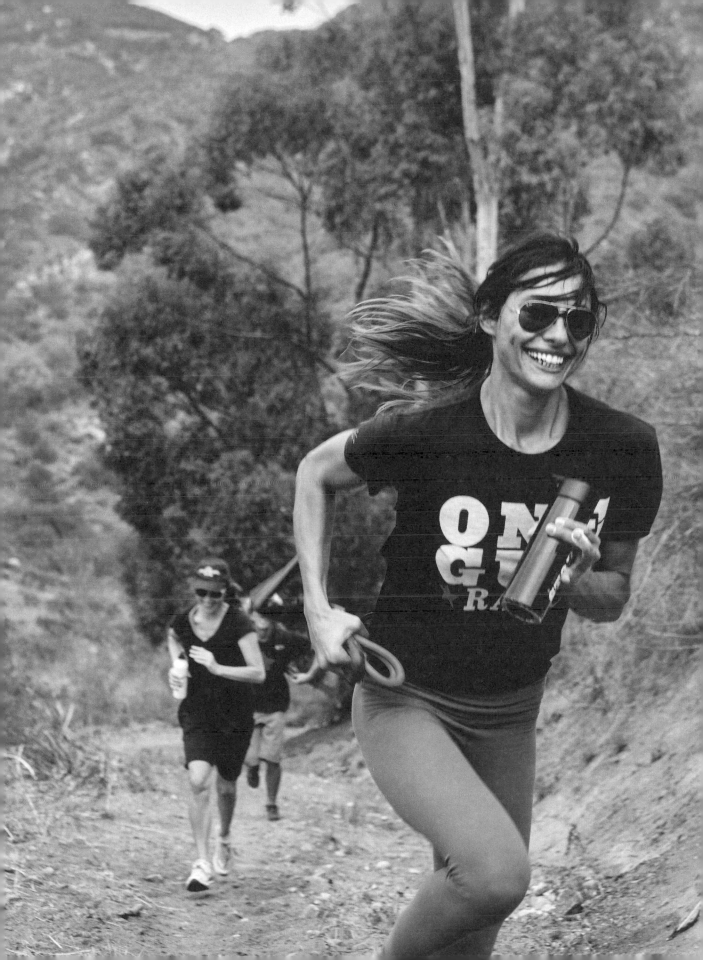

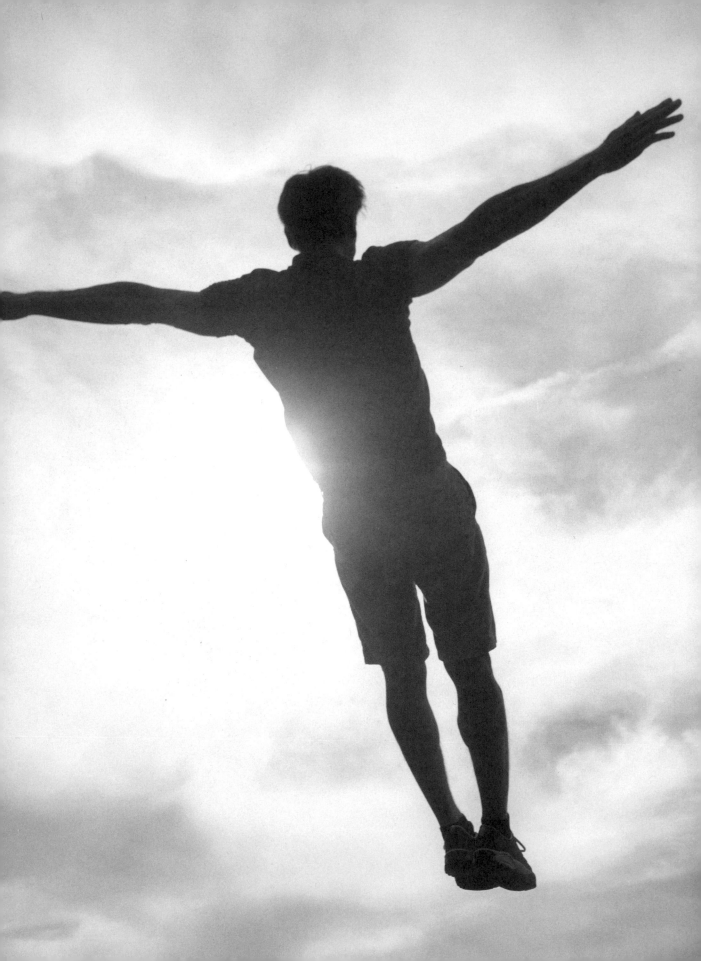

Multi-Planar Lunge (page 123)

* 2 to 3 sets, 12 to 20 reps

Bent-over Rows/Dumbell Pull (page 124)

* Using barbell or dumbbells
* 2 to 3 sets, 12 to 20 reps

Plank Up-Down

* 2 to 3 sets, up to 10 each side, alternating, or 30 to 60 second intervals

THE COOL-DOWN AND STRETCH

NOW THAT YOU'VE BALANCED, stabilized, bent, twisted, jumped, run, squatted, lunged, pushed, and pulled, it's time for a good cool-down and stretch. Post workout, or after any strenuous activity, is a great time to check that flexibility and range of movement, because your body temperature is up and the muscles have been moving. The key is to pay attention to muscle groups that tend to shorten, like calves, hip flexors, the TFL muscles in the thighs, your abdominals, and the lats on either side of your back. Also pay attention to whether one calf, quad, or lat might be tighter than the other. This is a very basic, yet important, form of body awareness that will help you move better.

1. **Child's Pose:** Hold for 60 seconds.

2. **Lying Calf Stretch:** Lie on your back and lift one leg up as close to 90 degrees to the hip as possible. Try to keep your knee extended as you pull your toes down by engaging your shin muscle (anterior tibialis). Don't use your hands to assist. Hold for 25 breaths, then switch legs.

3. **Piriformis Stretch:** Cross either foot over the opposite knee and pull that knee up until you feel a good glute stretch. Pull with your hip flexor and try not to assist with your hands. Hold for 25 breaths, then switch legs.

4. **Lying Oblique Stretch:** Lie on your back, bend your knees, and place your feet flat on the floor. Lower both knees and your hip to one side. Hold the stretch. Return to center, then repeat on the opposite side. Keep both shoulders on the floor or mat. Allow the foot of your top leg to rest on the foot of your lower leg. Your arms can be extended out to the sides. Hold for 25 breaths on each side.

5. **Half-Kneel Hip Flexor Stretch:** From a kneeling position, bring the right foot forward, making sure that the right knee is directly over the right ankle. Place both hands gently on the right thigh to help maintain a straight, tall spine. Keep your pelvis stable and lean forward into your right hip while keeping your left knee pressed into the ground. Hold for 25 breaths on each side. Bend laterally to get a stretch in the TFL, obliques, and lats.

THE ONE GUN RANCH HIKE WORKOUT

HIKING IS EXPERIENCING A real resurgence in California right now, and for good reason. A truly versatile workout, a hike can be as easy or as hard as you want it to be. Anyone, young or old, can hike. You can carry an infant along in a hiking carrier and bring the dogs along, too. Just like going for a long walk with the family after an indulgent Sunday lunch, hiking is a great social activity and between the conversation, the new discoveries we make along the way as we spot interesting plants and wildlife, and the amazing

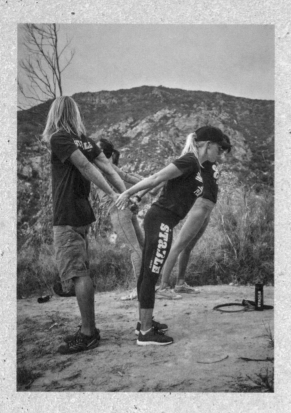

We always make sure to get a good dynamic warm-up in before setting out for a hike. Stretching and core stabilization work is a must, and if it's to be a more intense hike, we do some side shuffles, crossovers, side lunges, and step-ups to prepare the ankles, knees, and hips. A good solid ten-minute warm up is the key to injury prevention.

Set out at a moderate pace, then get into a light jog, then a run, and then back to a jog to recover. The goal is to hit intervals of fatigue, recover, and hit it again. The steeper the hill, the harder your body has to work.

Use the landscape around you. Sometimes there will be a run of obstacles, so I'll treat that section as an obstacle course: Jumping on and off rocks, running across a log, jumping over a creek . . . whatever is in the way! This is fun and really tests your fitness.

I also like to add upper-body exercises, since hiking and trail running are so lower-body centric. I often bring along some resistance bands or a TRX for the journey, because they're compact, lightweight, and versatile. We will stop at a good tree at some point for some rows and chops. Logs can be used for tricep dips, and if I see a nice boulder, maybe we throw in a set of push-ups.

The health benefits of hiking or taking a walk in the park are also much more substantial than those of doing something similar on a treadmill in the gym. Numerous studies show that walking among trees, or even just looking at the trees, reduces blood pressure and cortisol and adrenaline production, thus lowering stress. Scientists believe that, unlike natural environments, urban environments are filled with stimulation that capture our attention dramatically, making them less restorative. Walking in nature or viewing pictures of nature can therefore

views that we are rewarded with at the end, we often have so much fun that it hardly seems like exercise.

That said, hiking is a fantastic cardiovascular and strength workout that burns calories and builds muscle. Walking uphill at a steep or steady incline engages multiple muscle groups in the lower body, works your abdominals, and improves your balance and coordination. The rugged terrain forces your body to stabilize itself, which increases your aerobic threshold and cardiac function, and improves lung capacity. At the Ranch, we often switch between trails, change up the pace, and stop to do some push-ups or sit-ups along the way. The landscape is never the same, changing with the time of day and the season, and providing endless variety and motivation so that a hike never gets boring.

improve our ability to direct our attention. In Japan, the practice of *Shinrin-yoku*, or "forest bathing," was introduced by the Forest Agency in 1982 to encourage the population to adopt a more healthy lifestyle. This practice of guided walks through the forest is now a scientifically recognized stress-management activity.

A FORAGING HIKE AT ONE GUN RANCH

THERE ARE MANY NATIVE plants that grow wild in the Santa Monica Mountains around the Ranch, and as we started hiking the trails, we became fascinated with discovering more about how the Chumash had used these plants traditionally and how we might use them now.

A hike makes for a great workout, and we loved the idea that we might also pick up some ingredients for lunch along the way, so we enlisted the help of Pascal Baudar. Pascal is a wild food expert who has spent the past twelve years studying the flora and fauna in Southern California and integrating this wild food into a sustainable lifestyle, while creating what he calls "an authentic California cuisine."

We now like to organize a wild-food hike around the property for friends and family several times a year, ending with a tasting at the Wild Edible Saloon of all that we find. The best time for foraging in Malibu is in January. Here is what we commonly find and how we use it:

Black and Purple Sage: These perennial shrubs are common in the coastal sage scrub of Southern California and cover the mountains surrounding the Ranch. The Chumash brewed sage into teas to relieve pain, as it contains anti-inflammatory compounds.

Sage can be used in so many recipes, from soups to stuffings to compound butters as well as a garnish, but we particularly like to infuse raw local honey with sage leaves and add sage to tea, or spike some hot chocolate with a couple of leaves.

California Bay Laurel: The leaves of this tree can be dried and used as you would any bay leaf, but be aware that the California Bay has a much stronger flavor, so you may want to use less than normal in recipes. Bay leaves jump-start the immune system, so are perfect used in a warming winter soup.

California Mugwort: Because of its mild sedative properties, the Chumash called mugwort "dream sage" and would burn it to promote good dreams and heal the spirit. The stems and leaves were also tied in bundles to make smudge sticks used for cleansing and purification, and infusions were used to treat stomach complaints. Pascal also taught us to save the larger stems for use as skewers, as they infuse food with their aromatic flavor.

Curly Dock: Also known as sheep sorrel, this sour green is loaded with vitamin C and has more iron than spinach. It is wonderful with fish, sautéed with olive oil and garlic and served with eggs, or on a wood-fired pizza.

Dandelion: A common weed, dandelion leaves are easy to spot and make for a delicious salad green. They can also be sautéed and used in an omelette or soup, and are packed with vitamin A, vitamin C, and beta-carotene, as well as minerals, flavonoids, and omega-3s. The bright yellow flowers are an excellent source of lecithin, which helps maintain good brain and liver function, and are also edible and make a beautiful addition to a salad.

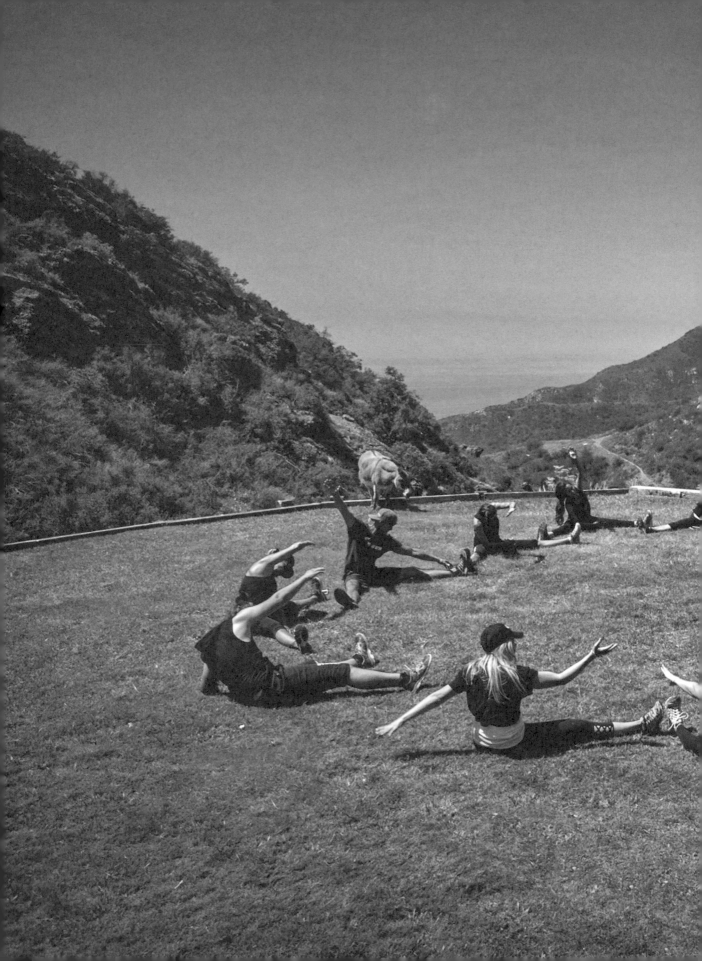

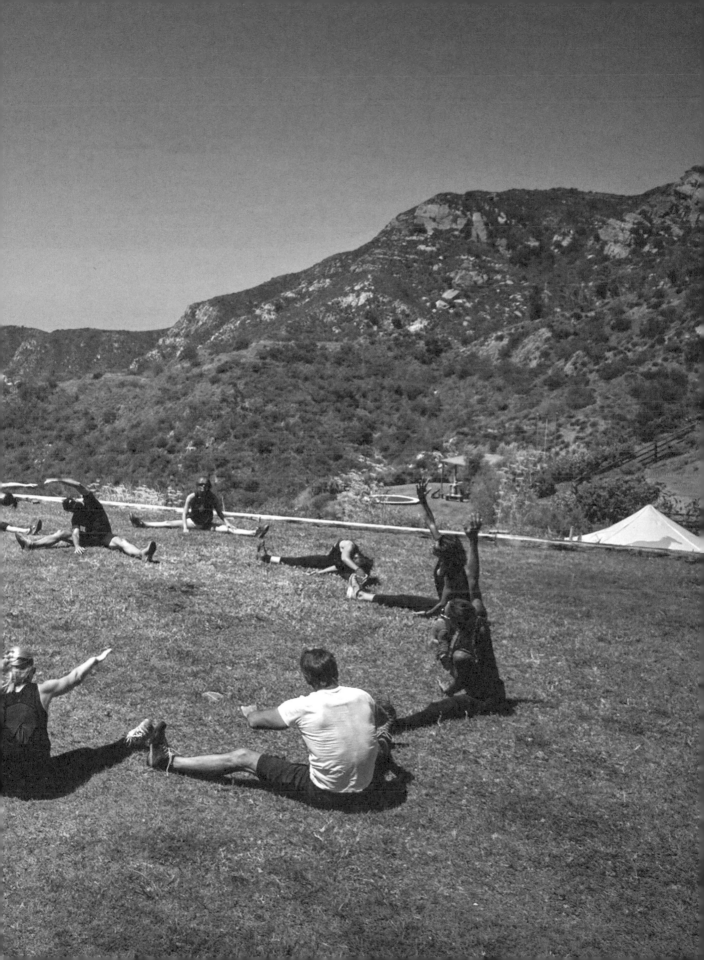

Eucalyptus: While not native to California (the blue gum tree was brought over from Australia in the 1870s when there was a high demand for wood), there are a lot of eucalyptus trees on our property and the fresh, camphorlike scent they give off as the wind blows through the leaves is really lovely. To make a eucalyptus infusion to treat coughs, colds, congestion, and throat infections, pour 1 cup of boiling water over 2 teaspoons of crushed eucalyptus leaves. Steep for 10 minutes and then strain before drinking or inhaling the vapors.

Pink Peppercorn: Pink peppercorns are not true peppercorns; they are, in fact, the aromatic berries of the Brazilian pepper tree and the Peruvian pepper tree, which grow wild in Southern California. Pink peppercorns are light and fluffy, almost hollow, and have a citrus flavor. They go well with fruit and in desserts and can be used to infuse oils and vinegars.

Piñon Pine: Pine needles are very high in vitamins C and A, resveratrol, quercetin, flavonoids, tannins, anthocyanins, and proanthocyanin and make for a wonderful antioxidant-rich tea. Simply collect a handful of young green needles, remove the brown sheaths at the base, wash the needles thoroughly, and chop them into small pieces. Pour boiled water over a tablespoon of the needles and allow it to steep until most of the needles have settled to the bottom of the cup. Strain and drink. We also infuse oils and vinegars with pine needles for 3 to 6 weeks.

Wild Fennel: The wild fennel that grows in Southern California is *Finocchietto selvatico*, the same variety that grows on the coastal areas of Southern Italy. Wild fennel does not produce a significant bulb, so we gather the fronds and use them to stuff into fish or sprinkle in salads, and harvest the blossoms for pollen (just shake the flower heads into a bag to dislodge the creamy, yellow powder) and dust it onto fish, cioppino, or roasted vegetables.

Wild Mustard: Part of the *BRASSICA* family, in the spring, bright yellow mustard flowers pop up all over the property. They can be used raw, along with the young leaves, in salads. Later in the summer you can sauté the greens with olive oil and garlic and use them as you would broccoli rabe.

Yarrow: A soft herb similar to tarragon, you can substitute the two for each other in any dish, or mix yarrow and tarragon with other soft herbs like chervil and parsley in a compound butter or infused oil. Yarrow is used extensively in herbal medicine as it has antibacterial and anti-inflammatory properties; the Chumash chewed on yarrow leaves to relieve toothaches.

Yucca: The white petals from the flowers of the tall, spiky yucca are edible and can be sautéed with olive oil and lemon, while the tough leaves are perfect for tying up food before putting it on the grill. The leaves and roots can also be used to make handy natural soap simply by grinding them up and mixing with water.

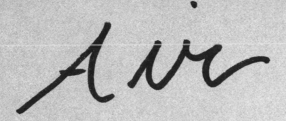

THE STABLE FITNESS

Biodynamic Programs

BECAUSE FEELING FIT and healthy is paramount and exercise is an integral part of our day, we decided to create some fun workouts that could be done outdoors at the Ranch. The Stable happened organically, as Annie and I both love working out in the open air and we love collaborating with the community. It's something that we've always done. When we are traveling, we always work out with friends and family in a group. The yoga program at Daylesford in the UK was inspired by my invitations to practice yoga with me on the farm. When we bought the Ranch, we inherited a dressage ring filled with sand; what is now the Secret Garden was a volleyball court; we found a huge trampoline, which we sank into a piece of land overlooking the Pacific Ocean and we converted a grassy area also overlooking the ocean into an outdoor gym so that we could work out with friends.

Because our athletic pursuits change with the seasons, we asked Chris Chandler, the Stable's resident holistic personal trainer and health coach, who is also an avid surfer, to design four seasonal programs to help improve our conditioning and athletic performance in the ocean and the sand, on the slopes and the trails, and on the court and the field. The goal of the programs is to improve posture, stability, mobility, gait, muscular endurance, muscular strength, speed, power, and overall athletic performance, while correcting muscle imbalance and reducing chance of injury.

The Warm-up

For better performance, I recommend warming up prior to any workout, physical activity, or sport. This warm-up is a combination of isometric stabilization and dynamic movement. The goal here is to raise your core temperature, get those core muscles firing, address muscle imbalances, establish some joint range of motion (ROM), and generally prepare your body for the work ahead. Visually preparing yourself is also crucial. Whether you're warming up for a good workout, a surf session, a trail run, or a tennis match, always visualize yourself feeling good and performing your best.

This general warm-up will get you ready for most performance-based workout sports. I like to spend at least 10 minutes just warming up. As you go along, try to be aware of any muscle imbalances. They are the key to how efficiently you move and perform and whether you're likely to be injured. Most of us have a more dominant leg, are stronger on one side, or twist to one side more easily than the other, because we throw, swing, or twist (football, baseball, tennis, golf, volleyball) repetitively; have a dominant foot forward (surfing, waterskiing, snowboarding, wakesurfing, and wakeboarding); or are repetitive in the same plane of motion (cycling, cross-country skiing, running, and hiking). We also sit too much and for too long, so bridging the gap between your desk and your sport is crucial.

1. **One-Foot Balance:** Maintain your balance for 30 seconds on each leg.

2. **Six-Point Stance:** Drop onto your hands and knees, with your toes down. Put one hand behind your head. Maintain a neutral spine and hold for 30 seconds. Extend the opposite leg. Hold for 30 seconds. Switch sides and repeat.

3. **Six-Point Dynamic:** Still on all fours, lift one arm and pull in your elbow, raising the opposite knee to meet it. Keep the head neutral and at 12 o'clock. Do 12 to 20 reps.

4. **Take a Child's Pose for a short recovery.**

5. **Plank Pose:** With extended arms, a neutral spine, head neutral, and core tight. Control for 30 to 60 seconds before progressing. It's okay to start from the knees if needed. Stability before mobility.

6. **Plank with an Upper Body Twist:** Tight core; feet straight; breathe. Turn your head to the right and look up to the sky, twisting your upper body and raising your right arm above the shoulder using your full range of motion. Keep the hips neutral and use a controlled tempo. Do 12 to 20 reps on each side.

7. **Plank with Alternating Leg Raises:** This really fires up the glutes. Pick up one hand and the opposite foot and control for up to 30 seconds, then switch sides. 12 to 20 reps.

8. **Side Plank:** Neutral spine. Control for 30 seconds on each side before progressing.

9. **Side Leg Raise (Hip Abduction):** Again, you can start from knees and progress to extended legs. Do 12 to 20 reps on each side.

10. **Overhead Squat:** The focus is on lower body stability and posture. Maintain a neutral head and spine, keep the arms extended, heels loaded, and the knees tracking with the feet. Breathe and squat, hold for 30 second intervals.

11. **Leg Swings (or Toy Soldiers):** Walk forward, fully extending one leg; extend the opposite arm and touch your toes. You can also do this stationary, stabilizing yourself by holding on to the back of a park bench or a tree with one hand while swinging the opposite leg backwards and forwards, then switching sides. 30 to 60 second intervals.

12. **Lateral Shuffle, Skipping with High Knees, or Crossovers:** 30 to 60 second intervals.

At this point you are ready to rock! Make sure that water canteen is full . . . but take care to sip as you go.

Water

SURFING,

Wakesurfing/Wakeboarding, Waterskiing, and Stand-up Paddleboarding

WATER IS AN UNSTABLE and spontaneous medium, and therefore water sports require a great deal of balance, overall stability, and specific conditioning. Training on an unstable medium like a Bosu, a stability ball, or even on one leg is a great way to prepare and will help keep you dialed in when you're out of the water. If you're a paddler, or are being pulled by a rope, left foot forward, right or sometimes parallel, it's important to be aware of and to compensate for resulting imbalances. This alone is a game changer.

The Warm-up

Single-Leg Romanian Dead Lift or Warrior III

- Using your bodyweight and a kettle bell or dumbbell
- 10 to 12 controlled reps on each side

Target: These really get your glutes firing, which is crucial to lower-body stability. Balance, coordination, and total body awareness (proprioception) are emphasized.

Single-Leg Romanian Dead Lift

1. Grab the weight in one hand. Lower your upper body by bending at the hip. Let the leg and foot on the same side as the weight travel back at the same rate as your head lowers, in a hinge movement. Keep your back straight and head neutral; let your arm hang below your shoulder.

2. Push your hips back and slightly bend the knee on your supporting leg during the descent. Swing your free leg back so it stays in line with your torso. Continue lowering your upper body until a mild stretch is felt in the hamstrings.

3. Return to the starting position.

OR

Warrior III

Inhaling deeply, extend your arms over your head with palms facing each other. As you exhale, stretch the arms forward, hinging at the hips, and lift your left leg behind you until your body is at a 90º angle to the standing leg. Stretch through the toes, the fingers, and the crown of the head to make a straight line, keeping the hips in line. Take three controlled breaths. Return to a standing position and repeat on the other leg.

1. Hold Warrior III on each side for 30 seconds. This exercise builds strength in the legs and the hips while improving balance and stability throughout the core.

2. Stand on a Bosu ball to challenge your stability more. Add load to make it even more difficult.

Monster Steps and Side Steps

* Using resistance bands
* 2 to 3 sets, 30 to 60 second intervals

Target: This exercise improves hip stability, strengthens the hip abductors, and increases stability in the knee joints. Both steps can also be performed standing up in place.

1. Place a resistance band around both ankles. Add another around both knees for an additional challenge. If you have knee issues, place the band just above the knees only. There should be enough tension that they are taut when your feet are shoulder-width apart. I prefer medium resistance.

2. Take 10 short steps forward, alternating your left and right foot, then take 10 steps backwards to where you started. These should be big steps forward and back, with feet parallel and wider than normal.

3. Recover briefly, then start stepping laterally. 10 in one direction, 10 back.

Box Jumps

* 8 to 10 explosive reps, 2 to 3 sets

Target: This exercise increases lower body power, strength, and speed, and also improves coordination and core stability. If you are jumping, focus on landing softly to minimize the impact on your knees. It's also important that you don't land deeper than your starting point.

1. Stand in front of a secured box or bench at an appropriate height for your ability. Bend down into a squat position, then quickly explode your hip and legs upward while swinging your arms in the air to propel yourself on top of the box. Land softly on the box and come to a standing position.

2. Slowly step off the box back into starting position. Alternate legs for your dismounts.

3. When you feel ready, jump back down as well, focusing on a smooth landing with good form.

4. Also when you're ready, try starting on the box, jumping down and right back up, to challenge your reactive strength, which most sports require.

5. Rest for 3 to 5 minutes between sets.

OR

Squat Jumps

* 8 to 10 explosive reps, 2 to 3 sets

1. Stand with your feet shoulder-width apart. Bend into a squat, loading your heels. Keep your knees in line with your toes, hands in front with good posture.

2. Engage your core and jump up explosively. Fully extend your arms overhead into full extension.

3. Land softly with control and lower your body back into the squat position. For a reactive-strength challenge, don't pause at the bottom.

Ice Skaters

* 2 to 3 sets, 30 to 60 second intervals

Target: This exercise works the glutes and improves core stabilization, mobility, speed, and stamina.

1. Start by standing on one leg. Hop from side to side, switching legs as if you were speed skating.

2. Swing your arms from side to side, touching the opposite arm to the opposite standing leg, lowering your body down to do so.

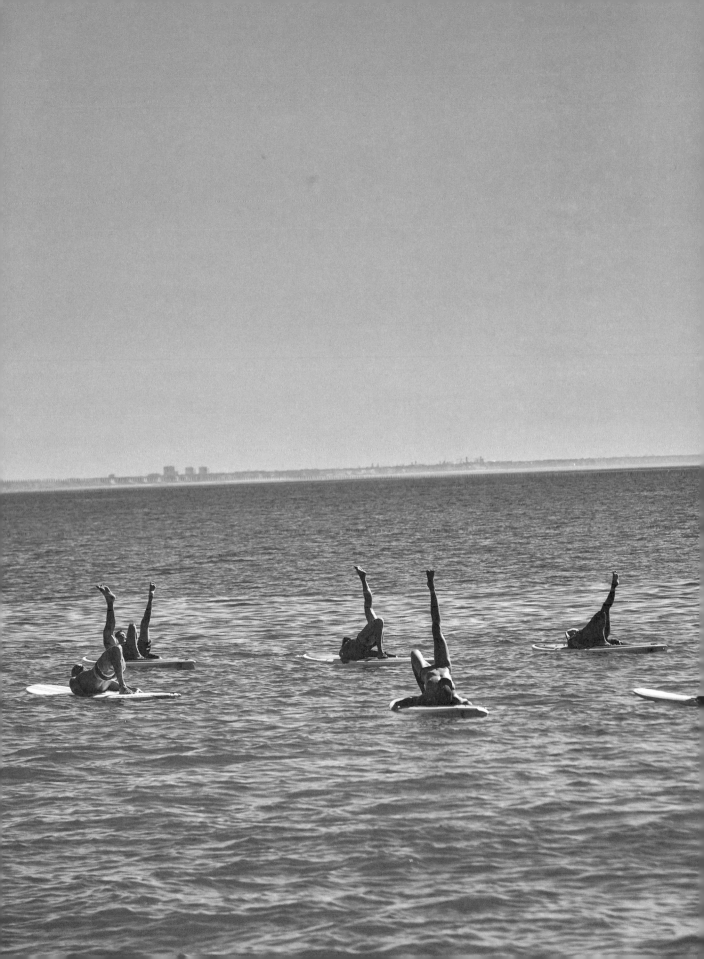

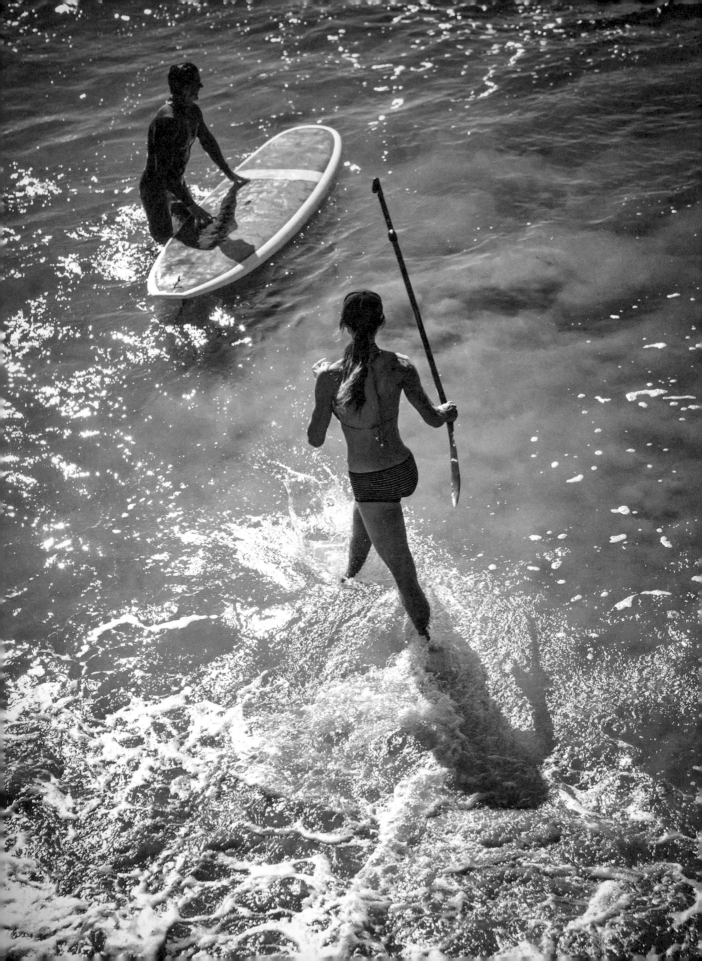

3. Maintain good posture with a straight back, tight core, and neutral head. Use your legs, not your lower back. Get those steps wide. I like to use cones as a guide. This is a sprint, so take a few minutes between sets.

Sprints

* 2 to 3 sets, 20 to 30 second intervals

Target: Any cardiovascular challenge is beneficial for athletes, and even more so for surfers and swimmers, who need to hold their breath for a length of time. High-intensity intervals are also the most efficient way to rev up your metabolism and turn your body into a fat-burning machine.

At the Ranch we use the horse paddock, which is filled with sand, for sprints, as well as grass and even dirt trails. It's good to change up terrain, as that provides the maximum benefit to your workout and really reduces chance of injury—so mix it up! The beach, a field in the park, or a local running track are also good places to get some sprints in. Add in some hills for an increased challenge.

1. Sprint for 30 to 60 seconds at 60 to 80 percent, or for 20 to 30 seconds all out. Take 5 minutes to recover between sets.

Multi-Planar Lunge

* 12 to 20 reps each side for each direction

Target: This exercise, which is broken into forward, side, and back moves, improves hip mobility while strengthening the hip muscles, and improves balance and stability. Emphasize loading the heel of the loaded leg. Your knees should track with your toes, not pass them. Maintain good posture and ensure that your feet are parallel in the side lunges.

Forward Lunge

1. Take a big step forward with one leg.
2. Once your front foot touches down, lower your body down towards the ground until your back knee taps the floor.
3. Push strongly off the front foot to move back to the starting position.

Lateral Lunge

1. Take a big step to the side, much wider than your normal base.
2. As your foot touches down, sit all your weight onto the heel and push your butt back.
3. The stationary leg should straighten out.
4. Push strongly off the lateral leg to move back to the starting position.

Back Lunge

1. Same as Forward Lunge above, but step back, tap your knee, and drive off your forward foot back to the starting position.
2. Breathe. Repeat.

Overhead Squats

* Using bodyweight, barbell, dumbbells, or kettle bells.
* 2 to 3 sets, 10 to 12 reps

Target: This is a compound, full-body exercise that emphasizes lower-body strength, mobility, core stabilization, and postural strength. This is a fundamental compound movement that should be performed by all athletes. Squatting is also vital for day-to-day functional movement and everyday tasks. Hold a barbell, dumbbells, or kettle bells of appropriate weight overhead for increased challenge. Try one hand (offset) for additional core challenge. Compare sides.

1. Begin in a standing position, feet straight, with arms extended overhead. Your upper arms should be beside your ears, head neutral, with thumbs facing behind you.

2. This movement starts by moving the hips back and bending the knees and hips to lower your torso. Maintain posture and arm position as you descend.

3. Load your heels and track your knees with your feet.

4. Try to get your thighs parallel to floor. Use a bench as a reference point until you can control descent, then progress lower if needed.

5. Return to standing position.

6. Repeat.

Horizontal Wood Chops

- Using a weighted ball (medicine) or resistance band
- 2 to 3 sets, 12 to 20 reps or 30 to 60 seconds each side

Target: This exercise works your obliques and core muscles as you twist, for increased mobility and power. Compare sides and look for imbalances. Add an extra set to your less dominant side.

1. Rotatory strength is very important. I like to start people at chest level with an emphasis on the obliques. Perform a couple of sets with the band beside you and a couple with the band straight ahead of you, hitting both the anterior and posterior oblique chains. Keep the hips stable. Increase your range of motion as you improve and correct imbalances.

2. Wrap a resistance band around a tree or post at eye level. Grab the band and step away until it's taut. Your outstretched arm should be aligned with the band, feet positioned shoulder-width apart.

3. Reach upward with your other hand and grab the handle with both hands, with arms fully extended.

4. In one motion, pull the handle across your body horizontally while rotating your torso. Minimize hip movement, using your core to produce and reduce force. Keep your back and arms straight and core tight.

5. Return to the starting position, slowly and with control.

6. Repeat. Breathe.

7. If using a weighted ball, start with your feet a little wider than hip distance apart, keeping the knees slightly bent and the hips stable, and bring the weighted ball to your left shoulder.

8. Chop the ball down diagonally across your body toward your right knee while rotating your torso, but keep your hips stable and maintain good posture.

9. Control the ball back up to the starting position. The more speed, the more torque generated, the harder the core works.

Bent-Over Rows/Dumbbell Pull

- 2 to 3 sets, 12 to 20 reps each side

Target: These exercises target the back muscles and improve upper body strength, core stabilization, and shoulder range of motion. If your sport is lower-body dominant, it's crucial to train your upper body, especially with pulling exercises.

1. Holding a dumbbell in one hand, place your opposite hand and knee on a bench. Chin down, shoulders down—no shrugging.

2. Keep your back flat as you let the dumbbell hang down to your side and line up your arm in front of your shoulder.

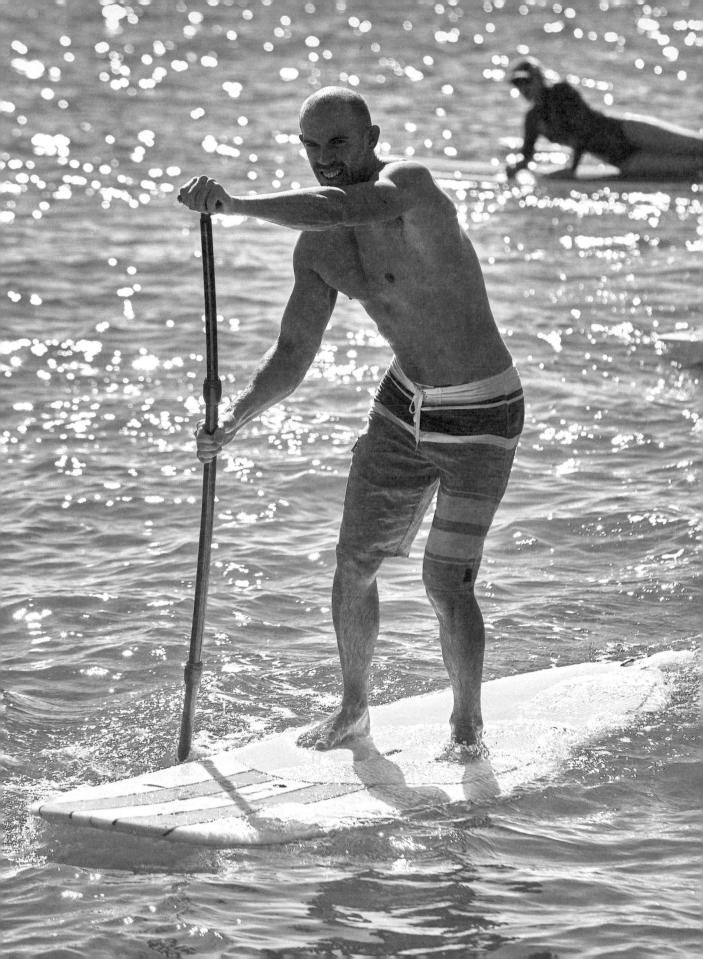

3. Using your upper-back muscles, pull the dumbbell up and back toward your hip, keeping your elbow close to your body.

4. Pause, then slowly return to the starting position.

5. Switch sides and repeat with the other arm.

AND

Straight-Arm Pull

♦ 2 to 3 sets, 12 to 20 reps each side

1. Use a medium tension band anchored to a tree or post at waist level. Grab a handle in each hand, hands shoulder-width apart, and walk back until band is barely taut.

2. With arms extended, bend at the hip with a straight back, chin down, and slowly pull your hands to your hips. Don't round the back when you pull.

3. Maintain form as you return to the starting position.

Tucks

♦ 12 to 20 reps, or 30 to 60 seconds

Target: Mountain Climbers and Tucks are full-body exercises that engage most muscles in the body, improving core stabilization and muscular endurance.

1. Begin in a plank position with arms straight and hands directly under your chest, shoulder-width apart.

2. Lift your right foot off of the floor and pull your knee up to your chest.

3. Explosively reverse the positions of your legs as if you are running with high knees.

4. You can also tuck one knee up into the chest and alternate slowly.

5. For an added challenge, hold a plank with your feet on a Bosu ball, chin down, and pull your knees up into your chest, squeezing your abdominals. Keep your core tight as you return to the starting position.

OR

Mountain Climbers

♦ 12 to 20 reps, or 30 to 60 seconds

1. From a plank position, put your shins hip-width apart on a stability ball.

2. When stable, slowly pull both knees and ball under your chest, squeezing your abdominals.

3. Return to the starting position with control.

4. Breathe. Repeat.

Burpees

♦ 2 to 3 sets, 8 to 10 explosive reps

Target: Burpees are another a full-body exercise that engages most muscle groups, with an emphasis on explosiveness. The basic movement is performed in four steps. Pause briefly between each step if needed to ensure stability.

1. Begin in a standing position, with feet shoulder-width apart.

2. Drop into a squat position, placing your hands on the ground, shoulder-width apart.

3. Kick your feet back into a plank while keeping your arms extended. More advanced athletes tap their chest to floor.

4. Immediately explode your feet into the squat position, hands in front.

5. Jump up from the squat position, extending your arms overhead.

6. Breathe. Repeat.

The Cool-down and Stretch (page 111)

STAND-UP PADDLEBOARDING

ON A HOT DAY in Southern California, there is nothing better than being on the water, so on such a day we like to head down to the beach via the winding road that connects One Gun Ranch to the Pacific Coast Highway and get out the paddleboards.

Stand-up paddleboarding started out in Hawaii and has become incredibly popular over the last few years because it is, as our great friend Mickey Eskimo has dubbed it, the ocean's bicycle. Our neighbor, pro surfer Laird Hamilton, has also compared the experience to walking on water, as standing on a board in the middle of the ocean is a spectacular way to see ocean life up close. Dolphins have joined us on several occasions, and it's a lovely way to explore the coastline without the noise of a boat's engine.

Not only is paddleboarding one of the best ways there is to enjoy the water, it is also a great full-body workout, as almost every muscle in the body is used at some point. Much larger and more stable than a surfboard, an SUP board is basically a giant balance board, so just standing on the unstable platform engages your core muscles and legs, while paddling works the upper body. From there it's up to you how hard you want your workout to be. You can paddle slowly and tour, taking in the views and chatting to friends, or you can work in sprints and intervals along with some yoga poses. And similarly, if you are paddling in the ocean and there are a lot of waves and a strong current, your workout will be more intense than on a relatively calm day.

THE STABLE SUP WORKOUT

WE START WITH A WARM-UP on the shore to address all of the muscle groups we will use while paddleboarding. There are certain movements and stretches that SUPers should do to warm up and cool down and to compensate for repetitive movement patterns to reduce the risk of injuries.

Next, we go over some of the yoga poses and movements we will be doing once we're on the water, and the basics of the board, such as how to enter the surf safely and how to hold the paddle properly.

Once we are out on the water, stance, paddle technique, and posture are covered before the group sets out on a quick little tour to get the feel of the board. When we're nice and loose, I throw in some paddle sprints and get the group fired up.

When our heart rates are up, we find a good spot and have the group form a circle. Now that giant balance board provides a great challenge for any yoga poses, including Down and Up Dog; Warrior 1, 2, and 3; Crescent Pose, and even headstands. We like to mix these in with lunges, squats, push-up variations, and we might even throw in some Burpees (opposite page).

Interval training on paddleboards is also a great workout, so we might do some sprints to the buoy and back, working on quick turns and switching our footing.

We finish off with a restorative paddle cruise and a few stretches, lying on the boards again before a quick talk about getting back in to shore safely. A few good stretches on the beach for the lats, oblique systems, hip flexors, and calves round out the session nicely.

BIODYNAMIC HEROES:
GABBY REECE & LAIRD HAMILTON

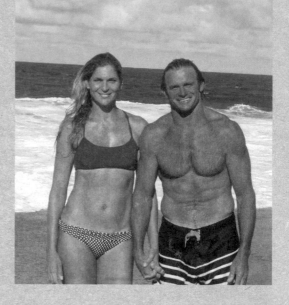

GABBY REECE AND LAIRD HAMILTON ARE world-famous athletes who work tirelessly with organizations such as Heal the Bay, the Surfrider Foundation, and the American Heart Association Teaching Gardens. They are also neighbors of ours in Malibu. They are a couple who we hugely respect and enjoy spending time with, as we have many shared interests, including growing our own food and working out in nature. Both local heroes, Laird is now also part of Malibu folklore thanks to the day he shot the Malibu Pier on Big Wednesday in 2014.

Was there a defining moment that set you on this path?

For both Laird and me, coming from a sports background, a lot of what we do with food is to improve our performance. But as we went along, we both began to realize: When I eat cleaner and closer to the source, I feel better, I have more energy, I sleep better, my recoveries are better—so I think that's how we began to connect to this in a bigger way.

A few years ago, we made a berm on our land in Hawaii, and because the soil is so rich there, in six months we had seven-foot apple trees, bananas, and papaya trees. In Hawaii, if you have an excess of something growing on your trees, you bring it over when you go to a friend's house. This is a culture where people gather over food; it's part of life. We fish and farm and yes, we go to the grocery store, but we're still connected to the process.

Why is the health of our soil so important in the age of modern farming?

Living in Hawaii, you learn a lot about the wider effects soil has on our health. We have a lot of golf courses here spraying Roundup, which causes a lot of destruction to the reef and the ecosystem. Kauai is the only island in Hawaii with navigable rivers that lead straight into the sea, so there is a direct relationship with what is happening on the land and how it affects the water, the reef life, fish, and turtles. You're so close to it that you can see how it's directly impacting the ocean.

What is your approach to growing, buying, and eating food?

We don't grow anything at our house in California because of the drought. We only have succulents on the property. In Kauai, one of the wettest spots on Earth, we have avocados, papayas, and bananas, but it's not dry enough for citrus. Farther up from where we are, I have friends with Meyer lemon trees, and we give them our fruit in exchange. On Kauai, we buy our beef from the gas station because it's meat from a local farm two miles away. We know the guy who raises the cows and what they eat. That is a luxury—although it shouldn't be. Everyone I know on the island grows something, but it could be an even bigger part of the culture. It's funny to me that something so elemental has become exotic, and I hope it will just become a normal part of life again, growing food and such.

If we are training really rigorously, sometimes we're just trying to get food into our bodies within 30 minutes and we might not have time to prepare a meal. So for us, our diet really depends on the day. The way I grew up, meat was the focal point, with everything else around it. My palate has really shifted though; now we start with the vegetable, and maybe some form of a starch like sweet potato. We don't really eat that many grains, but maybe some beans or a smaller piece of animal protein. I have children, so while we try to be a good example to the children, we also try not to make anything taboo so that they don't develop any issues or feel like they've been denied anything.

What are you working toward?

In the work I do with the American Heart Association Teaching Gardens, what is essential is bringing the process [of growing food] to young children who don't have access to that. Connecting them with where their food comes from layers in that love. It exposes them to a lot of foods they've never eaten, and they learn to grow and to prepare food. With my kids, I've seen it's not just about growing food but also about preparing the food that makes them want to eat it. If I make it and it just appears, their love and understanding of it is different. Planting the seeds and playing in the dirt is fun and it's cooperative. [It] creates harmony in our very compartmentalized and separated lives. For both Laird and me, everything we do is about promoting a sense of community and cooperation because we've been impacted so positively by our own community.

What is something you tell people they can do to make a difference?

Keep it simple and go back to basics. A hundred years ago, we didn't have as many options. Think about how many steps it took for something to get to your plate and try to step it back. . . . There are so many simple, delicious ways to make healthy food. Get your children involved in the process even though it may take longer and create more of a mess. Plan ahead so that if you're stuck at work and you only have a pizza joint downstairs, you have something healthy available. Make extra food the night before and take it to work for lunch.

It isn't about being perfect; it's about putting systems in place to be successful. If you have the opportunity to buy from the people that are growing in your area, do it. The commerce has to be connected. It's a change in habits and it can be a little more inconvenient. We've been groomed to want more, faster, for less, but you have to ask, just because this system is in place, is it the right system? We are too willing to put things that don't serve us in our bodies and we need to rethink that. Laird always says that the coolest machine you own is your body, because you can drive a car or fly a plane, but your body is the starting point.

People are busy, they don't want to be inconvenienced, and many are just scraping by; so we need to take into account everything that people are dealing with when we have this conversation. It's a real cultural shift, but if we make it a priority, we can help each other. This is a time for all hands on deck, so let's get serious.

"7" THE MALIBU Biodynamic Eating Plan

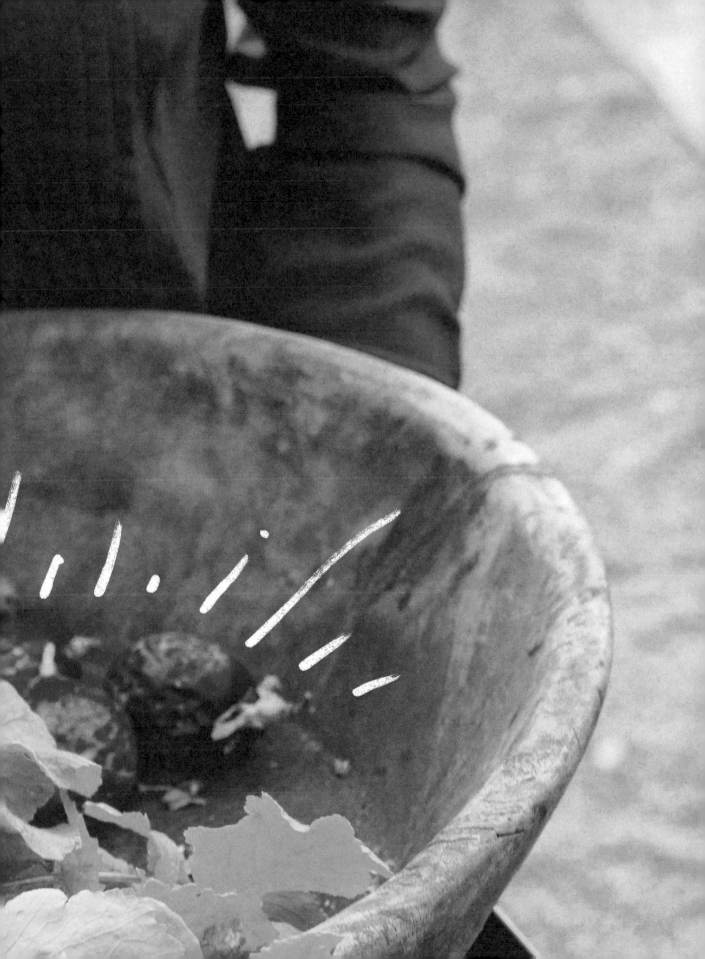

The way we eat at One Gun Ranch
is a diet for life.

IT'S A CELEBRATION of good food and good health, not about sacrifice. Eating well means being well, and for us this is not a diet that we resort to when we feel that we need to lose weight, or detox—it is a joyful way of living, always.

The Malibu Biodynamic Eating Plan is about embracing health: seasonal, local eating and the rhythms of nature, not restriction. The plan encourages us to understand our food—where it has come from and when and how it should be eaten. We avoid processed and genetically modified foods, and stick to organically, sustainably grown food.

We believe in eating *more* types of fresh, healthy, seasonal, delicious, and nutrient-packed foods instead of cutting foods out. With the advent of industrial farming and processed foods, we now eat a far smaller variety of foods than our ancestors and have limited the range of nutrients in our diet. It is believed that ancient hunter-gatherer tribes ate up to 700 types of plants and animals each year, with marked seasonal differences. Today, by shopping at the supermarket, we eat the same types of foods again and again out of habit, reaching for tomatoes or asparagus in the dead of winter rather than in-season pears or Swiss chard.

The greater variety of foods we eat, the greater chance we have of eating our daily vitamins and minerals, the healthier our guts, and the stronger our immune systems. Processed foods have plenty of ingredients in them, but we want our food to have just the one ingredient. With simple, ripe, organically grown produce, the quality shines through, providing plenty of flavor without additives, artificial flavorings, preservatives, and added sugars and salts. We all have a choice: Do we eat to nourish ourselves and cause good or do we eat mindlessly, putting convenience over all, even if it makes us unwell?

We follow the old saying "Breakfast like a king, lunch like a lord, dine like a pauper." That means starting the day with filling, nourishing, and fat-burning foods such as warming quinoa or oatmeal, bananas, nuts, eggs, and breads. Lunch should feature proteins, including grilled chicken or fish, legumes, and grains, while dinner is the lightest meal of the day, consisting of soups and salads.

We also eat cyclically, using the lunar cycle as a guide. The human body is approximately 60 percent water and so, as with the tides and Earth's water table, it is affected by the phases of the Moon. Each new moon kicks off a cleansing diet of juices, soups, and broths to give our digestive systems a chance to renew and heal. With every full moon, we feast, celebrating the bounty of the season—the abundance of the harvest, friendship, and community.

In addition, when planning our menus, we use the biodynamic calendar to guide us. On a Leaf Day, we incorporate salads, spinach, leaf herbs like mint and basil, leeks, cabbages, and cauliflower into our diet. On a Fruit Day, we focus on strawberries, raspberries, apples, plums, and fruiting vegetables like tomatoes, cucumbers, zucchini, beans, peas, peppers, and pumpkins. On a Root Day,

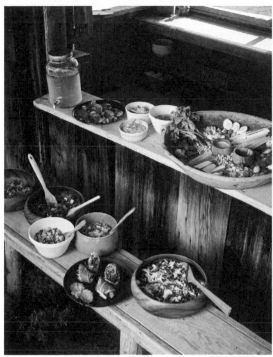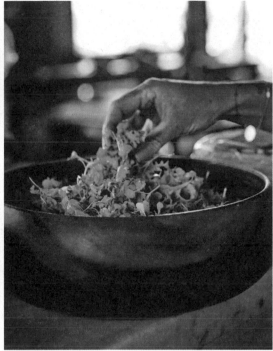

we play with carrots, parsnips, onions, garlic, and radishes. In the pages that follow, in addition to sections devoted to breakfast recipes, snacks, proteins, sauces, drinks, and more, we also created groups of recipes organized by Root, Fruit, Leaf, and Flower days.

We are empowered when we grow, shop, and eat mindfully. Shop at local farmers' markets and educate yourself about what is in season so you know what you should be looking for in your local supermarket, too. Start to experiment with new ingredients and find recipes that you love. Ours follow the rhythm of the seasons. This way of eating—in sync with the Earth, Moon, Sun, and stars—puts us more in tune with our natural and instinctive needs. We have found that eating along these biodynamic principles makes us feel more vital and connected to our bodies and the earth. Our energy levels are higher and everything flows and grows better!

A lot of the recipes in these pages are ones that Annie and I have grown up with, firm favorites that we've cleaned up and cut out any unnecessary additions. A lot are from my travels in India, Thailand, and France, and of course there are new additions I've adopted since being in America. All are gluten free. We believe in taking time to spoil ourselves and cooking is a wonderful way to do that.

All of these recipes are meant to be super easy to make and even easier to adapt, depending on what is in season or available at the farmers' market. I never really follow a recipe to the word. I'm not afraid of swapping out ingredients based on what is perfectly ripe and ready to be eaten that day.

FAVORITE ONE GUN
BIODYNAMIC MENUS

AS WE KNOW, THE SOIL and all crops planted in that soil are affected by the cycle of the Moon. Just as there are days in that cycle that are better for planting roots, flowers, leaves, and fruit, so are too there optimum days to harvest and eat that produce, and we have designed our eating plan accordingly. Using the One Gun Biodynamic Calendar, you can establish whether it is a Root, Flower, Leaf, or Fruit day and find a corresponding recipe.

Root Day recipes might feature an abundance of root crops, such as carrots, beets, parsnip, onion, garlic, and radishes or highlight just one that can be enjoyed at the peak of the season. Flower Days can include flowering vegetables like cauliflowers and broccolis along with flowering herbs and edible flowers. Leaf vegetables like kale, spinach, and lettuces are the most versatile as they can also be harvested and enjoyed on Fruit and Flower Days. In addition to fruit, Fruit Days include all the fruiting vegetables, like tomatoes, cucumber, peppers, and pumpkins, and are also great for enjoying a glass of biodynamic wine!

For lunch and supper, if you feel you want more than a salad, there is a range of vegan protein and lean organic meat and fish options to choose from. We eat local and sustainable fish three or four times a week, organic free-range chicken and turkey a couple of times week, and red meat once or twice a month. Get to know your fishmonger and butcher, so that you know where your meat is coming from and that it has been raised as humanely and sustainably as possible.

SPRING NEW MOON
CELEBRATION

Each spring new moon we start anew. It's a time to set new intentions and celebrate new birth and new beginnings. After a New Moon Meditation session with friends (page 104), we serve this lean but nourishing menu, which uses the best of the season and makes for an elegant dinner.

Beetroot Soup 165

Parisienne Leek Vinaigrette 180

Chicken Paillard with Lemon & Herbs 265
OR One Gun Quinoa with Tomatoes,
Cilantro, and Basil 197

SUMMER LUNCH

Celebrating all that summer has to offer, this menu uses colorful, seasonal produce to a beautiful effect and is delicious, to boot.

Gazpacho 185

Avocado, Carrot, & Radish Salad 175

Beet Carpaccio with Cumin 162

Salt-Baked Fish 248

Grilled Corn with Sage 205

Barbecued Watermelon 188

CAMPFIRE KITCHEN
HARVEST LUNCH

We often serve this to school tours and on education days or days when we have the community coming up to make the compost. This is served as an easy, nourishing grab-and-go lunch after a long day working on the Ranch.

One Gun Crudités with
Raw-Nasturtium Pesto 228

Collard Wraps 216

Beef Consommé with Ginger 273

Dark Chocolate and Beet Brownies 303

WINTER
WELLNESS LUNCH

This lunch, evocative of warmer climes, makes for the perfect antidote to a bleak winter afternoon.

Roasted Butternut Squash
& Ginger Soup 161

Yellow Dal 286

Turmeric Tofu Curry 283

Ranch Veg 177

Gluten-Free Jamaican Ginger Loaf 305

FALL
FULL MOON FEAST

The full moon is all about abundance and enjoying the fruits of one's labor. This time of year is when the biggest, brightest Super Moons come out and we like to eat outside, illuminated by the Moon, enjoying the One Gun Ranch harvest with friends.

Grilled Tuscan Kale 207

Roasted Carrots with Carrot-Top Pesto 172

Halloween Stew 183

Celery Root Purée with Thyme, Rosemary, and Lemon 166

One Gun Spinach and Pomegranate Salad 212

Poached Figs 301

Honey, Sage, and Rosemary Ice Cream 314

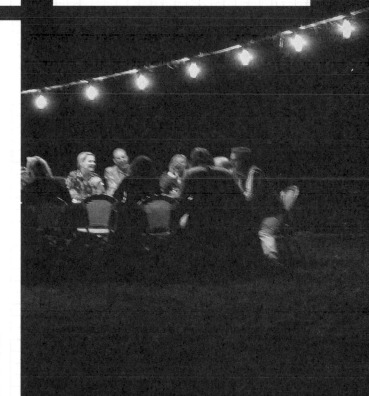

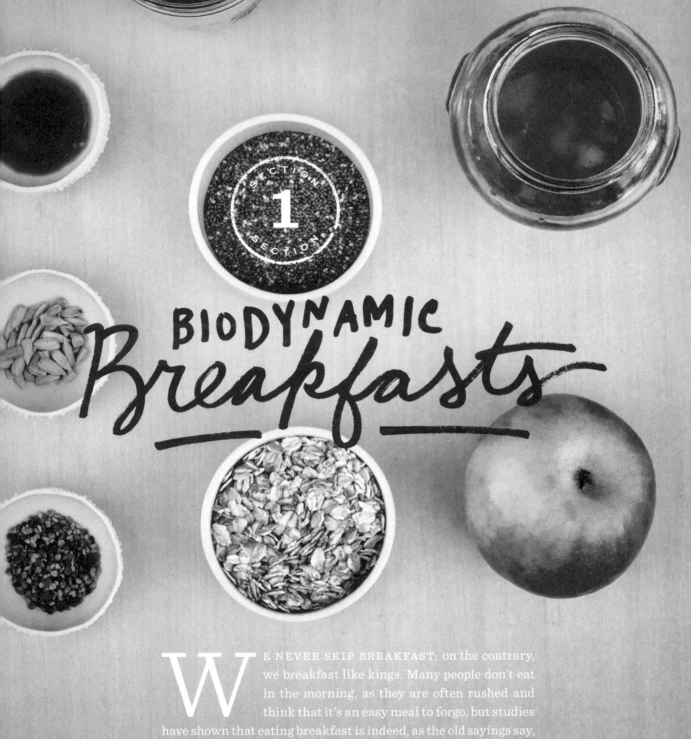

BIODYNAMIC
Breakfasts

W E NEVER SKIP BREAKFAST; on the contrary, we breakfast like kings. Many people don't eat in the morning, as they are often rushed and think that it's an easy meal to forgo, but studies have shown that eating breakfast is indeed, as the old sayings say, vital to a healthy diet, because it energizes you for the day ahead by jump-starting your metabolism.

In the recipes that follow, there are plenty of vegan, vegetarian, and simply simple options—for example, a plate of ripe watermelon or peaches is an easy-to-prepare, delicious start to the day.

CHIA
BREAKFAST BOWL

Serves 1

Chia seeds are full of protein, fiber, calcium, and omega-3 and -6 fats, so a chia pudding makes for super nutritious breakfast. It is very important to always soak chia seeds before eating them as they are hydrophilic and can hold nearly twelve times their weight in water. If you ingest dry chia seeds they will draw that water from your body instead. Chia absorbs liquid very quickly. In just 10 minutes the pudding should have a consistency similar to tapioca. Add more liquid as needed. You can pick up bee pollen in your local health food store or on an artisanal honey producer's website.

2 tablespoons organic gluten-free rolled oats

2 teaspoons chia seeds

1 cup coconut water or raw almond milk, or more if needed (start with 1 cup and add more if the mix looks dry; you want it quite wet so the chia and oats can swell)

1 teaspoon vanilla extract or paste

1 organic apple, grated

1 teaspoon each lucuma powder, maca powder, unsweetened cacao powder, bee pollen, and/or almond butter (optional)

1 teaspoon sunflower seeds, toasted

Combine the chia seeds, oats, coconut water, and vanilla extract together in a bowl. Cover and refrigerate overnight.

In the morning, give the mix a stir and add more liquid if needed. Stir in the apple and any of the optional powders or the bee pollen or almond butter. Top with the toasted sunflower seeds and enjoy.

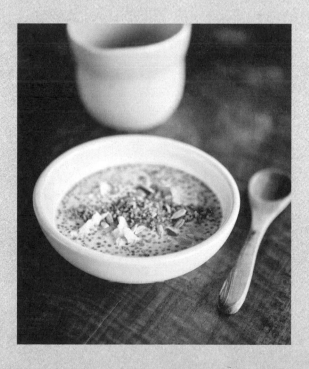

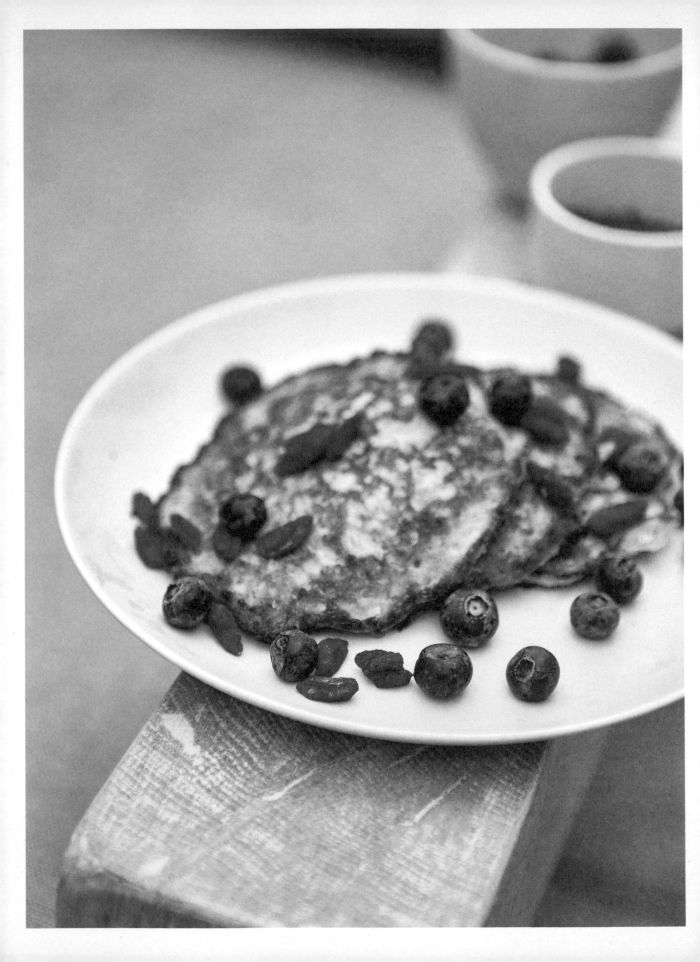

HEALTHY
OAT PANCAKES

Serves 4

These pancakes are a weekend staple at the Ranch. Oats are a slow-burning carbohydrate that the metabolism digests and absorbs over several hours, providing your body with a steady source of energy. They're a great start to the day before a long hike or ride along the trails like the ones surrounding the Ranch.

1 cup organic gluten-free rolled oats

¼ cup almond flour or other gluten-free flour

1½ tablespoons coconut nectar or raw sugar

1 teaspoon baking powder

Large pinch of sea salt

2 large organic free-range eggs

1¼ cups almond milk or buttermilk

2 tablespoons coconut oil, melted, plus more for the pan

1 teaspoon vanilla extract or paste

Fresh organic berries or sliced bananas and dried goji berries for serving

In a large bowl, combine the oats, almond flour, coconut nectar, baking powder, and salt and stir to mix well. Make a well in the center of the ingredients and set aside.

In a medium bowl, combine the eggs, the almond milk or buttermilk, the 2 tablespoons melted coconut butter, and the vanilla. (Make sure the butter has cooled a little or it will scramble the eggs.) Combine the mixture roughly with a fork, then tip it into the well in the dry ingredients and continue to mix until just combined.

Cover the mixture, transfer to the refrigerator, and let rest for at least 1 hour or up to 8 hours. (This allows the buttermilk and rising agents to get to work while the oats soak.) The batter is ready when it is the consistency of runny paint or light cream. If it seems to have thickened too much, whisk in filtered water as needed.

Smear a griddle or a sauté pan over medium heat with a little coconut butter and let heat to smoking hot. Pour the batter onto the hot pan in ¼-cup scoops and let the pancakes cook until golden, about 2 minutes per side. Transfer to a platter and place in a low oven when done. Repeat to cook more pancakes, smearing the pan with more coconut butter between each batch as needed. Keep them warm in the oven, or eat straight out of the pan as you work.

Serve warm, with a mixture of fresh berries or bananas with goji berries.

BANANA-BEE POLLEN SPLIT

Serves 2

We make this when we need a super-energizing breakfast. Raw honey is specified because this ensures it has not been heated or pasteurized, which destroys the live enzymes, antioxidants and nutrients in the honey. Local honey is also preferable, as it can help reduce allergy symptoms caused by plant pollen in your area. Bee Pollen, on the other hand, is packed with protein, amino acids, vitamin B, and folic acid.

When buying tropical fruits like bananas, always look for sustainability hallmarks like "Fair Trade" and "Rainforest Alliance," and always buy organic to ensure the fruit was grown without pesticides. Putting them in the refrigerator overnight will give them the ideal chill.

2 large organic bananas, well chilled

1 (6-ounce) container sheep's-milk yogurt

1 tablespoon raw local honey

1 tablespoon bee pollen

½ tablespoon hempseed (optional)

Remove the cold bananas from the refrigerator and split lengthwise on a large plate.

Spoon on the yogurt, then drizzle with the honey and sprinkle the pollen and hemp seeds over the top. Serve immediately.

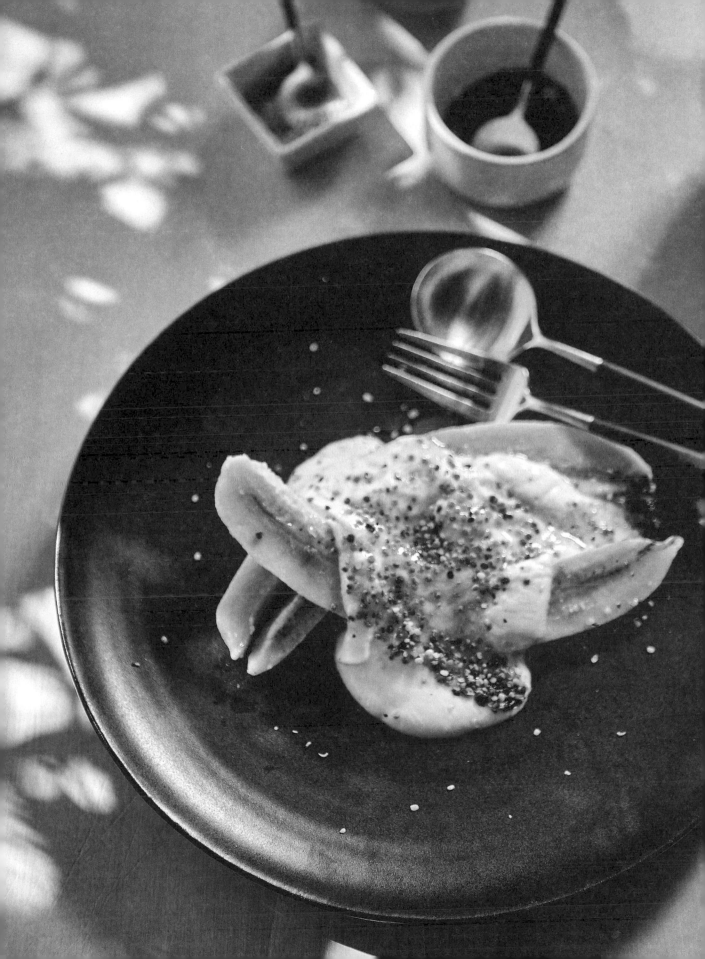

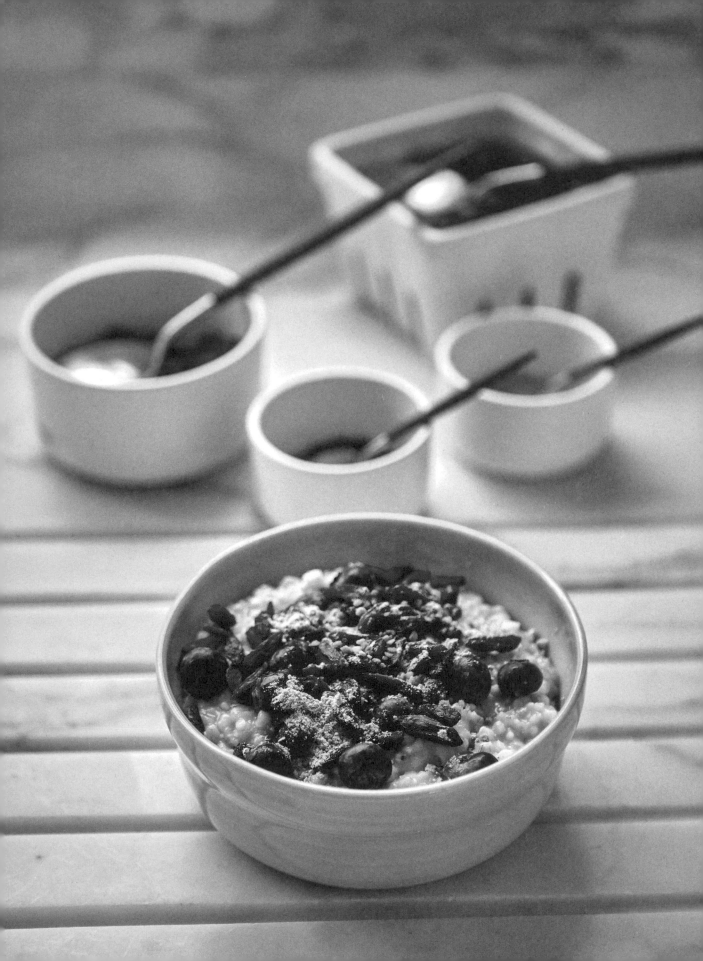

STEEL-CUT
OATS
WITH GINGER, BEE POLLEN & GOJI

Serves 1

We also call these Superfood Oats: A warming, filling start to the day, oats provide hours of steady energy, while ginger stimulates the metabolism and nutrient-rich bee pollen and goji berries provide plenty of protein, fiber, and B vitamins.

1 cup cooked organic gluten-free steel-cut oats

1 tablespoon ground ginger

½ tablespoon bee pollen

Handful of dried goji berries

Handful of fresh or dried organic blueberries

Top the warm bowl of oats with the ginger, bee pollen, and berries. Serve.

EGG WHITE
SCRAMBLE

Serves 2

You can use basil, parsley, cilantro, or whatever looks good and fresh from the garden that day to scent this scramble. Feel free to add some minced jalapeño or chopped mushrooms for added bite or bulk.

1 to 2 teaspoons coconut oil

6 large organic free-range egg whites

¼ cup coarsely chopped mixed fresh herbs, plus more for garnish

3 young curly kale leaves, tough stems and spines removed, chopped

8 colorful cherry or grape heirloom tomatoes (or 2 medium tomatoes), diced

Guacamole for serving

In a large frying pan over medium heat, melt the coconut oil. Stir in the egg whites, then add the herbs, kale, and tomatoes. Sauté until the egg whites are set.

Serve garnished with more fresh herbs and a side of guac.

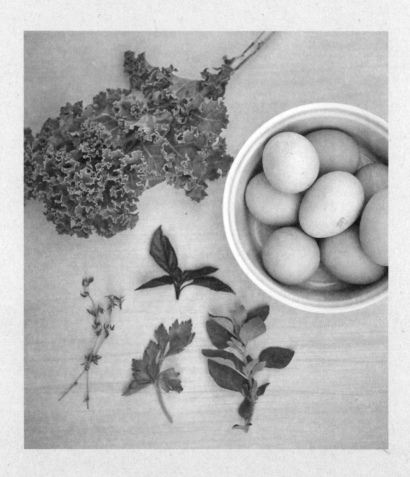

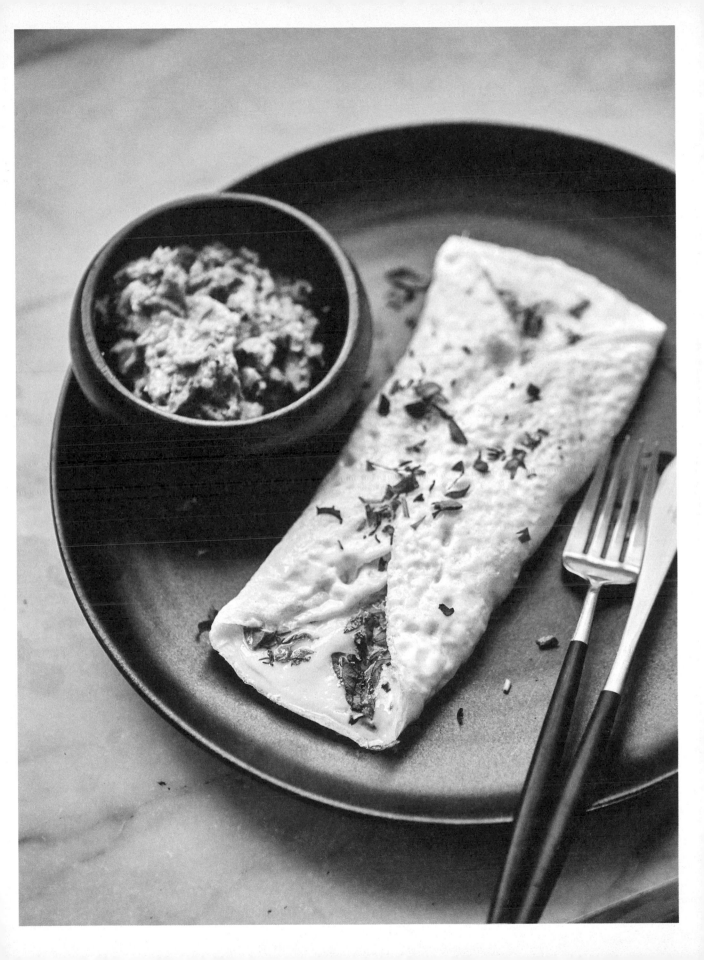

AVOCADO TOAST

Serves 1

A healthy breakfast or any-time-of-day snack, avocados are packed with healthy fats and vitamins.

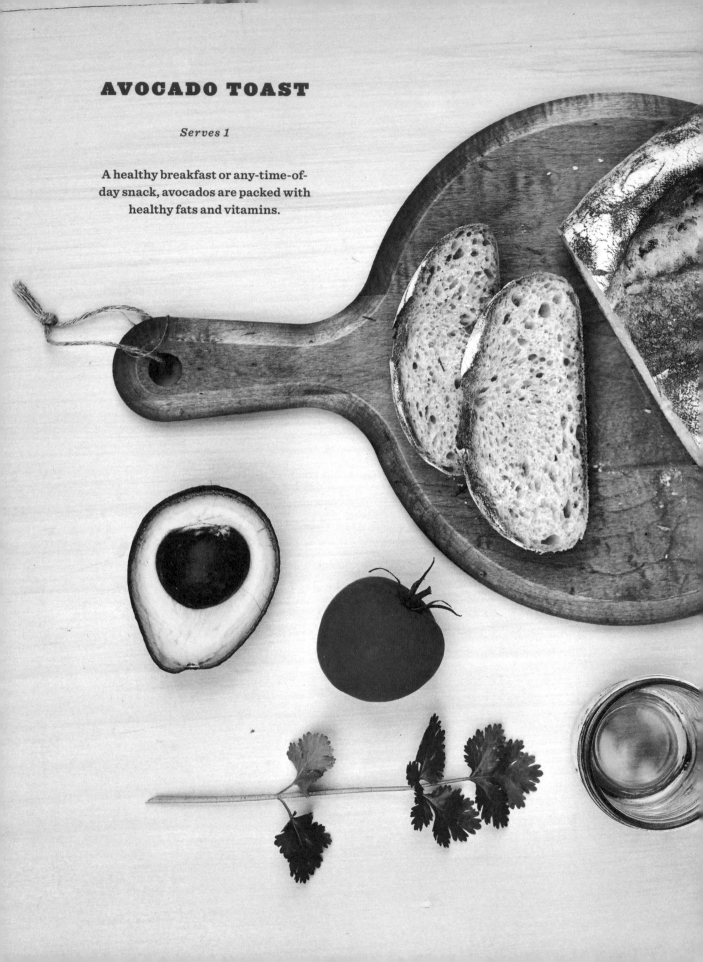

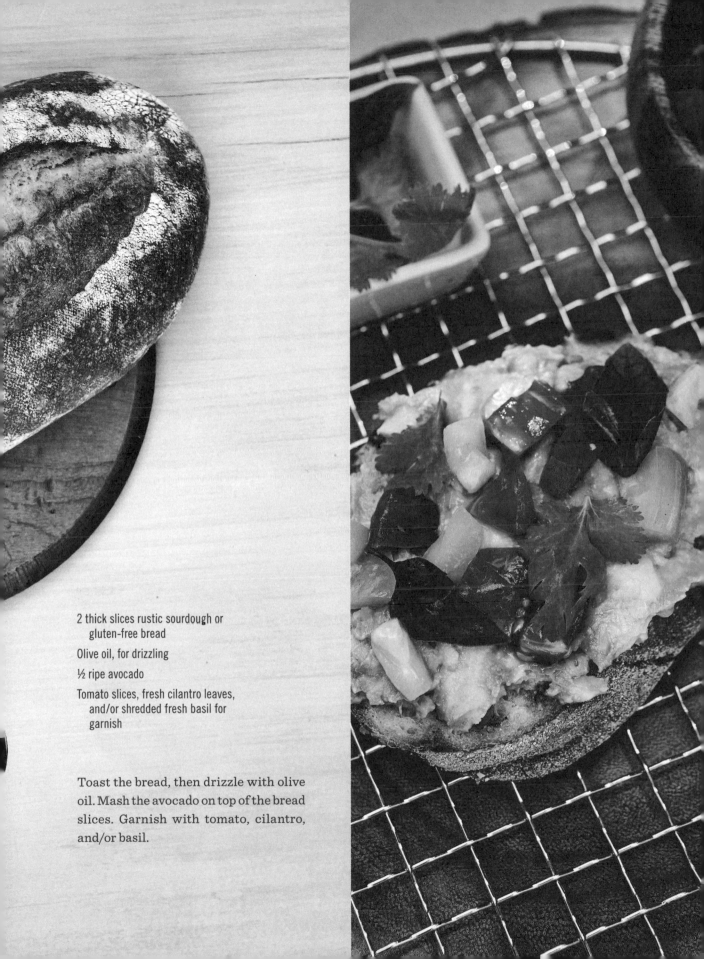

2 thick slices rustic sourdough or
    gluten-free bread

Olive oil, for drizzling

½ ripe avocado

Tomato slices, fresh cilantro leaves,
    and/or shredded fresh basil for
    garnish

Toast the bread, then drizzle with olive
oil. Mash the avocado on top of the bread
slices. Garnish with tomato, cilantro,
and/or basil.

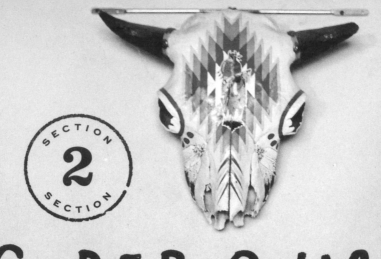

SUPER SNACKS

These snacks are delicious and packed full of
energy to have on the go during the day, while on the
road, or for a nutritious snack at home.

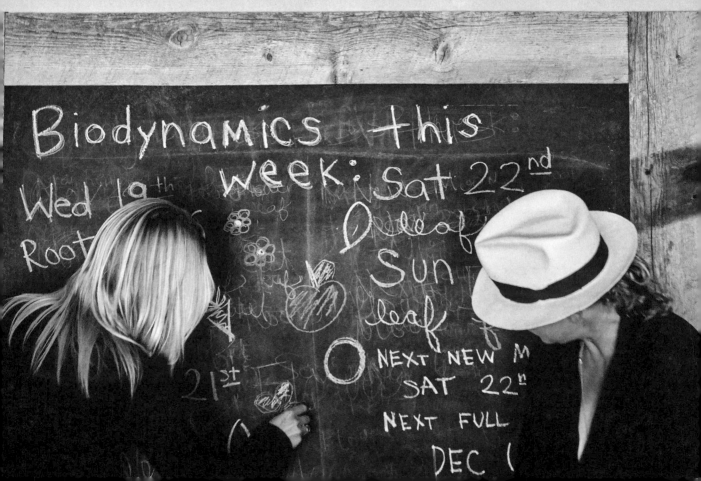

ENERGY BALLS
(ONE GUN BULLETS/AMMO)

Makes approximately 12

Packed full of goodness and energy, these are perfect for an on-the-go snack or an afternoon pep-up. Dates are high in fiber; the flax and hempseed are packed with protein and omega-3s and -6s; and the maca gives an added boost of energy.

½ cup raw almonds

½ cup dates

1 tablespoon coconut oil

4 tablespoons unsweetened cacao powder

1 tablespoon flaxseed

1 tablespoon hempseed

1 tablespoon dried goji berries

1 teaspoon ground ginger

1 teaspoon maca powder

In a food processor, combine the almonds, dates, coconut oil, and three-fourths of the cocoa powder and process until a sticky paste forms. Add the flaxseed, hempseed, goji berries, ginger, and maca and give the quickest whizz, just until everything is blended.

Roll the mixture into 3-inch balls, coating them with the rest of the cacao powder. Arrange the balls on a parchment paper–lined baking tray and put in the freezer for an hour to set.

When all of the balls are done, put the pan in the freezer for at least 1 hour to set, or up to 12 hours, before serving.

For a super snack with anti-inflammatory properties and that's high in antioxidants, combine the almonds, dates, and coconut oil with ½ cup organic gluten-free rolled oats, 1 teaspoon each of ground turmeric and ground cinnamon, ½ teaspoon vanilla extract, and ⅓ cup unsweetened coconut, and follow the remaining instructions above.

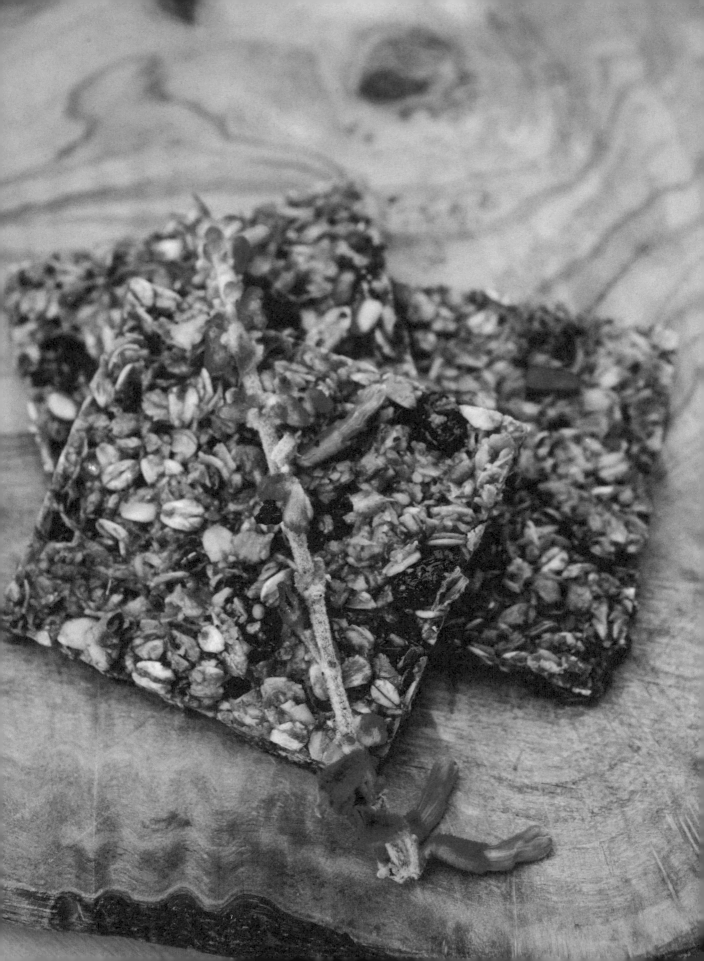

HEMPSEED
MEXICAN SAGE FLAPJACKS

Makes sixteen 2-inch squares or about 12 bars

These handy bars, full of protein, are a fantastic, energizing snack. We always pack these on long hikes to provide plenty of fuel.

2 cups organic gluten-free
  rolled oats

3 tablespoons raisins

2 teaspoons flaxseed

2 teaspoons hempseed

2 teaspoons dried Mexican sage
  flowers, plus more for garnish

½ cup raw local honey

⅓ cup coconut oil

Preheat the oven to 325°F. Generously grease an 8-inch-square baking pan or small baking sheet, and line with parchment paper.

In a bowl, combine the oats, raisins, flaxseed, hempseed, and 2 teaspoons sage flowers. Set aside.

In a small saucepan over medium heat, melt the honey with the coconut oil. Heat the mixture, stirring often, until it boils and begins to foam. Boil for 15 to 30 seconds longer, then pour over the oats mixture and stir to combine well.

Spread the mixture in the prepared pan with a wooden spoon, pressing to flatten well in an even layer.

Bake until the top is golden, 15 to 20 minutes. Remove from the oven and let cool. Cut into sixteen 2-inch squares or rectangular bars in any size you like for packing a snack. Garnish each with a few Mexican sage petals.

CACAO
ALMOND BUTTER

Makes about 1¼ cups

Almond butter is itself a great source of protein, but we've elevated this recipe to superfood status with the addition of raw cacao, which is high in magnesium and super antioxidant flavonoids; maca, which is loaded with amino acids; and lucuma which is a wonderful, naturally low glycemic sweetener that is also high in iron. You should be able to find all of these in powdered supplement form at your local health food store and online.

Spread this on rye bread or dollop onto porridge.

1 cup almond butter

1 to 3 tablespoons raw local honey

2 heaping teaspoons unsweetened cacao powder

A good pinch of sea salt

1 heaping tablespoon *each* maca powder and/or lucuma powder (optional)

Simply blend the ingredients by hand or in a food processor until combined.

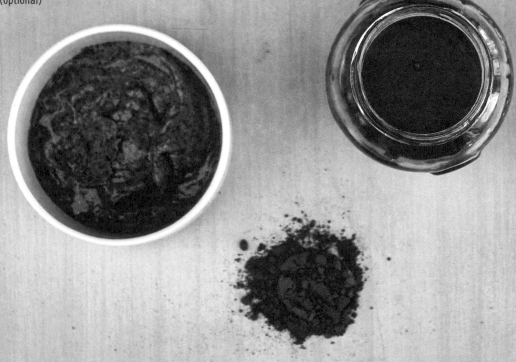

PERFECT POPCORN

Makes about 4 cups popped popcorn; serves 4 to 6

Popcorn is such a great healthy snack. We just love to make it on the go when traveling or in big batches to be shared at home. It's a lot of fun to play with flavor combinations, and these are some of my favorite ones we've developed at the Ranch.

1 tablespoon coconut oil or olive oil

¼ cup organic popcorn kernels

Generous pinch of sea salt

In a large pot over medium-high heat, melt the oil. Add a few kernels of popcorn to make sure the oil is hot enough. Once the kernels start popping, add the rest and cover the pot.

Shake the pot gently, then reduce the heat to medium and cook until all the popcorn pops, shaking the pot every few seconds. Pour into a big bowl, season with salt, and serve immediately.

Experiment with adding flavors to your popcorn— whether by adding spices or herbs to the pot before popping or using infused coconut or olive oils.

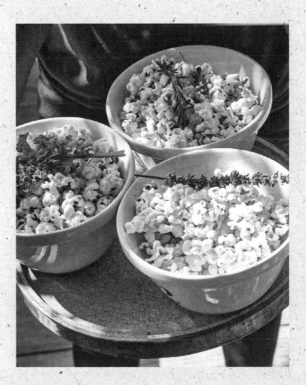

BIODYNAMIC
Gluten-Free
BREADS

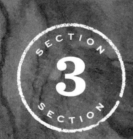

SECTION
3
SECTION

↗ GLUTEN-FREE
Banana Bread
(page 159)

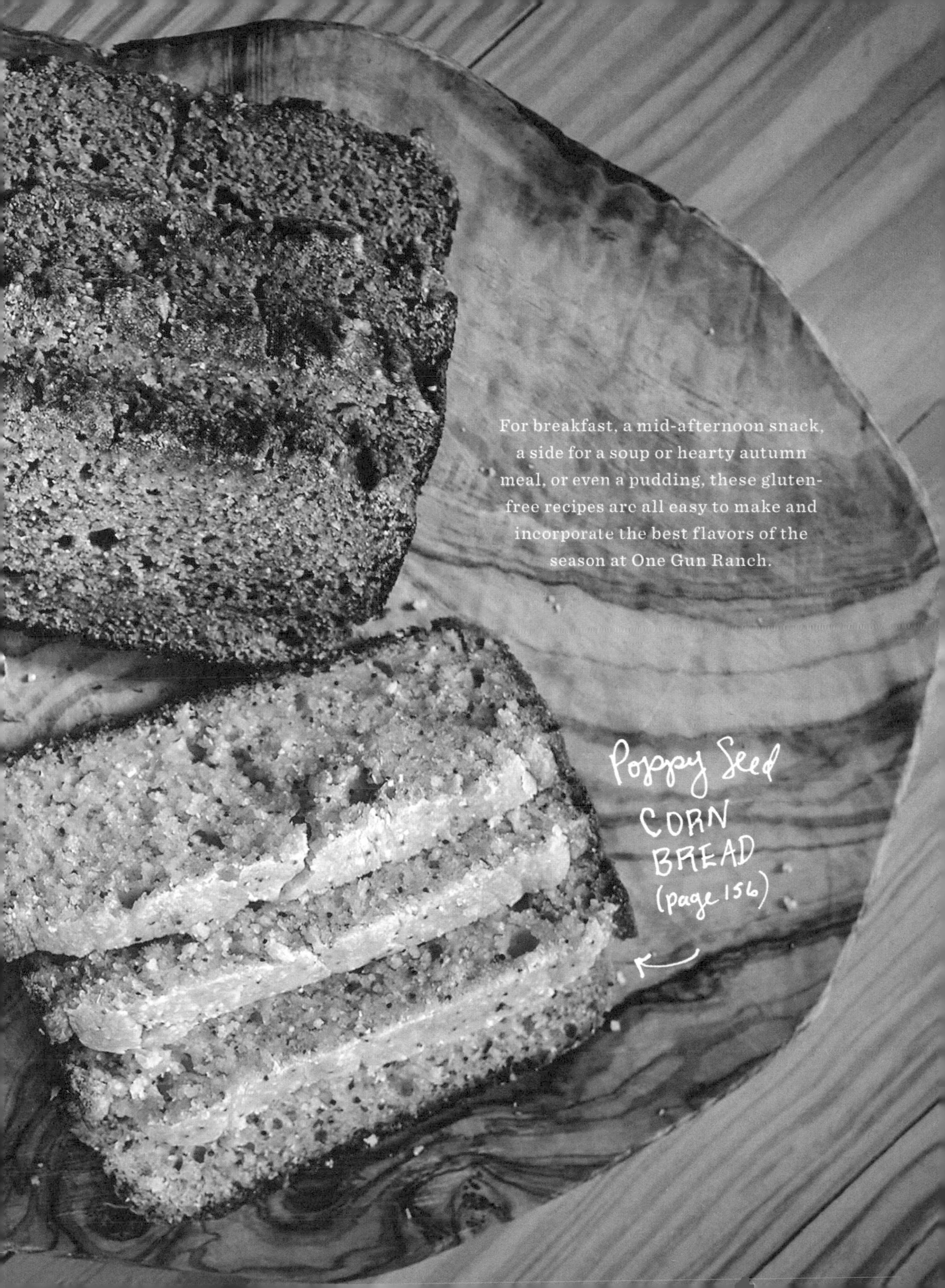

For breakfast, a mid-afternoon snack, a side for a soup or hearty autumn meal, or even a pudding, these gluten-free recipes arc all easy to make and incorporate the best flavors of the season at One Gun Ranch.

Poppy Seed
CORN
BREAD
(page 156)

POPPY SEED
CORN BREAD

Serves 4 to 6

I fell in love with the simple joys of corn bread while celebrating my first Thanksgiving in the United States. And I find that adding poppy seeds or rosemary makes it even more versatile. The former transforms corn bread into a polenta-style cake, while the latter is a more flavorful. A One Gun Ranch take on the classic!

1¼ cups cornmeal

1¼ cups gluten-free all-purpose flour

3 teaspoons baking powder

1 teaspoon baking soda

Pinch of sea salt

½ cup honey

1 (15-ounce) can coconut milk, shaken well

¼ cup coconut oil, plus more for serving

Zest and juice of 1 small Meyer lemon

2 teaspoons poppy seeds

1 teaspoon apple cider vinegar

Preheat the oven to 350°F.

In a large bowl, whisk together the cornmeal, flour, baking powder, baking soda, and salt.

In a small saucepan over very low heat, stir together the honey, coconut milk, and oil until they are gently melted together. Be careful not to let it come to a simmer; you only want to see a bit of steam coming off the top.

Using a wooden spoon, slowly stir the warm, wet ingredients into the dry ingredients. There will be a few clumps, but try to stir out as many as you can. Once you have a lovely thick batter, gently fold in the lemon zest and juice, poppy seeds, and vinegar.

Pour the batter into a 10-inch square baking pan or cast-iron skillet generously greased with coconut oil. Bake until the edges are golden brown, 25 to 30 minutes. Transfer to a wire rack and let cool slightly.

Cut into squares or wedges and serve with a touch of coconut oil on top.

VARIATION: ROSEMARY CORN BREAD

Make the Poppy Seed Corn Bread as directed, but omit the poppy seeds and lemon zest. Stir 1 tablespoon finely chopped fresh rosemary in with the lemon juice and vinegar.

BUCKWHEAT, CORN & ROSEMARY
BREAD

Serves 4 to 6

We like to serve this easy, gluten-free bread at Thanksgiving, although it works just as well as an accompaniment to a hearty soup. Buckwheat flour is really high in fiber and adds a lovely nutty flavor to this bread.

1 cup buckwheat flour

3½ tablespoons cornmeal

2 teaspoons baking powder

1 teaspoon Himalayan pink sea salt

1 teaspoon finely chopped fresh rosemary

1 cup water

1½ tablespoons grapeseed or melted coconut oil

Preheat the oven to 350°F. Line a baking sheet with parchment paper.

In a bowl, whisk together the flour, cornmeal, baking powder, salt, and rosemary. Add the water and oil and whisk to mix well.

Scoop the dough into a sturdy plastic bag (or a piping bag fitted with a large round tip). Snip off the tip of one corner of the bag and squeeze to pipe the dough onto the prepared pan, making sticks about 3 inches long and 1 inch wide and spacing them 1 to 2 inches apart.

Bake until golden, 15 to 20 minutes. Serve warm.

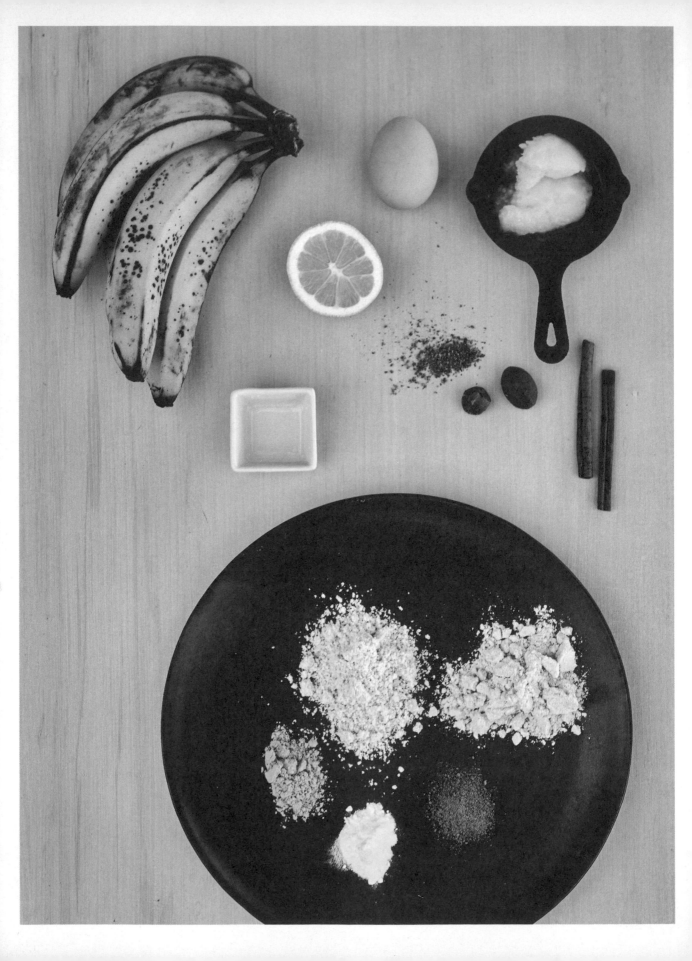

GLUTEN-FREE
BANANA BREAD

Serves 4 to 6

The smell of bananas always reminds me of Barbados, where I spent a lot of time growing up. This gluten-free version is a nice treat to have in the afternoon when sugar cravings hit. The riper your bananas, the better.

4 ripe bananas

Zest and juice of ½ lemon

1½ teaspoons coconut oil

½ cup coconut sugar

4 large organic free-range eggs

½ teaspoon banana extract

½ cup coconut flour

½ cup almond flour

1 teaspoon baking soda

Pinch of freshly grated nutmeg

Pinch of ground cinnamon

Pinch of ground ginger

Preheat the oven to 325°F.

In a bowl, mash the bananas with a fork, then stir in the lemon zest and juice and set aside.

In a large bowl, cream the coconut oil and sugar together with a wire whisk. Beat in the eggs one at a time, then the banana extract.

In separate bowl, whisk together the flours, baking soda, nutmeg, cinnamon, and ginger.

Slowly add the flour mixture to the wet ingredients, mixing just until all the flour has been combined. Fold in the banana mixture.

Spoon the batter into a 1-pound nonstick or greased loaf pan and bake 35 minutes. Remove the pan from the oven and cover with aluminum foil. Place the covered pan back in the oven and bake until golden brown, about 15 minutes longer.

Transfer to a wire rack and let cool slightly in the pan, then turn out on the rack. Serve warm, or let cool completely.

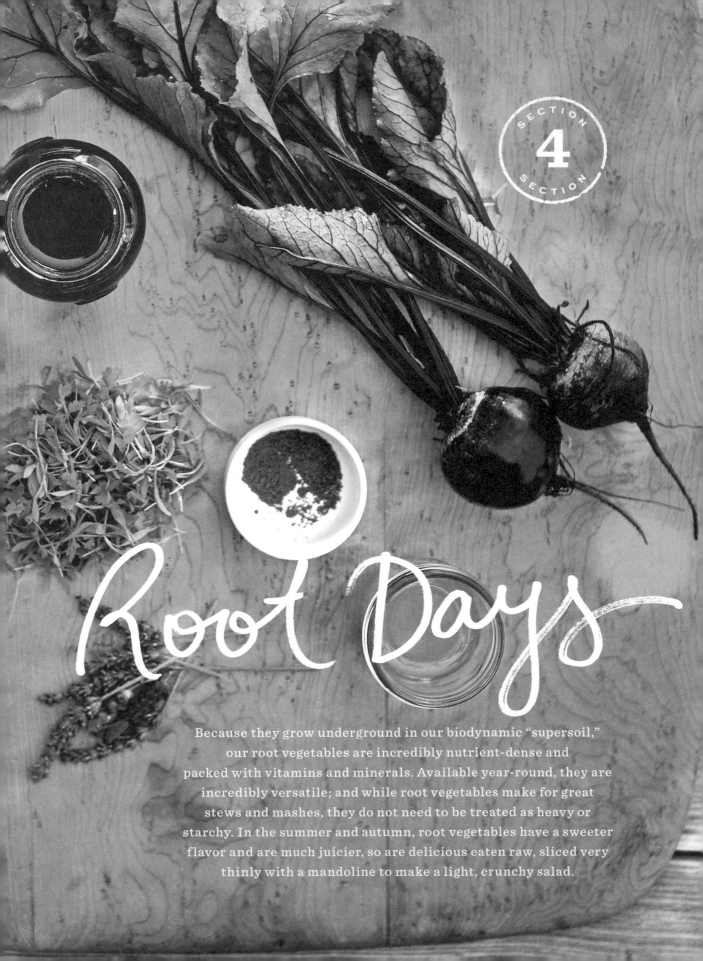

Root Days

Because they grow underground in our biodynamic "supersoil,"
our root vegetables are incredibly nutrient-dense and
packed with vitamins and minerals. Available year-round, they are
incredibly versatile; and while root vegetables make for great
stews and mashes, they do not need to be treated as heavy or
starchy. In the summer and autumn, root vegetables have a sweeter
flavor and are much juicier, so are delicious eaten raw, sliced very
thinly with a mandoline to make a light, crunchy salad.

ROASTED
BUTTERNUT SQUASH
& GINGER SOUP

Serves 4

This warming winter soup, thanks to the addition of ginger and jalapeño, is hearty enough to be a simple lunch or supper. We love spicy food, but you can, of course, cut down on the jalapeño (especially the seeds, wherein most of the heat lies), or leave it out altogether.

1 medium butternut squash, peeled, seeded, and cut into big chunks

3 tablespoons olive oil

Leaves from a few sprigs of fresh thyme, plus sprigs for garnish

Sea salt and freshly ground black pepper

1 large white onion, quartered

1 clove garlic, unpeeled

4 cups chicken or vegetable stock, plus more if needed

Squeeze of lime

1½-inch piece fresh ginger, peeled and finely grated

2 jalapeño chiles, one seeded and finely grated, one diced

Preheat the oven to 400°F.

Pile the squash on a large baking sheet. Season with the olive oil, thyme, and salt and pepper. Tuck the onion and garlic on the pan and roast until the squash is tender and the onion is soft and golden, about 35 minutes.

In a saucepan over medium-high heat, warm up the stock with the lime juice, ginger, and the grated jalapeño.

Working in batches, combine the squash, onion, garlic, and stock mixture in a blender and blend to a lovely, thick soup texture. Pour each batch into a medium pot as you work. When everything is blended, heat over medium-low heat until hot, adding more stock if the soup becomes too thick.

Ladle into bowls and serve, garnished with a sprig of thyme and some diced jalapeño.

BEET
CARPACCIO
WITH CUMIN

Serves 4

With the addition of cumin, this delicious, simple dish is infused with a flavor of India. It's beautiful made with either all purple beets or any of the colorful varieties we grow at the Ranch.

2 large beets, trimmed and scrubbed

2 tablespoons olive oil

1 tablespoon apple cider vinegar

2 teaspoons raw local honey

Large pinch of cumin seeds

Handful of micro cilantro or fresh cilantro leaves

Preheat the oven to 400°F.

Roast the beets whole with the skins on—no need to add oil—until tender, about 45 minutes. Set the beets aside to cool.

Using a vegetable peeler, thinly slice the beets into carpaccio strips and lay the strips across a large plate.

In a jar, combine the olive oil, vinegar, and honey. Close tightly and shake well. Drizzle the vinaigrette over the beets and let marinate for 10 minutes. Garnish with the cumin seeds and cilantro and serve.

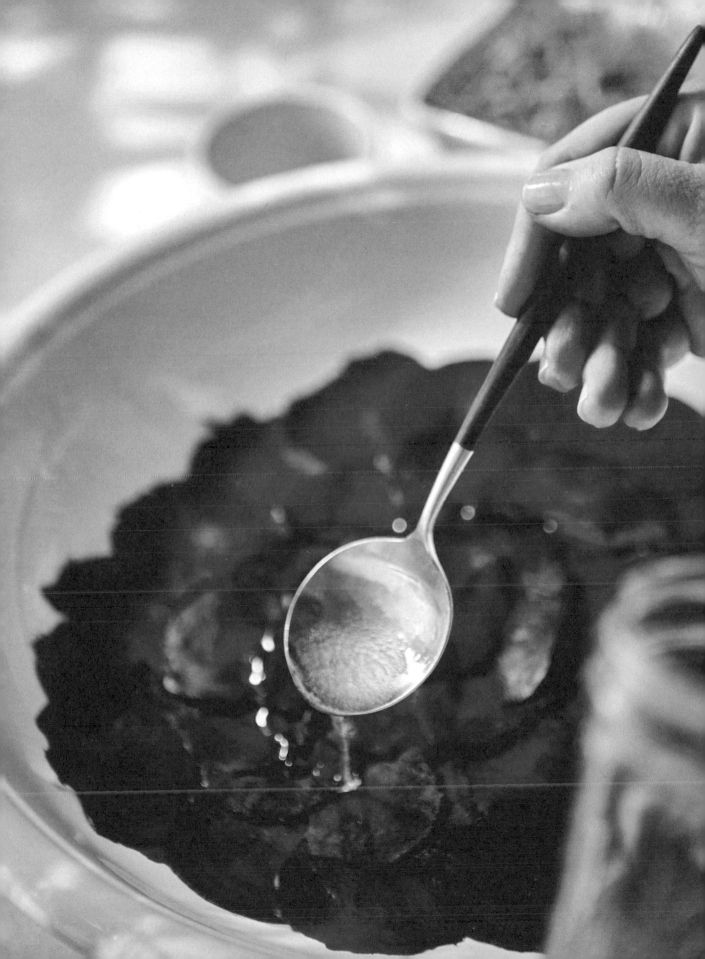

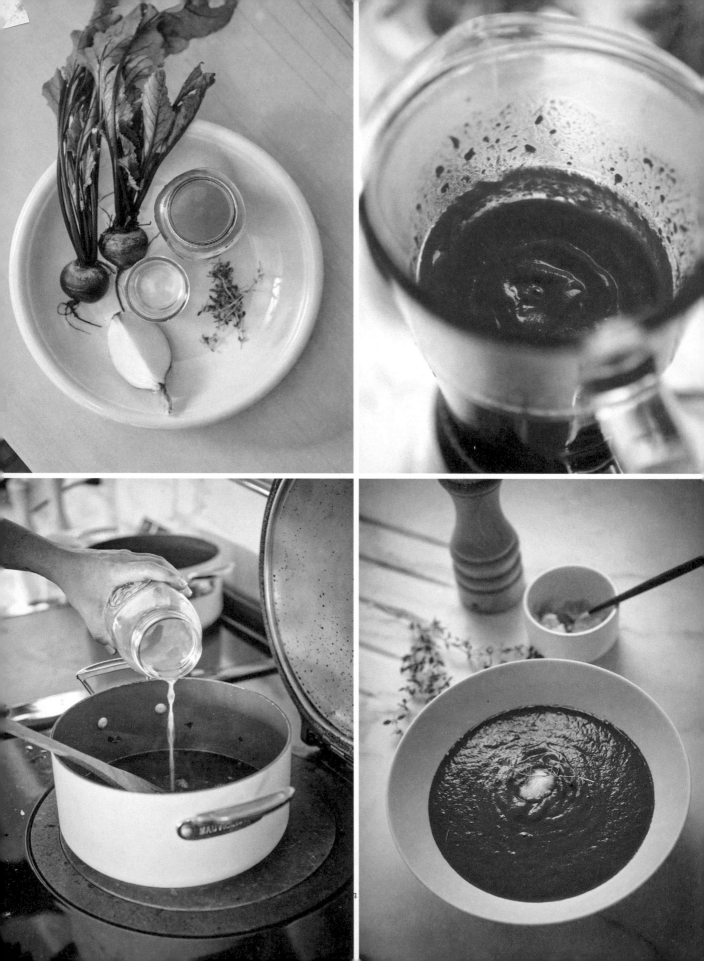

BEETROOT
SOUP

Serves 4 to 6

This soup is a favorite that I grew up with. It's a great way to eat your beets and the color is incredible. It's fantastic either hot or cold. For a more decadent winter soup, add bacon.

2 tablespoons olive oil

2 white onions, finely chopped

1 pound beets, trimmed, peeled, and cut into ½-inch cubes

1 quart chicken stock

Juice of 1 lemon

1 sprig fresh thyme

Sea salt and freshly ground black pepper

Prepared horseradish for serving

Heat the olive oil in large pot over medium-high heat. Add the onions and cook until soft, about 2 minutes. Add the beets to the pan, cover, and cook for another 10 minutes, stirring often to prevent sticking.

Add the stock, lemon juice, and thyme to the pot and bring to boil, then reduce the heat to low and simmer until the beets are very tender, about 25 minutes.

Remove from the heat and let cool slightly before transferring to a blender. Working in batches if necessary, blend until smooth. Season with salt and pepper.

Serve hot or cold, garnished with a dollop of horseradish.

CELERY ROOT
PURÉE
WITH THYME, ROSEMARY & LEMON

Serves 4

Celery root is one of my favorite vegetables. Its ugly, nobbly appearance belies its delicate flavor. This makes for a healthy side dish, while still being comforting and hearty. Also known as celeriac, the smaller roots are more flavorful.

1 tablespoon olive oil

1 celery root, peeled and cut into ½-inch cubes

Handful of fresh thyme leaves, plus a sprig for serving

3 to 4 tablespoons chicken stock or water

Squeeze of Meyer lemon juice

Handful of fresh rosemary leaves, minced, plus a sprig for serving

Pinch of sea salt and freshly ground black pepper

Heat the olive oil in a saucepan over medium-high heat. Add the celery root and thyme leaves and sauté until soft, about 5–7 minutes.

In a separate saucepan, combine the stock, lemon juice, and minced rosemary and warm gently over medium-low heat.

Transfer the celery root and the warm stock mixture to a blender and blend until creamy. Add more stock if the purée seems too thick.

Transfer to a serving dish, garnish with thyme and rosemary sprigs, and serve. Add salt and black pepper to taste.

ONE GUN SUPERFOOD:
Celery Root

High in potassium, antioxidants, and vitamin K, celery root is also very high in fiber while being low in calories, unlike many other root vegetables.

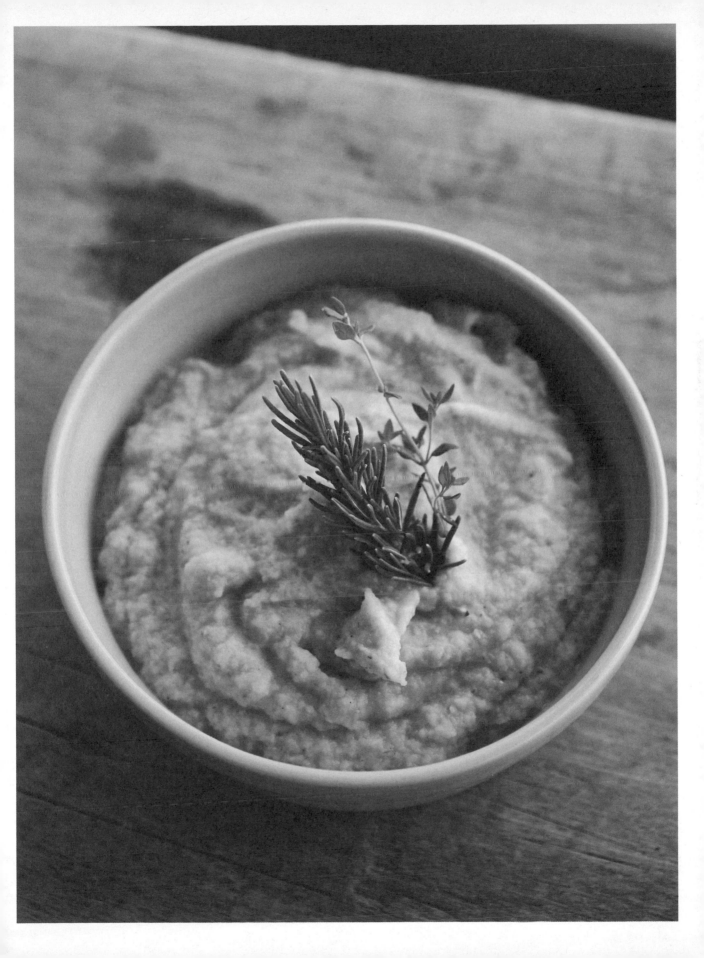

KALE & CELERY ROOT
SOUP

Serves 4 to 6

To me, this soup is pure wellness and warmth in a bowl. Perfect on a chilly winter day, it's packed with nourishing greens and lots of fiber. For a side of crunch, serve it with Turmeric Chia Seed Crackers (page 284).

1 bunch Tuscan kale, tough stems and spines removed, plus a few finely chopped leaves for garnish

3 celery roots, peeled

2 celery stalks, plus a few finely chopped leaves for garnish

1 carrot, peeled

1 white or yellow onion

1 quart chicken or vegetable stock

Roughly chop the kale (reserving the garnish), celery roots, celery, carrot, and onion. Working in batches, put all of the vegetables in a blender with the stock. Blend until thick and creamy.

Pour the purée into a pot and heat over medium-high heat until hot, stirring occasionally. Ladle into bowls and serve hot, garnished with the finely chopped kale and celery.

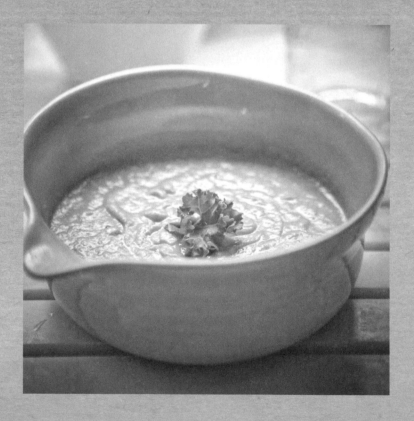

CARROT, ORANGE, & GINGER
MASH

Serves 4

This bright, sunny, vitamin C–packed dish delivers just the right amount of heat to warm up the coldest winter days—a healthy alternative to stodgy mashed potatoes using the best of the season.

2 pounds carrots, peeled and roughly chopped

2 cups chicken stock

1 tablespoon raw local honey

Sea salt and freshly ground black pepper

¼ cup olive oil

1½ tablespoons peeled and finely grated fresh ginger

1 clove garlic, minced

Juice of 1 orange

1 teaspoon ground ginger

Chopped fresh sage for garnish

Combine the carrots, stock, honey, and a pinch of salt and pepper in a saucepan over medium heat.

Bring to a simmer and cook until the carrots are tender, about 20 minutes. Drain the carrots, reserving ¼ cup of the cooking liquid.

Heat the olive oil in small saucepan over medium-high heat. Add the fresh ginger and garlic and cook, stirring, until softened, 2 to 3 minutes. Remove from the heat and pour into a blender. Add the carrots and orange juice and blend to a smooth purée.

Add 1 to 2 tablespoons of the reserved cooking liquid and blend until the purée is lovely and silky smooth. Season with another pinch of sea salt and pepper.

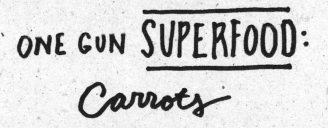

ONE GUN SUPERFOOD: Carrots

Packed with beta-carotene, which protects the skin from UV radiation, and the lesser-known alpha-carotene, which promotes healthy sleep, carrots are also a great source of potassium, vitamins B6 and A, and biotin for healthy hair.

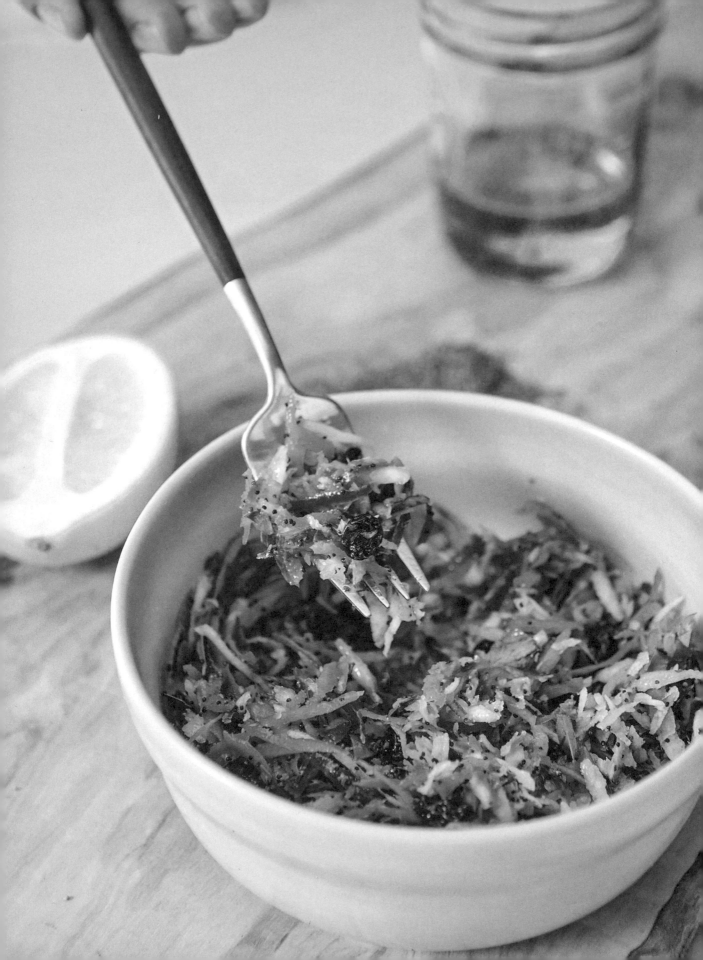

SHAVED
CARROTS
WITH RAISINS & POPPY SEEDS

Serves 4

This beautiful, simple salad puts the many varieties of carrots we grow at the Ranch to good use. I love to get as many colorful carrots in this salad as possible, so if you are at the farmers' market, keep an eye out for yellow, orange, scarlet, and purple carrots. When we have school groups up at the Ranch to learn about growing your own biodynamic vegetables, they always get a kick out of these rainbow-colored beauties, too.

2 bunches (about 1½ pounds) rainbow-colored carrots, trimmed, peeled, and grated

1 bunch fresh parsley, roughly chopped

1 cup raisins

1 tablespoon poppy seeds

1 tablespoon olive oil

½ tablespoon fresh Meyer lemon juice

In a large bowl, toss all of the ingredients together and serve.

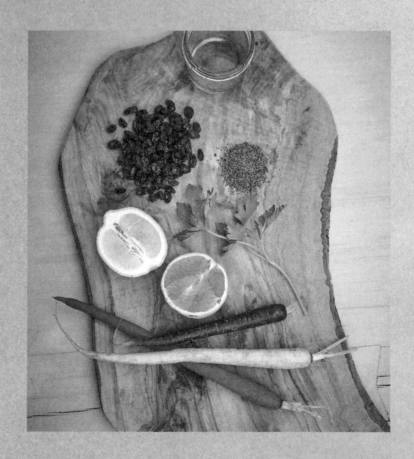

ROASTED
CARROTS
WITH CARROT-TOP PESTO

Serves 4

This can be vegan nose-to-tail-eating at its finest! Nothing goes to waste in this dish, as every part of the vegetable is used—biodynamics on a plate.

1½ pounds small bunch carrots, trimmed and peeled, carrot-top leaves and stems reserved

1 tablespoon vegetable oil or melted coconut oil

Pinch of minced fresh rosemary

Sea salt and freshly ground black pepper

1½ tablespoons pine nuts

½ clove garlic

¼ cup packed fresh basil leaves

2 tablespoons finely grated Parmesan cheese or Parma! (vegan Parmesan)

¼ cup extra-virgin olive oil

A pinch of ground ginger

A pinch of ground sage

Preheat the oven to 400°F.

On a large baking sheet, toss the carrots with the vegetable oil, rosemary, and salt and pepper to taste. Roast, stirring occasionally, until golden brown, about 25 minutes.

Remove from the oven and let cool.

In a food processor or blender, blend or pulse the pine nuts and garlic until you have a coarse paste. Add the carrot tops, basil, and Parmesan or Parma! and process to a coarse purée. Add the olive oil in a stream and blend until combined and smooth, scraping down the sides of the blender jar as needed. Season the pesto with salt and pepper.

Serve the roasted carrots with the pesto spooned on top.

Serve in a large bowl garnished with a few grindings of pepper, the ground ginger, and a sprinkle of sage.

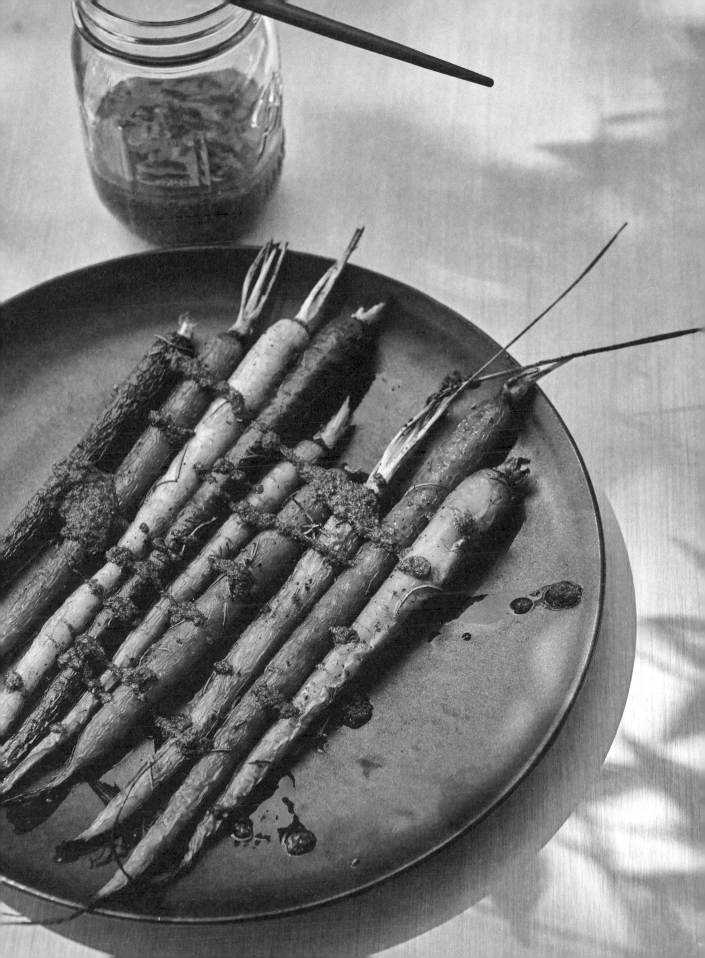

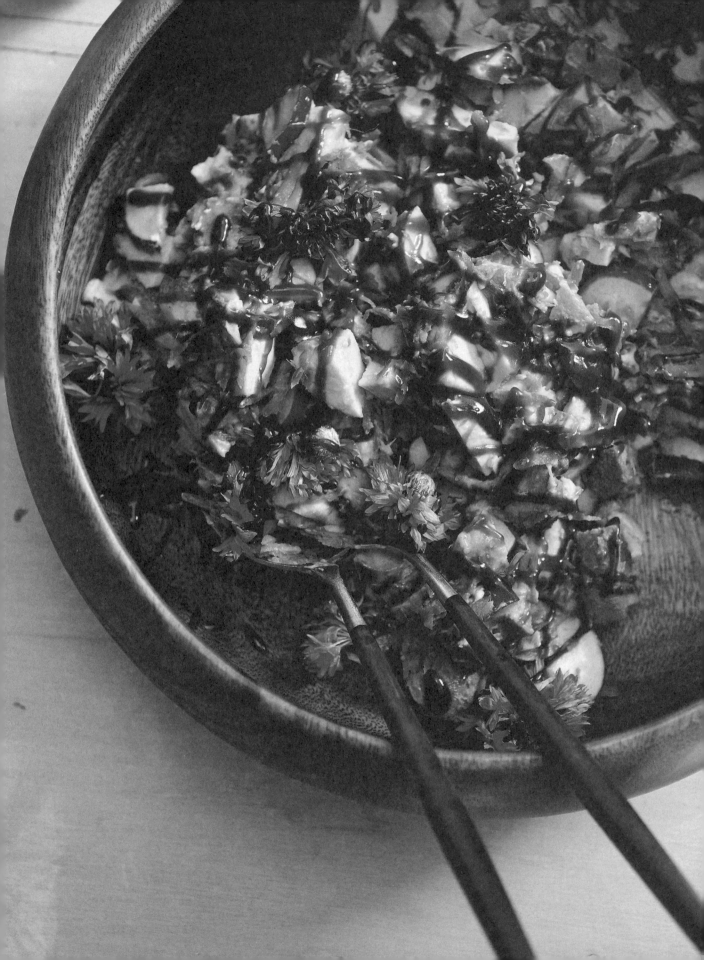

AVOCADO, CARROT & RADISH
SALAD

Serves 4

This simple One Gun Ranch salad perfectly blends spicy radishes and crunchy sweet carrots with creamy avocados, precluding the need for any oil or dressing—although a squeeze of lemon juice can be added to prevent the avocados from browning.

1 bunch (about 1 pound) carrots, trimmed and peeled

6 large or 10 small radishes, trimmed

3 ripe avocados, pitted, peeled, and chopped

Lemon juice (optional)

Roughly grate the carrots and radishes into a bowl. Gently fold in the avocados. Serve immediately, or squeeze some lemon juice over mixture, cover, and refrigerate for up to 8 hours.

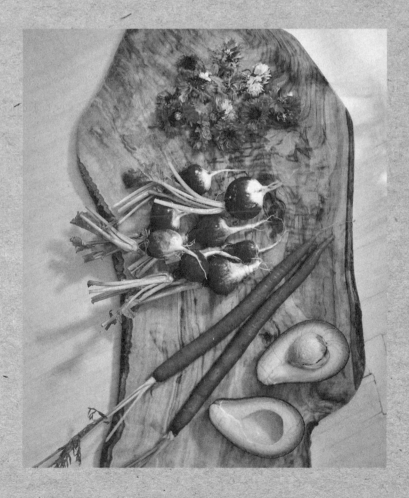

BALSAMIC-ROASTED
ONIONS

Serves 4 to 6

I love this dish because of the mix of sweet and sharp flavors that manage to work together wonderfully. If you are eating outside, these decadent onions are fantastic cooked on the grill, too.

3 white or yellow onions, cut into wedges

3 tablespoons olive oil

3 tablespoons balsamic vinegar

Leaves from 1 sprig fresh rosemary

Leaves from 1 sprig fresh thyme

Pinch of sea salt

Preheat the oven to 400°F.

In a large bowl, toss the onion wedges with the olive oil, vinegar, rosemary, thyme, and salt. Spread the onions on a roasting pan; reserve the dressing left behind in the bowl. Roast until tender and caramelized, 50 to 60 minutes.

Remove from oven and transfer the onions to a serving dish. Drizzle with the reserved dressing and serve.

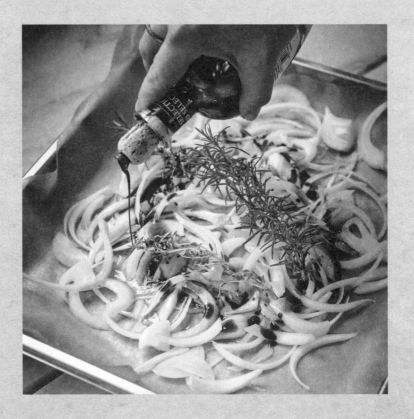

RANCH VEG

Serves 6

I have nicknamed this dish Simon & Garfunkel because of the herbs we use to season the vegetables. The lovely shades of orange make this a beautiful side dish for a harvest feast, or make it as a simple dinner served with a spicy arugula salad or some quinoa.

1 bunch (about 1 pound) slender carrots, trimmed and peeled

¼ pumpkin, seeded and cut into thick slices or wedges

1 sweet potato, scrubbed but not peeled, cut into thick slices or wedges

1 tablespoon olive oil

Sea salt and freshly ground black pepper

Handful of torn fresh sage leaves

Handful of fresh rosemary leaves, minced

Handful of fresh thyme leaves

Build a medium-hot fire in a charcoal grill, preheat a gas grill to medium-high, or preheat the oven to 400°F.

In a large bowl, toss the carrots, pumpkin, and sweet potato with the olive oil, a pinch each of salt and pepper, and the fresh herbs.

Grill or roast until golden and tender, about 45 minutes. Pile on a platter or into a bowl and serve.

ONE GUN SUPERFOOD: Sweet Potato

These root vegetables are high in fiber and packed with beta-carotene, vitamin C, and potassium. Note that the nutritional content of sweet potatoes is higher than yams, which they are often confused with, so make sure you know the difference between the two when shopping

ROASTED
SWEET POTATOES
WITH TURMERIC

Serves 4 to 6

The bright orange of fresh turmeric root combined with the deep orange of sweet potatoes makes for a gorgeous, vibrant dish that really brightens up the table while delivering a super-nutritious punch. You can use a small butternut squash in place of the potatoes; if you do, increase the roasting time to 45 to 50 minutes.

Serve with a green salad for a great meat-free lunch or dinner.

1 teaspoon olive oil

1 teaspoon peeled and finely grated fresh turmeric or 1 teaspoon ground turmeric

Sea salt

2 sweet potatoes

1 fresh red chile, thinly sliced

1 tablespoon roughly chopped fresh cilantro

Preheat the oven to 400°F.

In a small bowl, mix the olive oil and turmeric with a pinch of salt. Halve the sweet potatoes lengthwise and place, cut-side up, on a baking sheet or in a small roasting pan. Brush the cut sides generously with the turmeric and oil mixture and roast until golden and soft, 20 to 25 minutes.

Top with the chile and cilantro and serve immediately.

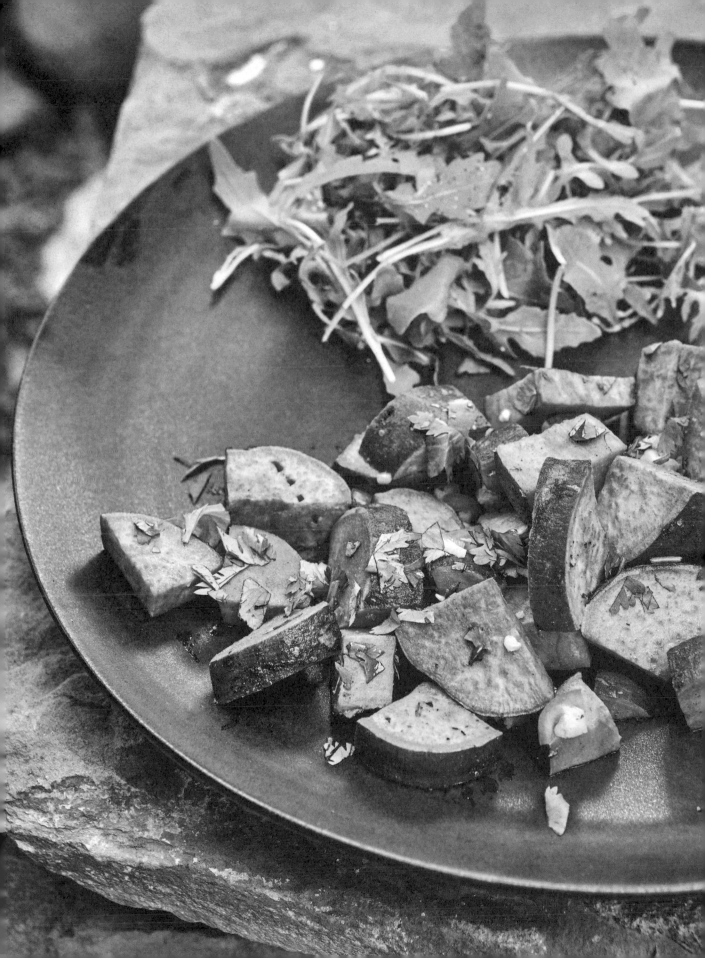

PARISIENNE
LEEK VINAIGRETTE

Serves 4

A One Gun version of the French classic, I fell in love with this dish while living in Paris, where it was served at my favorite bistro, Ma Bourgogne in the Place des Vosges. We like to eat it cold at lunch. In Southern California, we plant leeks in the fall and they are ready to eat in the spring.

12 young leeks

3 sprigs fresh thyme

Sea salt and freshly ground black pepper

2 tablespoons Dijon mustard

1 tablespoon red wine vinegar

3 tablespoons olive oil

2 large organic free-range eggs, hard-boiled, cooled, and peeled

1 tablespoon capers

1 small bunch fresh parsley, minced

Carefully wash and trim the leeks, taking off the roots at the bottom and leaving a small bit of green on the top. Slice each leek lengthwise halfway down in the middle.

Bring a medium pot of water to boil with the thyme sprigs and a pinch each of salt and pepper.

Add the leeks to the water and simmer until tender when tested with the tip of a sharp knife, 8 to 10 minutes. Using tongs, transfer the leeks to paper towels to drain.

Make a vinaigrette by combining the mustard and vinegar in a bowl or a large Mason jar. Whisk or cover and shake to mix well, then whisk or shake in the olive oil to make a thick, emulsified dressing. Season with salt and pepper.

Divide the leeks among 4 plates and spoon on the vinaigrette. Grate the hard-boiled eggs on top, garnish with capers and parsley, and serve immediately.

ONE GUN SUPERFOOD: Leeks

Packed with flavonoids, antioxidants, and vitamins A, C, E, K, and B6, leeks are also a great source of iron and folate. I ate lots of leeks throughout my pregnancy.

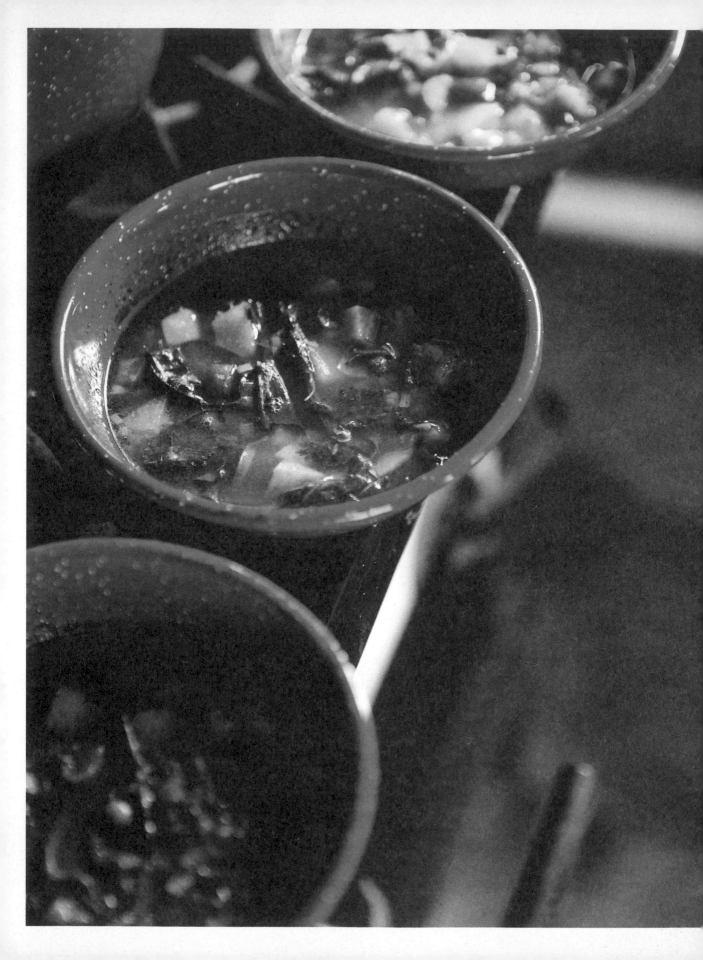

HALLOWEEN STEW,
OR SPICED PUMPKIN CASSEROLE

Serves 6 to 8

A true fall dish highlighting everything that's grown at the Ranch during this season, we like to eat it around the campfire while taking in the full moon. We've also often made huge pots of it to serve to the trick-or-treaters in Malibu Colony, as a welcome respite from all the candy.

1 tablespoon olive oil

1 teaspoon minced garlic

1 tablespoon peeled and minced fresh ginger

4 cups sliced leeks

4 cups peeled and diced carrots

2 cups peeled and diced celery root

6 cups diced ripe tomatoes

1 cup dried chickpeas or butter beans

1 cup dried red lentils

6 cups peeled and diced pumpkin or kombucha squash

1 teaspoon ground turmeric

1 teaspoon coriander seeds, toasted and ground (grind in a mortar using a pestle, a spice grinder, or a coffee grinder dedicated to spices)

6 cups water

3 cups torn red chard leaves, tough stems removed

2½ cups coarsely chopped fresh cilantro

Sea salt and freshly ground black pepper

In a large stockpot over medium-high heat, heat the olive oil. Add the garlic, ginger, leeks, carrots, and celery root and cook until the vegetables are soft, 5 to 8 minutes. Add the tomatoes, chickpeas or beans, lentils, squash, turmeric, coriander, and water and bring to a simmer. Cover, reduce the heat to low, and cook very gently for 2 hours.

Add the chard and cook until nicely wilted throughout the soup, 5 to 10 minutes. Add the cilantro and season with salt and pepper. Ladle into bowls and serve hot.

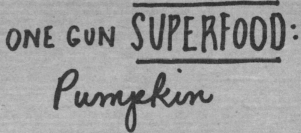

ONE GUN SUPERFOOD:
Pumpkin

Packed with fiber, pumpkin is also a great source of carotenoids and is high in potassium and vitamins A and C.

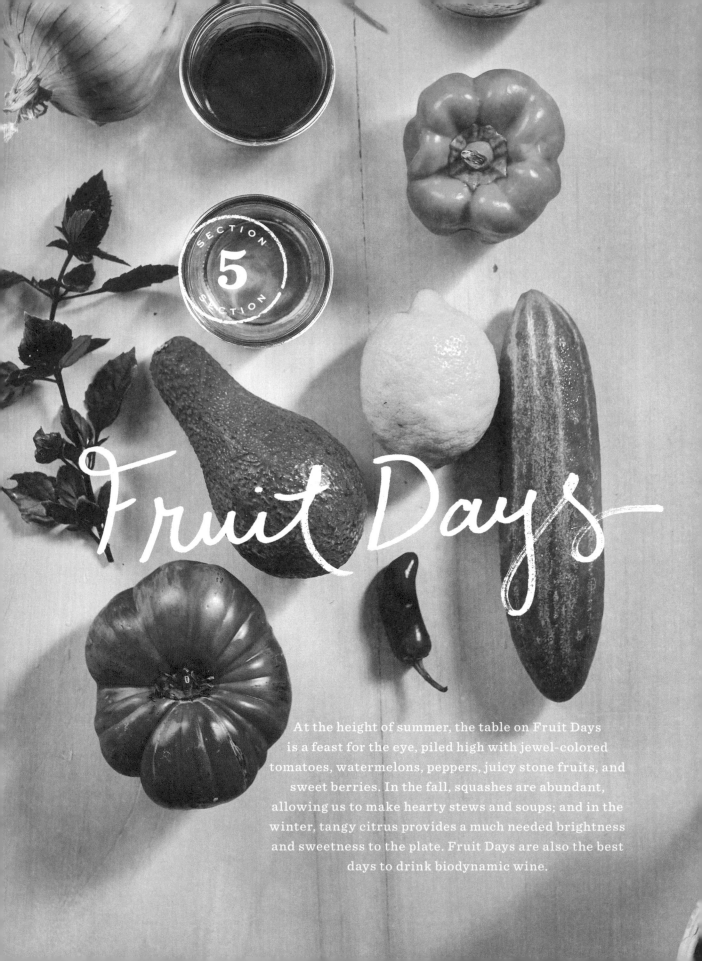

Fruit Days

At the height of summer, the table on Fruit Days is a feast for the eye, piled high with jewel-colored tomatoes, watermelons, peppers, juicy stone fruits, and sweet berries. In the fall, squashes are abundant, allowing us to make hearty stews and soups; and in the winter, tangy citrus provides a much needed brightness and sweetness to the plate. Fruit Days are also the best days to drink biodynamic wine.

GAZPACHO

Serves 4 to 6

One of my favorite go-tos, this healthy raw soup is so vibrant, you can just taste the freshness of the veggies bursting through. I first fell in love with this traditional Spanish dish when I was twelve, while staying with my best friend, Cristina, in Madrid. It was used as a daily staple as well as a fantastic lunch or supper dish. At the Ranch, I always keep a big jug of fresh gazpacho in the fridge, using the best of the season's tomatoes. The flavor is most delicious if you make gazpacho a day ahead.

1 pound tomatoes

½ pound sweet heirloom tomatoes

1 medium mild onion, roughly chopped

1 small green bell pepper, seeded and roughly chopped

1 medium cucumber, peeled and roughly chopped

⅔ cup chicken stock or water

1 tablespoon extra-virgin olive oil

1½ teaspoons red wine vinegar

1 to 2 tablespoons fresh lemon juice

Sea salt and freshly ground black pepper

FOR THE GARNISH:

1 jalapeño chile, finely chopped

Handful of fresh cilantro leaves

1 ripe avocado, pitted, peeled, and diced

4 sweet heirloom tomatoes, chopped

2 sprigs fresh purple flowering basil or cilantro flowers

One day in advance of serving, blanch all of the tomatoes in boiling water for 1 minute to loosen the skins. Drain, let cool, and peel, then squeeze the watery juices and seeds out and discard. Put the tomato flesh in a blender with the onion, bell pepper, and cucumber. Add the stock, olive oil, and vinegar and blend well.

Pour into a bowl and add lemon juice to taste. Season with salt and pepper. Cover and chill overnight.

When ready to serve the gazpacho, taste and adjust the seasoning. Pour into bowls and garnish with the jalapeño, cilantro, avocado, chopped tomatoes, and basil flowers. Serve cold.

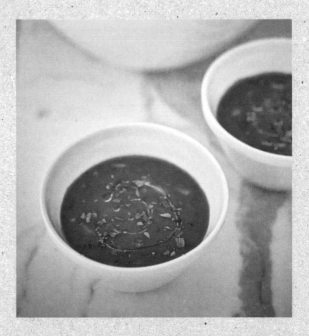

WATERMELON
GAZPACHO

Serves 4

Another way to enjoy gazpacho is to incorporate fresh, sweet watermelon. We have watermelon in abundance at the Ranch over the summer and this is a fun way to use it. This soup can also be served as a dessert.

8 to 10 cups cubed seedless watermelon (from about a 3-pound melon)

1 cup chopped tomatoes

1 large cucumber, peeled and diced, a few tablespoons finely chopped and reserved for garnish

½ red onion, chopped

½ cup packed fresh mint leaves, plus chopped mint for garnish

1 jalapeño chile, stemmed and seeded

2 tablespoons olive oil

Juice of 1 lemon

Juice of 1 lime

Sea salt and freshly ground black pepper

Working in batches, combine the watermelon, tomatoes, cucumber, onion, mint, jalapeño, olive oil, and lemon and lime juices in a blender. Blend until smooth. Pour into a large bowl and season with salt and pepper. Cover and chill overnight.

When ready to serve the gazpacho, taste and adjust the seasoning. Pour into soup bowls and garnish with the reserved cucumber and mint. Serve cold.

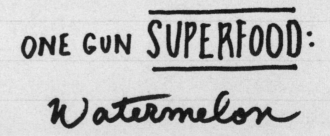

ONE GUN SUPERFOOD:
Watermelon

Containing even more lycopene than tomatoes, watermelon is a super antioxidant and is rich in vitamins A and C.

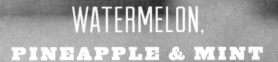

WATERMELON,
PINEAPPLE & MINT

Serves 6

This makes for a perfect summer dessert or party dish. When buying tropical fruits, such as pineapple, always look for sustainability hallmarks like Fairtrade and Rainforest Alliance, and always buy organic to ensure the fruit was grown without pesticides.

8 cups cubed seedless watermelon (from about a 3-pound melon)

4 cups cubed fresh pineapple (from about 1 medium pineapple)

Leaves from 1 bunch fresh mint, torn

Juice of 1 lime

Toss all of the ingredients together in a large bowl and enjoy!

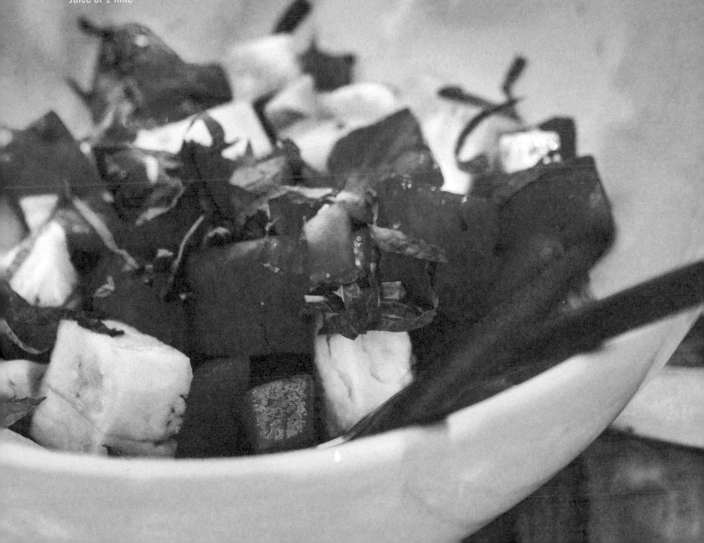

BARBECUED
WATERMELON

Serves 6

An unusual but delicious way to eat watermelon—make sure the melon you choose isn't too ripe or it will fall to pieces on the grill.

One 3-pound seedless watermelon

Juice of 2 limes

Aged, syrupy balsamic vinegar for serving

Chopped fresh cilantro for garnish

This is a great way to eat fresh peaches when they are in season; it makes a delicious dessert without any added sugar. Just substitute a few pinches of fresh mint leaves for the cilantro.

Build a medium-hot fire in a charcoal grill or preheat a gas grill to medium-high.

Cut the rind off the watermelon and cut the flesh into large (least 1 inch). Spread the cubes in a pan and brush on all sides with the lime juice.

Arrange the watermelon on the grill rack, working in batches if needed, and grill until lightly charred, about 5 minutes. Serve immediately, sprinkled with the balsamic and cilantro.

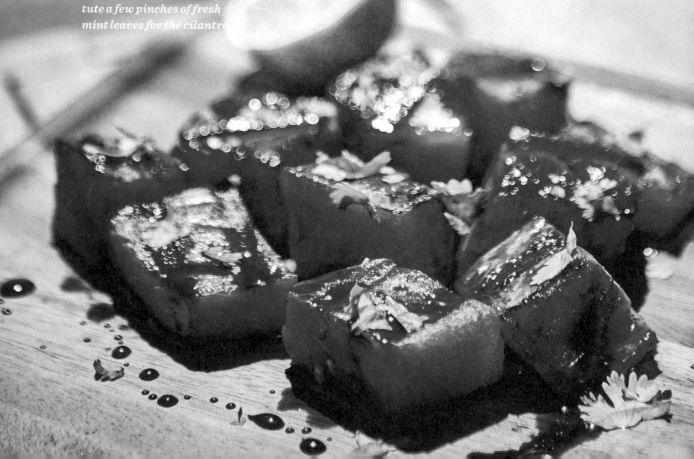

SLICED
PEACHES
WITH LIME & MINT

Serves 4

I am so happy when the first peaches come in season. We have a few young peach trees at the Ranch, but they do not produce any substantial fruit yet, so we buy ours from the specialist growers at the Malibu Farmers' Market. White peaches are best in this dish, as they are lower in acid and sweet even when they are firm. They look beautiful on the plate sliced super-thin like a carpaccio, and the lime really brings out their flavor while helping them keep their color when waiting to be served.

2 ripe peaches, very thinly sliced (carpaccio style; a vegetable peeler is a good tool for this)

Juice and grated zest of 1 lime

Leaves from 1 sprig fresh mint, torn

Lay the peach slices on a plate. Drizzle with the lime juice, sprinkle with the zest and mint, and serve.

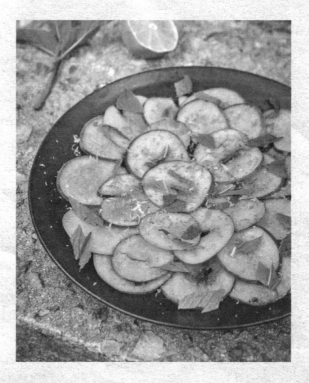

ROASTED
BEET, SQUASH & PUMPKIN

Serves 6

Using the best of the season's root vegetables and squash, this colorful dish is vividly evocative of fall at the Ranch. The rosemary really enhances the flavors and our Tamari Seeds give it a great crunch.

1 winter squash, such as butternut (about 2 pounds)

½ pumpkin (about 2 pounds)

4 medium beets, trimmed and peeled

2 tablespoons olive oil

Raw local honey for drizzling

Leaves from 1 sprig fresh rosemary, roughly chopped

2 tablespoons Tamari Seeds (recipe follows)

Preheat the oven to 400°F.

Halve the squash; peel and seed the squash and pumpkin. Cut the squash, pumpkin, and beets into roughly ½-inch cubes. Pile all of the veggies on a large baking sheet. Drizzle with the olive oil and honey and sprinkle on the rosemary. Toss to mix and coat well.

Roast, stirring once or twice, until tender, 45 to 50 minutes.

Let cool slightly, then toss with the Tamari Seeds. Serve immediately.

TAMARI SEEDS

Makes about ½ cup

A nutritious, crunchy, and gluten-free addition to any salad. Warning: these are addictive!

2 tablespoons raw sesame seeds

2 tablespoons raw sunflower seeds

¼ cup raw pumpkin seeds

1½ tablespoons Tamari Lite

1 teaspoon coconut oil, melted

In a bowl, stir together all of the ingredients. Set aside to marinate for several hours.

Preheat the oven to 300°F.

Line a baking sheet with parchment paper and spread the seed mixture in a single layer. Bake until lightly golden and aromatic, 1 to 2 hours.

The toasted seed mix will keep, stored in an airtight container, for up to 6 months.

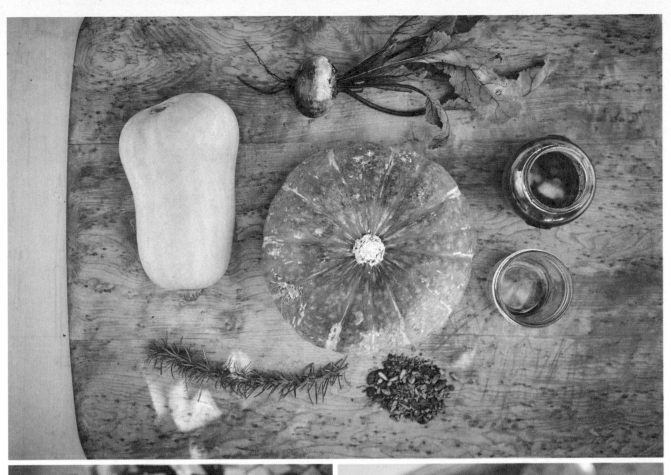

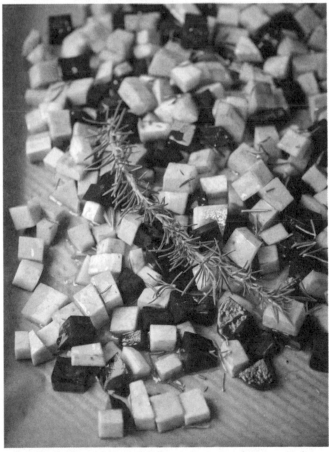

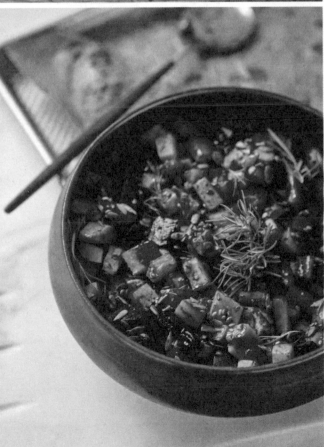

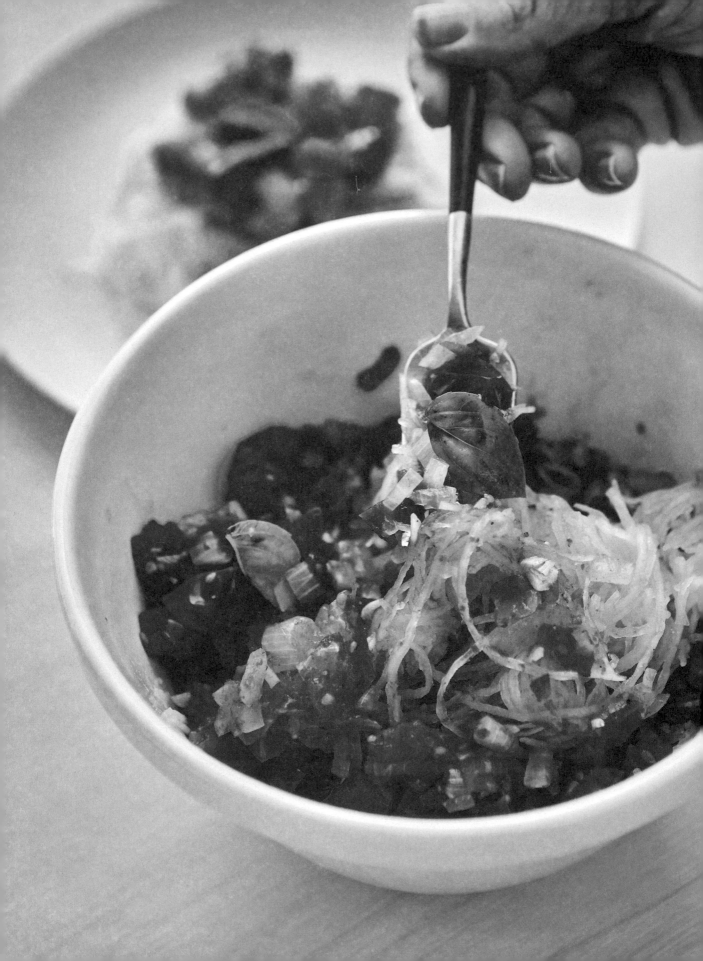

SPAGHETTI SQUASH
ARRABIATA

Serves 4

Try using spaghetti squash to make this super-satisfying, gluten-free, spicy "pasta" dish. You can also use zucchini, shaved into thin ribbons and quickly sautéed in olive oil, if you prefer. We forage the bay leaves for the sauce while hiking the trails around the Ranch and working up an appetite.

1 spaghetti squash (about 3 pounds)

Olive oil for brushing

Sea salt and freshly ground black pepper

FOR THE SAUCE:

½ yellow onion, diced

1 tablespoon minced garlic

1 cayenne chile, minced

1 or 2 jalapeño chiles, minced, a few pinches reserved for garnish

2 pounds vine-ripened tomatoes, diced

½ cup shredded fresh basil, plus basil flowers for garnish

1 tablespoon minced fresh oregano

2 bay leaves

Sea salt and freshly ground black pepper

Basil flowers for garnish

Preheat the oven to 375°F.

Cut the squash in half lengthwise. Scrape out the seeds and strings. Brush the cut sides with olive oil and sprinkle with salt and pepper. Place the halves, cut-side down, on a baking sheet. Bake until tender when pierced with a knife, about 40 minutes.

Let the squash rest. When cool enough to handle, using a fork, scrape out the spaghetti-like strands. Pile into a bowl as you work. Cover and set aside.

To make the sauce: In a saucepan over medium-high heat, sauté the onion, garlic, cayenne chile, and jalapeños to taste until soft, 2 to 3 minutes. Add the tomatoes, basil, oregano, and bay leaves, along with enough water to make a medium-thick sauce. Bring to a simmer and cook for 10 minutes, stirring occasionally. Season with salt and pepper. Discard the bay leaves.

Liberally cover the spaghetti squash "pasta" with the sauce, garnish with a sprinkle of the reserved jalapeño and the basil flowers, and serve immediately.

RAW
PAD THAI

Serves 4

A family adaptation of the Thai staple, we swapped out noodles for zucchini ribbons and kept it completely raw, so you can reap the full nutritional benefits of the biodynamically grown vegetables.

2 medium zucchini

2 medium carrots, peeled

½ head red cabbage

1 to 2 cups mushrooms, brushed clean

½ cup bean sprouts

1 jalapeño chile

FOR THE SAUCE:

Juice of 2 oranges

Juice of ½ lime

2 tablespoons raw local honey

1 tablespoon tamari

1 tablespoon almond butter

1 tablespoon unpasteurized miso

1 tablespoon peeled and minced fresh ginger

1 clove garlic, minced

Pinch of cayenne pepper

Chopped fresh cilantro for garnish

Chopped fresh mint for garnish

Using a vegetable peeler or a spiralizer, shave or cut the zucchini very thinly into long ribbons to create "noodles." Set aside.

Grate the carrots, cabbage, and mushrooms into a large bowl. Add the bean sprouts and toss to mix.

To make the sauce, in a bowl, whisk together the citrus juices, honey, tamari, almond butter, miso, ginger, garlic, and cayenne. Pour half of the sauce over the cabbage mixture, and toss to mix and coat completely.

Divide the zucchini "noodles" among individual plates and top with the cabbage mixture. Drizzle the remaining sauce on top. Sprinkle with the cilantro and mint and serve.

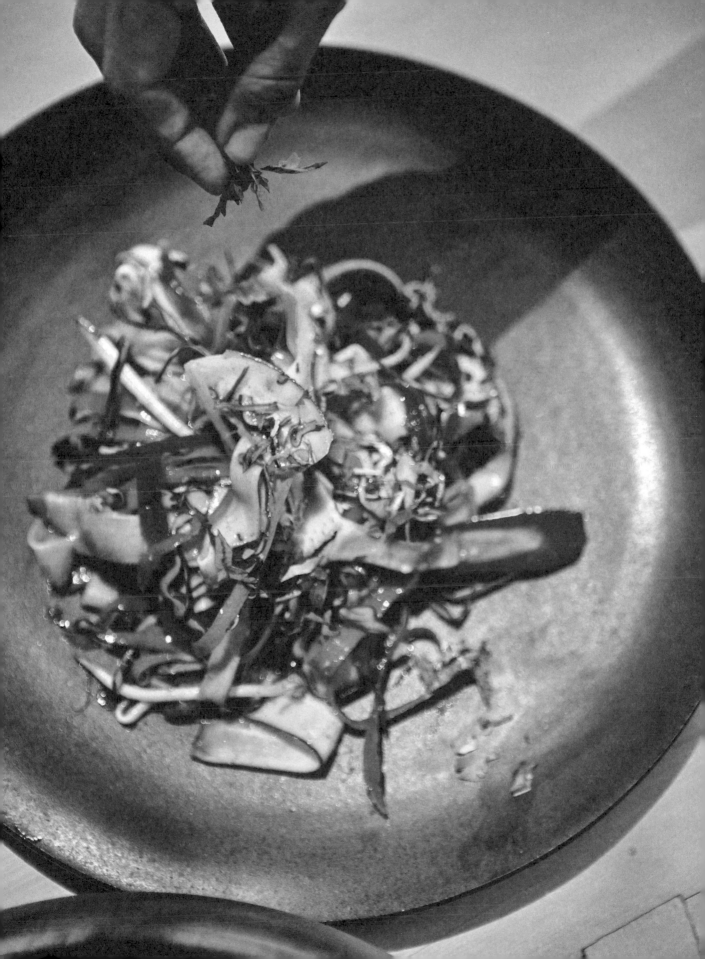

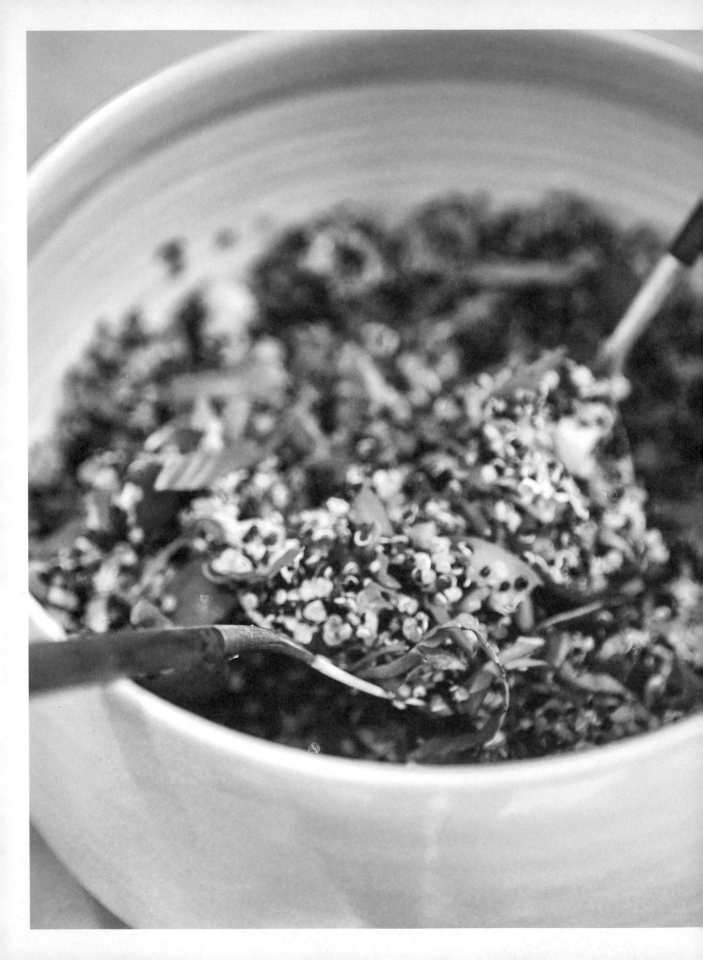

ONE GUN

QUINOA

WITH TOMATOES, CILANTRO & BASIL

Serves 4

A much-loved go-to at any time of year, this nutritious recipe is perfect as a main or side dish. Rinse the quinoa before cooking to remove some of the saponin, a chemical compound coating it that can make the cooked grains a little foamy and bitter.

1 cup tricolor quinoa

1 tablespoon chicken or vegetable stock

2 cups water

1 or 2 organic tomatoes, preferably biodynamic

1 jalapeño chile, minced

1 bunch fresh cilantro, chopped

Leaves from 1 large bunch fresh basil, chopped

Sea salt and freshly ground pepper (optional)

Edible flowers for garnish

In a saucepan, combine the quinoa, stock, and 2 cups water. Bring to a boil, then reduce the heat and simmer, covered, until the quinoa is tender and most of the liquid has been absorbed, 15 to 20 minutes. Drain, fluff with a fork, and set aside to cool.

Coarsely chop the tomatoes and stir into the cooled quinoa. Stir in the jalapeño and chopped herbs. Season with salt and pepper, if desired, garnish with edible flowers, and serve.

HEIRLOOM TOMATO &
BASIL SALAD

Serves 4

Summer is the time when tomatoes are at their most delicious. At the Ranch, we grow a variety of heirloom (more commonly called "heritage" in the UK) tomatoes that have been passed down over generations. Striped, purple, yellow, even green in color, some are large and almost pumpkin-like, others cherry or eggplant shaped, and all them flavorful beyond any greenhouse-grown tomato found on a supermarket shelf. We love to make a beautiful, large salad of mixed tomatoes sliced crossways to show off the array of colors, with green and purple basil layered on top.

1 pound mixed ripe heirloom
  tomatoes, thickly sliced
  crosswise

Leaves from ½ bunch fresh
  green basil

Leaves from ½ bunch fresh
  purple basil

Freshly ground black pepper

Balsamic Vinaigrette (page 295)
  for serving

Edible flowers for garnish

Arrange the tomato slices attractively on a platter. Layer the green and purple basil leaves over the top. Grind pepper over the salad and drizzle with the vinaigrette. Garnish with flowers and serve.

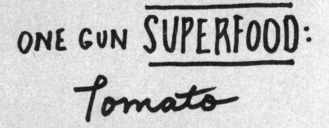

ONE GUN SUPERFOOD:
Tomato

Tomatoes are high in lycopene, which can lower the risk of Alzheimer's disease, stroke, and cancer, as well as minerals, antioxidants, and vitamins C and A.

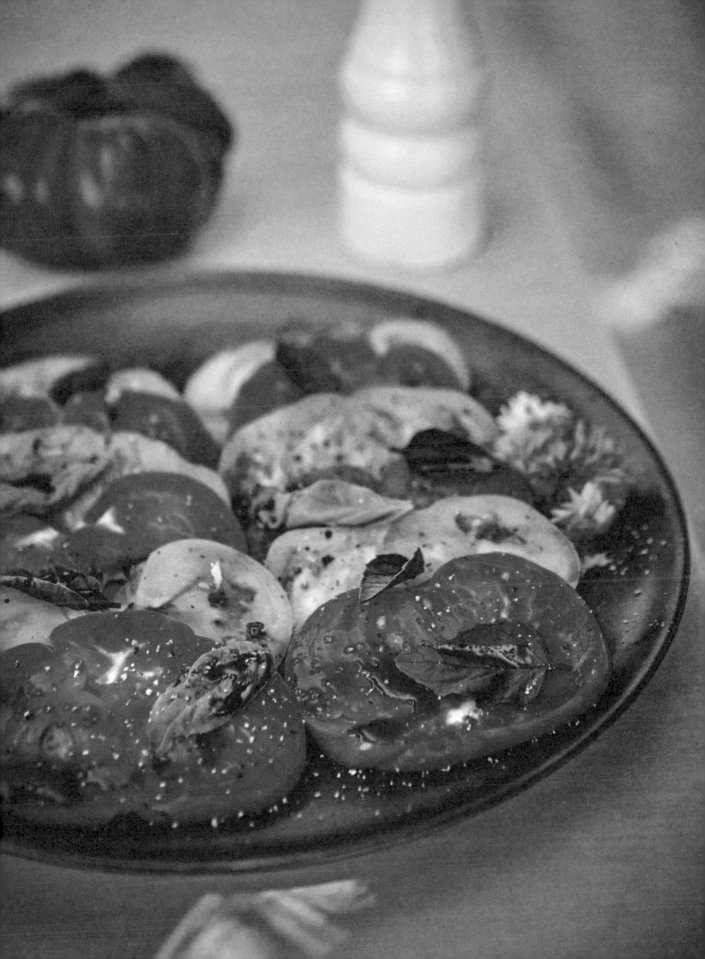

TOMATO CONSOMMÉ

WITH BASIL SORBET

Serves 4

This is the embodiment of a seasonal summer dish. The delicate flavor of the tomatoes and the cold freshness of the sorbet, which I absolutely love, is so simple but so fabulous—and a novel spin on the age-old and beloved pairing of tomato and basil. This dish is really the perfect refreshing summer lunch.

About 14 large ripe heirloom tomatoes

Sea salt and freshly ground black pepper

1 sprig fresh basil

Basil Sorbet (recipe follows)

Basil flowers for garnish

Cut the tomatoes into rough dice. Pile into a large bowl with their juices. Add a big pinch of salt, a few grindings of pepper, and the basil sprig. Blend with a hand blender until pureed, or process in batches in a blender. Let sit at room temperature for 1 hour to allow the flavors to marry.

Set up a strainer lined with a double layer of cheesecloth over another bowl or a small pot. Pour the tomato juice through the strainer and let stand until every drop has dripped through.

To serve, ladle the consommé into bowls and place a scoop of the sorbet in the middle of each. Garnish with a few basil flowers and serve.

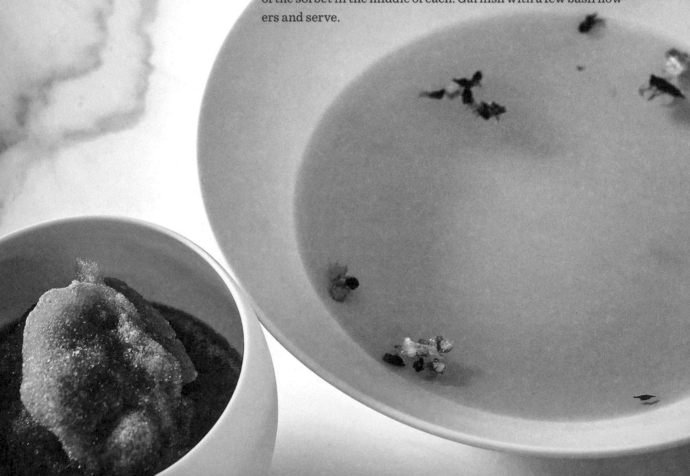

Basil Sorbet

Makes 2½ cups

Below are my methods for making sorbet with or without an ice-cream maker. A third way, the Italian granita method, is to stir the base in its dish in the freezer every 30 minutes to 1 hour or so, using a fork to help break up the ice crystals. I think my blender method is easiest. It takes a bit more prep time, but creates a beautiful sorbet or ice cream.

20 large fresh green basil leaves, minced

1 cup apple juice

1 cup water

½ cup fresh lime juice

¼ cup raw local honey

Combine all of the ingredients in a blender and blend until smooth. Strain the base through a fine-mesh strainer into a baking dish.

To make the sorbet in a blender: Cover the base and freeze overnight, or until completely frozen. Remove from the freezer, carefully break it up into large pieces, and quickly add to a blender. Give it a quick whizz in the blender until the sorbet has a soft, creamy texture. Transfer to an airtight container and return to the freezer for another 1 to 2 hours, or until the sorbet is completely frozen.

To make the sorbet in an ice-cream maker: Freeze the ice-cream maker freezer bowl overnight. Cover the base and refrigerate until well-chilled, 2 to 3 hours, or overnight. Freeze in the ice-cream maker according to the manufacturer's instructions. The sorbet will have a soft, creamy texture. Transfer to an airtight container and freeze until firm, about 2 hours.

Remove from the freezer about 15 minutes before serving.

CHILLED
TOMATO, CUCUMBER & FENNEL SOUP

Serves 6

Another soup which uses the best seasonal produce, this is a heartier take on a gazpacho with the addition of fennel, celery, and red and yellow bell peppers. Easy to prepare, all you need is a blender. This makes for a perfect late summer lunch.

1 jar or can (28 ounces) tomato passata or crushed tomatoes

⅔ cup roughly chopped cherry tomatoes

4 red vine-ripened cherry tomatoes, cut into ¼-inch dice

6 tablespoons olive oil

2 tablespoons balsamic vinegar

Juice of ½ lemon

¼ fresh red chile, seeded and finely chopped

1 clove garlic, crushed

1 teaspoon sugar

2 cups water

1 cucumber, seeded and cut into ¼-inch dice

1 fennel bulb, cored and cut into ¼-inch dice

½ red bell pepper, seeded and cut into ¼-inch dice

½ yellow bell pepper, seeded and cut into ¼-inch dice

½ green bell pepper, seeded and cut into ¼-inch dice

1 stalk celery, cut into ¼-inch dice

3 tablespoons chopped fresh cilantro

2 tablespoons chopped fresh flat-leaf parsley

Sea salt and freshly ground black pepper

Extra-virgin olive oil for drizzling

In a large bowl, combine the passata, fresh tomatoes, olive oil, vinegar, lemon juice, chile, garlic, sugar, and 2 cups water.

Pour the tomato mixture into a blender, working in batches if necessary, and blend until smooth.

In another large bowl, toss together the cucumber, fennel, bell peppers, and celery. Pour in the tomato mixture and stir gently. Cover and refrigerate until well-chilled, 1 to 2 hours.

Just before serving, chill 6 bowls. Take the soup out of the fridge and stir in the cilantro and parsley. Season with salt and pepper. Ladle into the chilled bowls, drizzle with a little extra-virgin olive oil, and serve.

CHILLED
AVOCADO & CUCUMBER SOUP

Serves 4

Serve this elegant green-of-summer soup when you plan to eat outside on a hot day or balmy evening. It's a gorgeous way to showcase everything grown at the Ranch, as the only thing added is water, and a little yogurt, if you like. Skip the yogurt for a vegan version.

1 ripe avocado, pitted and peeled

1 cucumber, peeled and roughly chopped

1 green onion, roughly chopped

½ jalapeño chile, finely chopped

2 tablespoons fresh cilantro leaves

2 tablespoons fresh lemon juice

½ cup cold water

1 cup sheep's-milk yogurt (optional)

Micro cilantro for garnish

Combine all of the ingredients except the garnish in a blender and blend until smooth and creamy. Refrigerate until well-chilled, 1 to 2 hours. Serve cold, garnished with the micro cilantro.

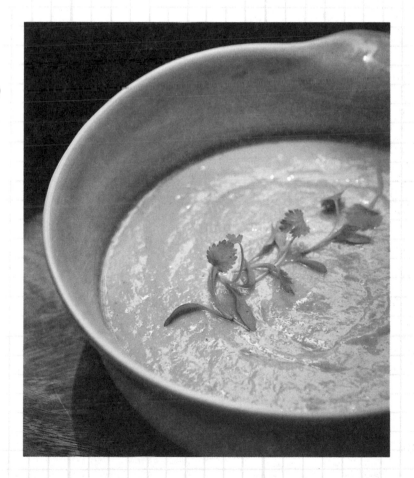

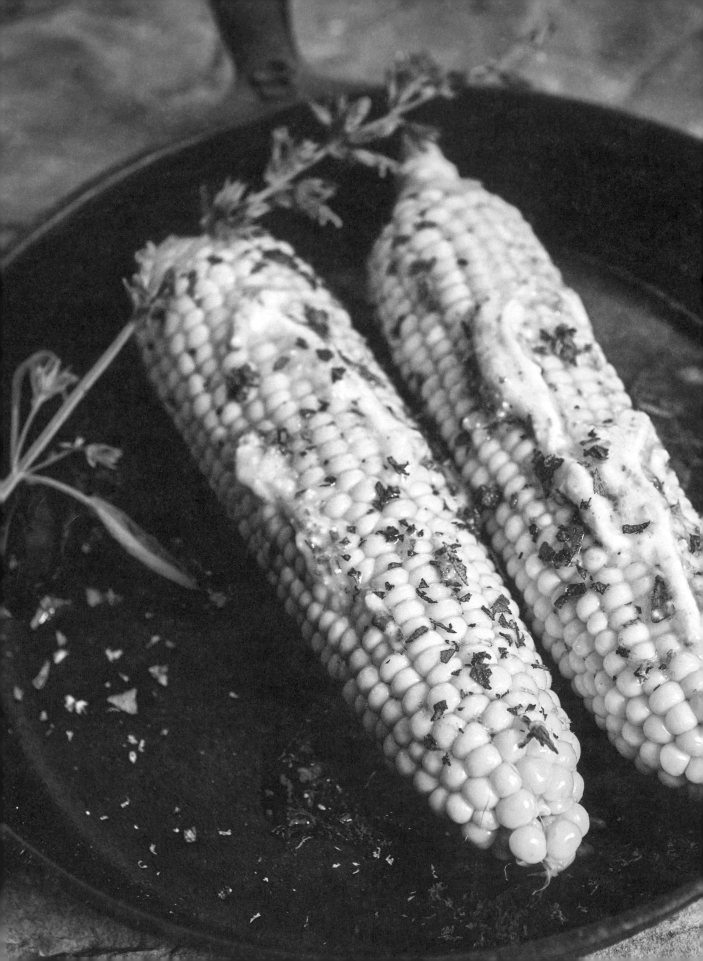

GRILLED CORN
WITH SAGE

Serves 4

At the Ranch, we grow both blue and yellow corn. While there are far too many cornstarch and corn by-products in most processed foods these days, I love fresh corn; and I think it's at its best when very simply prepared. This dish is great as a side and the perfect accompaniment for any grilled meat or fish. The addition of fresh sage—at One Gun, we forage for it, and there may be some near you, too!—elevates this easy recipe, making it melt-in-your-mouth delicious.

¼ cup coconut oil, melted

1½ tablespoons chopped fresh sage

Juice and zest of 1 lime

4 ears of corn, husks and silk removed

In a small bowl, stir together the coconut oil, sage, and lime juice and zest.

Build a medium-hot fire in a charcoal grill or preheat a gas grill to medium-high.

Grill the corn until lightly charred, 7 to 8 minutes. (Alternatively, boil the corn until the kernels are still tender, about 10 minutes.)

Spread on the sage oil while the corn is still hot. Serve immediately.

Leaf Days

Leaf Days are our favorite days, because we have so
many delicious salad mixes, kales, chards, and
roots with green tops growing on the Ranch, all of which
we incorporate into bright, vibrant, nutrient-packed
salads or simple sautéed side dishes. Serve alongside a
protein or quinoa, as needed.

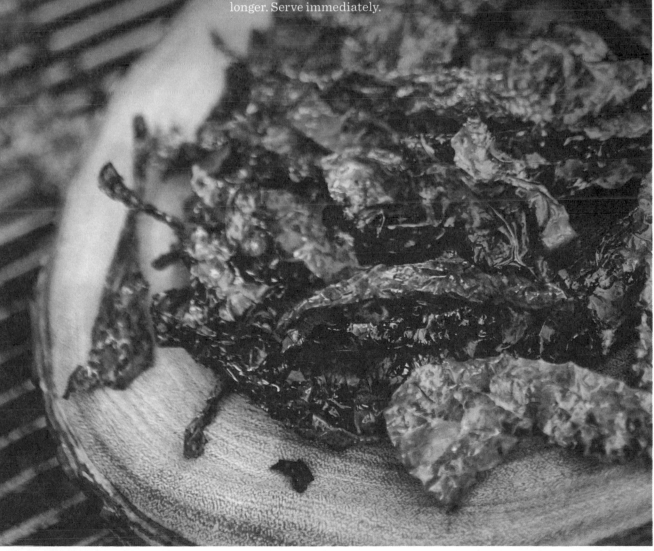

GRILLED TUSCAN KALE

Serves 4

This is our barbecued version of oven-baked kale chips. Super-healthy and more-ish, the plate will be finished in minutes!

2 bunches Tuscan kale
2 tablespoons olive oil
Sea salt

Build a medium-hot fire in a charcoal grill or preheat a gas grill to medium-high.

Remove the center spines and stems of the kale and rip the leaves into big pieces. In a large bowl, toss the kale with the olive oil and a few pinches of salt.

Grill for about 4 minutes on one side, allowing the kale to burn a little before turning over and cooking for about 2 minutes longer. Serve immediately.

ANNIE'S VEGGIES

WITH QUINOA

Serves 2

One of Annie's signature dishes, I always look forward to this—especially as it's so lovingly prepared, and it means I have a night off cooking. This Asian twist on quinoa is packed with leafy greens, highly nutritious mushrooms, and a spicy kick. Shrimp or chicken can also be added to this dish if you are craving some protein.

1 teaspoon coconut oil

1 white onion, thinly sliced

2 heads broccoli (about 3 pounds), trimmed and roughly chopped

2 heads bok choy, cored and roughly chopped

1 packet enoki mushrooms, roughly chopped

2 to 4 shiitake mushrooms, stemmed and roughly chopped

2 handfuls fresh cilantro leaves, roughly chopped

1 jalapeño chile, minced

1 tablespoon peeled and thinly sliced fresh ginger

1 tablespoon tamari

2 cups cooked quinoa (white, red, or tricolor)

Sambal for serving

In a large pan or wok over medium-high heat, melt the oil. When the oil is very hot, add the onion, broccoli, bok choy, enoki, shiitake, cilantro, jalapeño, and ginger to the pan. Sauté until the vegetables are softened but still crunchy, about 8 minutes. Stir in the tamari.

Add the cooked quinoa and stir until all the ingredients are well combined. Divide between 2 plates and serve with a side of sambal.

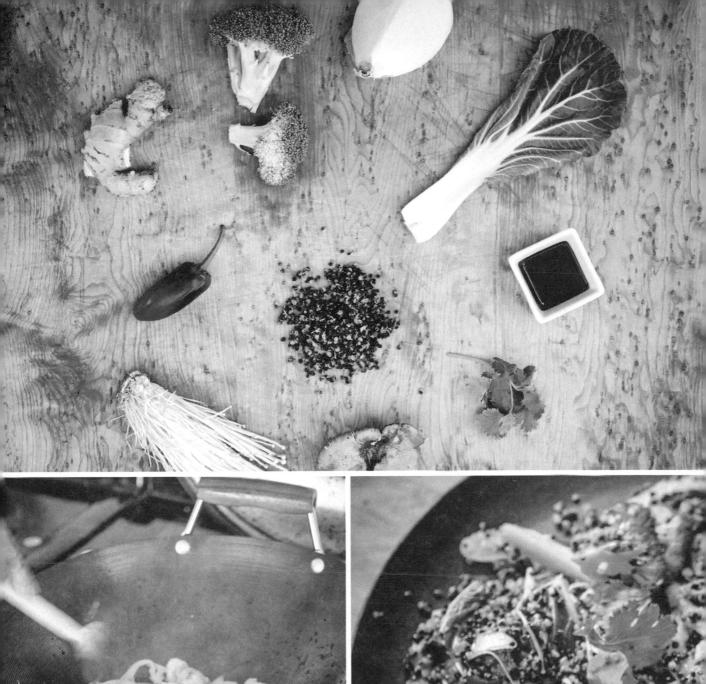

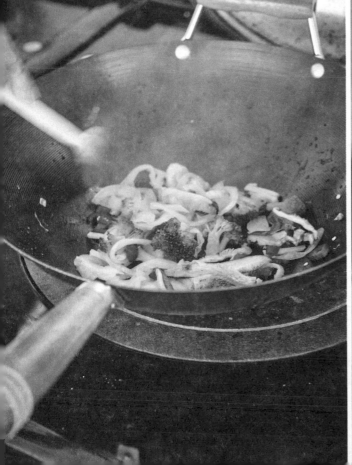

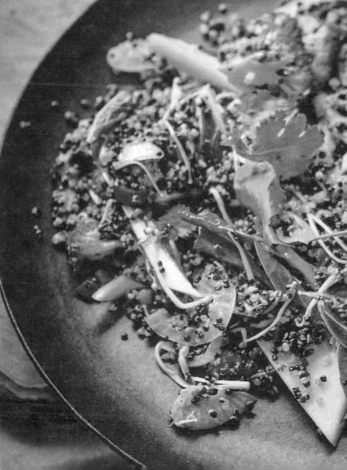

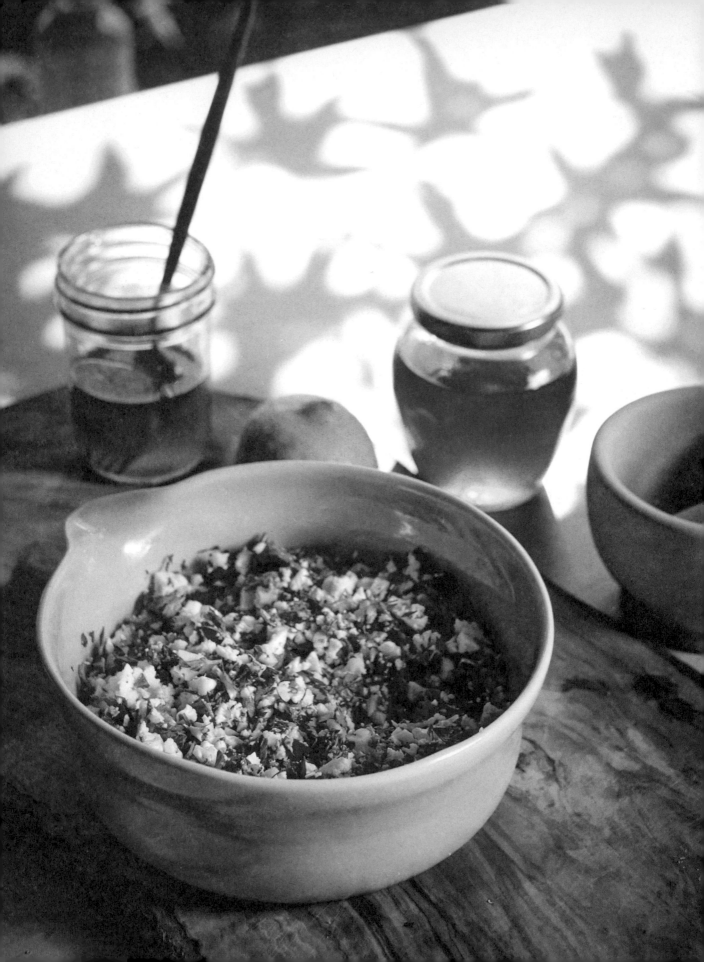

RAW
TABOULI

Serves 4

I love this healthy, raw, and gluten-free spin on the classic Middle Eastern dish, which uses cauliflower in place of bulgur wheat. This is also a perfect way to showcase the delicious parsley grown at the Ranch.

Juice of ½ lemon

2 tablespoons olive oil

1 tablespoon raw local honey

Dash of cayenne pepper

Pinch of sea salt

½ head cauliflower, cored and finely chopped

2 large ripe tomatoes, finely chopped

1 bunch fresh parsley, finely chopped

1 bunch fresh cilantro, finely chopped

½ cup hempseed, coarsely ground (grind in a mortar with a pestle or use a spice grinder or coffee grinder dedicated to spices)

In a small bowl, whisk together the lemon, olive oil, honey, cayenne, and salt. Set the dressing aside.

In a large bowl, toss together the cauliflower, tomatoes, parsley, cilantro, and hempseed. Pour in the dressing, toss well, and serve.

ONE GUN SUPERFOOD: Parsley

Packed with flavonoids and chlorophyll, which gives it that bright green color, parsley is highly alkaline and builds red blood cells. High in vitamins A, C, and K, it's also great for the digestion.

ONE GUN
SPINACH & POMEGRANATE SALAD

Serves 4

Stunning to look at, this fall salad is also super-nutritious and satisfyingly crunchy. I get so excited when each new fruit or vegetable comes into season, and this is a fantastic way to celebrate the pomegranate. I just love slicing them open and letting the juice run out all over my hands. The dark blood red of the pomegranate seeds atop the deep green of the spinach makes a beautiful combination. This can be served as a side dish or can be beefed up with some quinoa to make a nourishing supper.

1 pound spinach, tough stems removed, rinsed and drained

¼ red onion, thinly sliced

¼ cup alfalfa sprouts

¼ cup raw almonds (or use sliced, if you like)

¼ cup Balsamic Vinaigrette (page 295)

Seeds from 1 pomegranate

Put the spinach in a large bowl and add the onions, almonds, and alfalfa sprouts.

Pour in the vinaigrette and toss well. Top with the pomegranate seeds and serve.

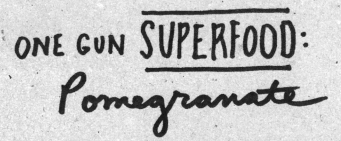

ONE GUN SUPERFOOD:
Pomegranate

Packed with antioxidants, polyphenols, and tannins, pomegranates are also high in vitamin C, folate, and potassium.

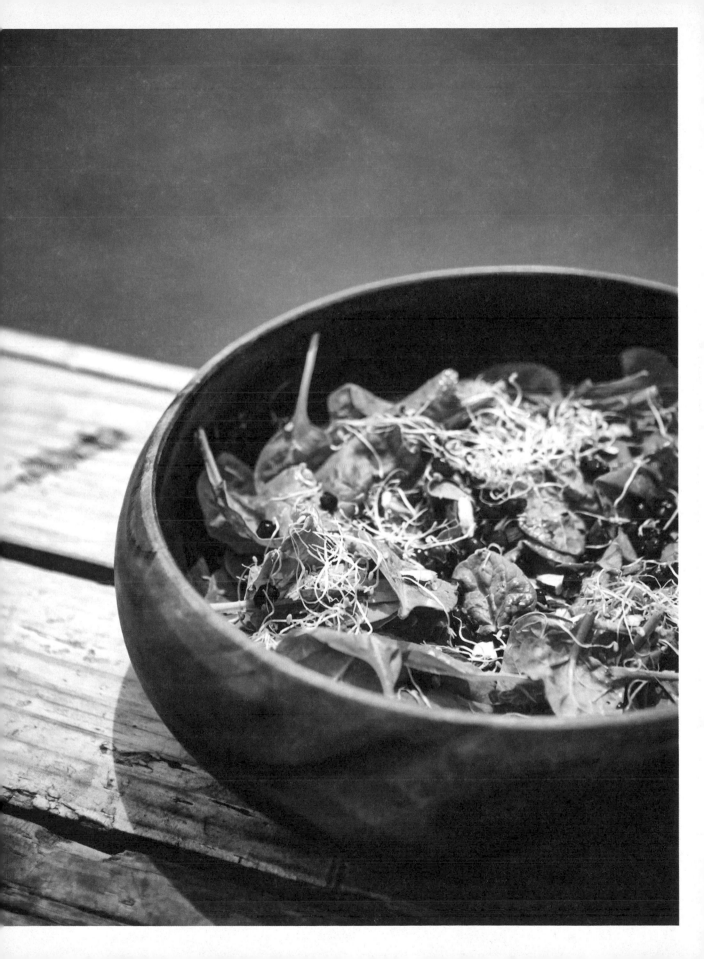

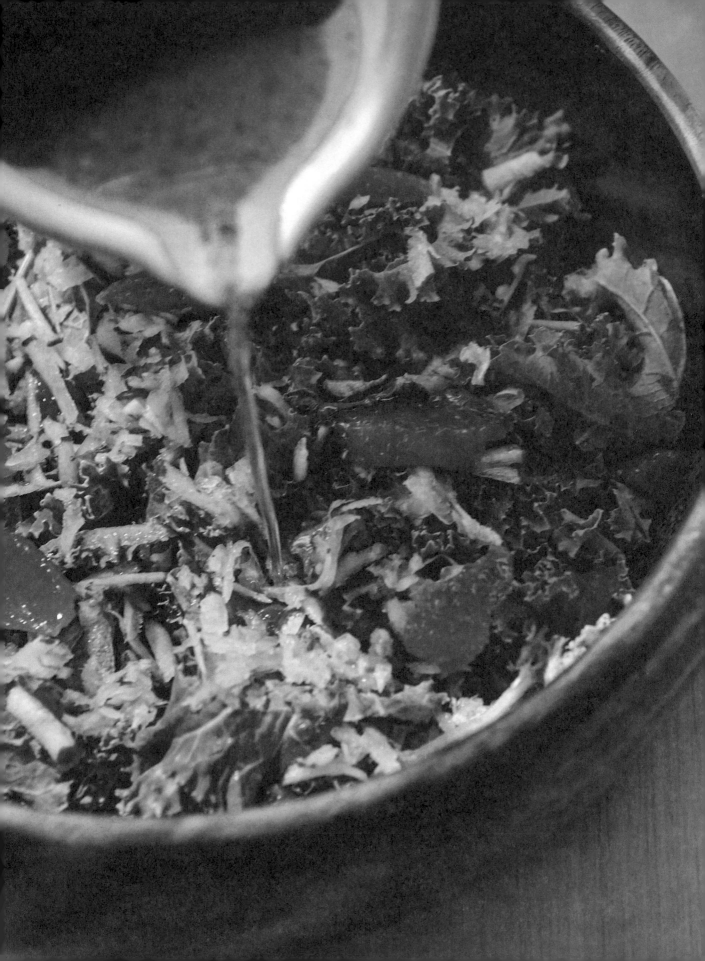

FENNEL, KALE & GRAPEFRUIT
SALAD

Serves 4

Fresh and zesty, this winter salad can brighten up even the dreariest day. If you have a mandoline, you can use that to make pretty, extra thin slices of fennel, but the easy grated version has a terrific texture.

FOR THE DRESSING:

Juice of ½ grapefruit

1 tablespoon extra-virgin olive oil

1 teaspoon raw local honey

Freshly ground black pepper

FOR THE SALAD:

2 bunches curly kale, tough stems and spines removed, leaves torn into bite-size pieces

1 fennel bulb, cored and grated

1 grapefruit, segmented, removed of pith, and cut into bite-size pieces

2 large radishes, trimmed and grated

Edible flowers for garnish

To make the dressing, in a bowl, whisk together the grapefruit juice, olive oil, and honey. Season to taste with pepper. Set aside.

In a large bowl or on a serving platter, layer first the kale, then the fennel, grapefruit, and radishes. Drizzle the salad with the dressing and serve, garnished with the flowers.

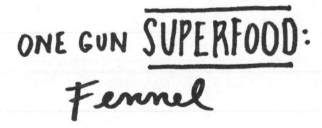

ONE GUN **SUPERFOOD:**
Fennel

A great source of vitamin C and potassium, fennel is also wonderful for the digestion. Breastfeeding mothers can eat fennel to increase their milk supply and soothe a colicky baby, as the digestive benefits are passed on through breast milk.

COLLARD
WRAPS

Serves as many as you have leaves for

This healthy, filling lunch is a staple at the Campfire Kitchen during compost making and our educational tours. Large collard leaves are used instead of tortillas to make the wraps gluten-free and super-healthy.

Lots of big fresh collard leaves

FOR THE SPREADS:

Carrot-Top Pesto (page 172) and
    Nasturtium Pesto (page 228),
    combined

Almond Pâté (recipe follows)

FOR THE FILLINGS:

Grated or shaved or spiralized
    cucumber, carrots, celery,
    zucchini, and/or beets

Sprouts and micro leaves

Chopped tomatoes

Chopped avocados

Raisins

Almonds

Hempseed

FOR THE SEASONING:

Lime, lemon, or orange juice

Cayenne pepper (optional)

Remove the stalk of each collard leaf.

Assemble to your and your diners' every desire (or let everyone make their own): Thickly spread with your choice of spreads. Layer the vegetables on top. Tuck raisins, nuts, or seeds in the very middle. Season with juices and cayenne pepper.

Roll the leaf up and over the filling and into a tight cylinder, and tuck in. These look great on the black plates!

Almond Pâté

Makes about 6 cups

A vegan pâté packed full of flavor, savory and sweet and highly beneficial with a perfect balance of protein and good fat.

1 cup raw almonds

Juice of 1 lemon

1 clove garlic

1 teaspoon honey

1 tablespoon peeled and minced fresh ginger

¼ cup water

Pinch of sea salt

Pinch of cayenne pepper

Combine all of the ingredients in a blender and blend until a hummus-type consistency is reached.

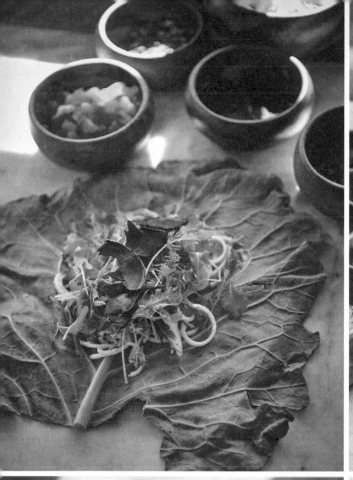

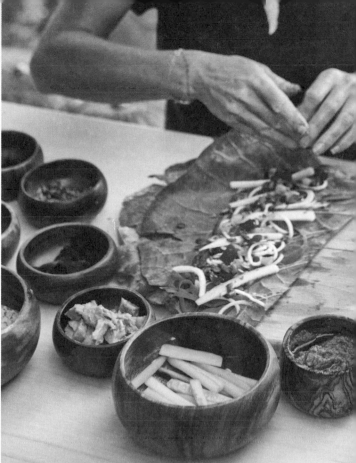

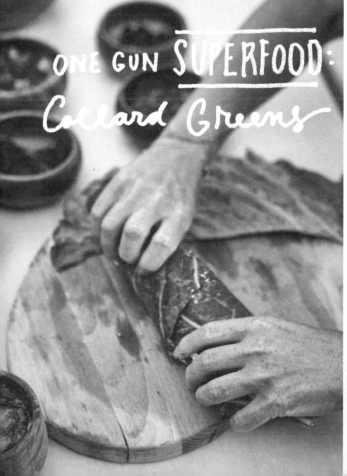

ONE GUN SUPERFOOD:
Collard Greens

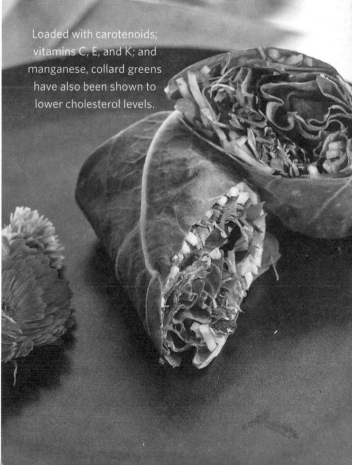

Loaded with carotenoids; vitamins C, E, and K; and manganese, collard greens have also been shown to lower cholesterol levels.

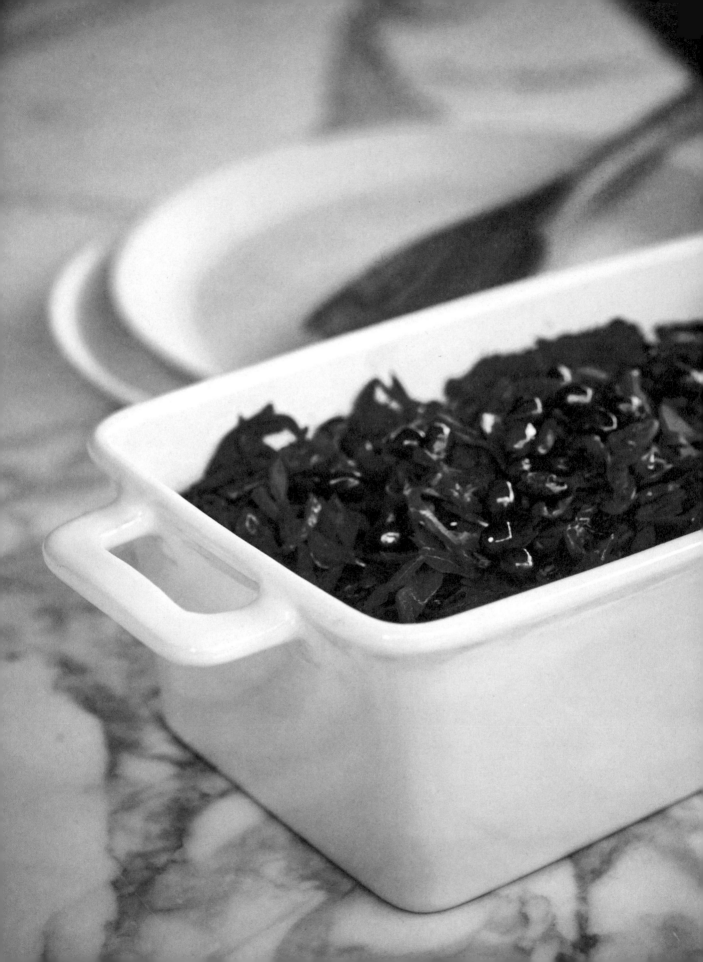

SPICED
PURPLE CABBAGE
WITH POMEGRANATE

Serves 6

We find this is a perfect side dish for the holidays, especially on Thanksgiving, when pomegranates are in season. The recipe is a healthy play on the traditional red cabbage dish that I grew up with, but with the added bite of pomegranate seeds, which glisten like little jewels in amongst the steaming cabbage.

- 1 medium head red cabbage
- 1 red onion
- 1 apple (any type of apple is fine; we like to use Braeburn)
- 2 teaspoons coconut oil
- 2 tablespoons maple syrup
- 2 tablespoons red wine vinegar
- 3 cups unsweetened pomegranate juice
- Pinch of ground cinnamon or allspice (optional)
- Seeds from ¼ pomegranate

Halve and quarter the red cabbage, then finely slice. Peel and finely slice the onion and the apple.

In a large sauté pan over medium-high heat, melt the coconut oil. Add the onion and cook, stirring, until it softens, about 5 minutes. Add the apple and cook until it has softened, about 5 minutes, making sure to scrape the bottom of the pan and not let the onion or apple burn. Slowly add the sliced cabbage, stirring after each addition. Allow it to cook down, making room for the next addition, before you add another handful. It may seem like there is too much, but it will all fit once everything wilts down!

Finally, add the maple syrup, vinegar, and pomegranate juice and give it a good stir.

Let everything come to a bubble, then turn the heat to low and put a lid on. Stir occasionally and cook gently on a very low heat for 2 to 3 hours.

Taste for seasoning; if it's a bit bland, add a pinch of cinnamon or allspice. Carefully spoon into a serving dish, garnish with the pomegranate seeds, and serve.

HEALTHY SLAW

Serves 6 to 8

A cleaned-up, guilt-free version of my favorite side! We've swapped out the mayonnaise for a tangy, pineapple-spiked dressing that lightens and brightens the dish. This is meant to be a versatile recipe to embrace what's ready to pick in the garden or is in season at the farmers' market, and we've found Chinese cabbage, Jicama, or broccoli are all great additions. I always like to include cabbage, available year round for a traditional taste and great crunch.

FOR THE DRESSING:

½ cup fresh pineapple juice, plus more if needed

¼ cup white wine vinegar

1 tablespoon fresh lime juice

½ cup raw almonds

1 tablespoon peeled and grated fresh ginger

½ teaspoon cayenne pepper

FOR THE SLAW:

½ medium green cabbage, grated

½ red cabbage, grated

2 large carrots, peeled and grated

1 small rutabaga, peeled and grated (optional)

¼ cup minced fresh parsley or cilantro

To make the dressing: In a blender, combine the pineapple juice, vinegar, lime juice, almonds, ginger, and cayenne and blend until super-smooth and creamy. Add more pineapple juice, if it seems too thick.

To make the slaw: In a large bowl, toss together the cabbages, carrots, and rutabaga, if using.

Pour the dressing over the vegetables and toss to mix thoroughly.

Serve with a sprinkle of parsley or cilantro.

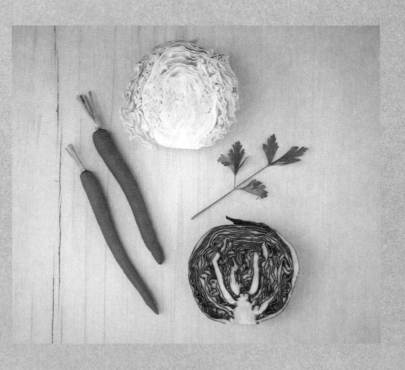

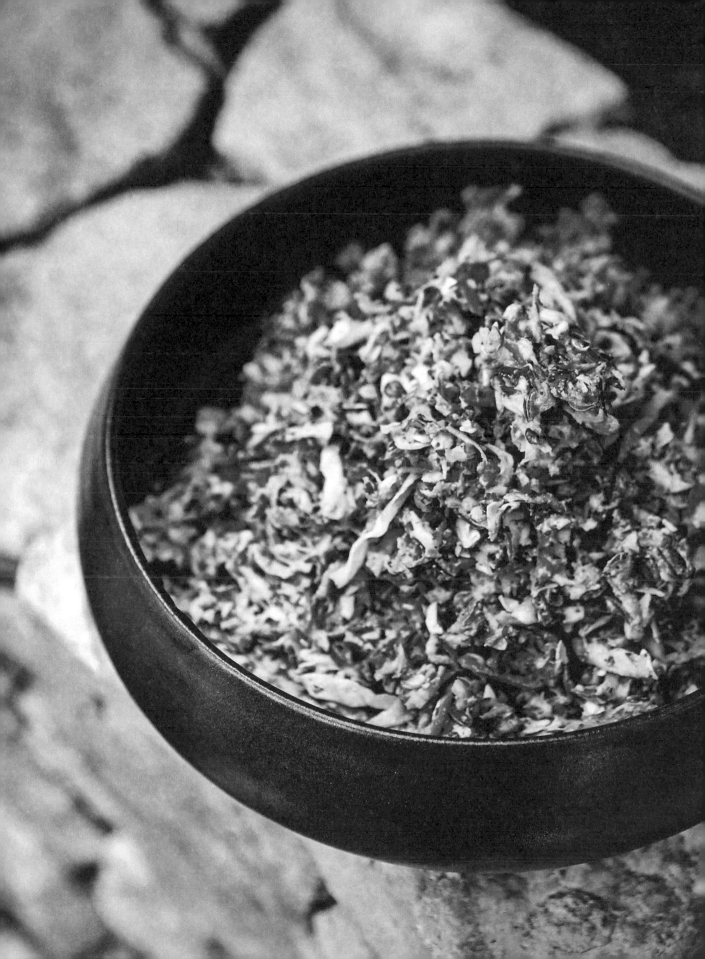

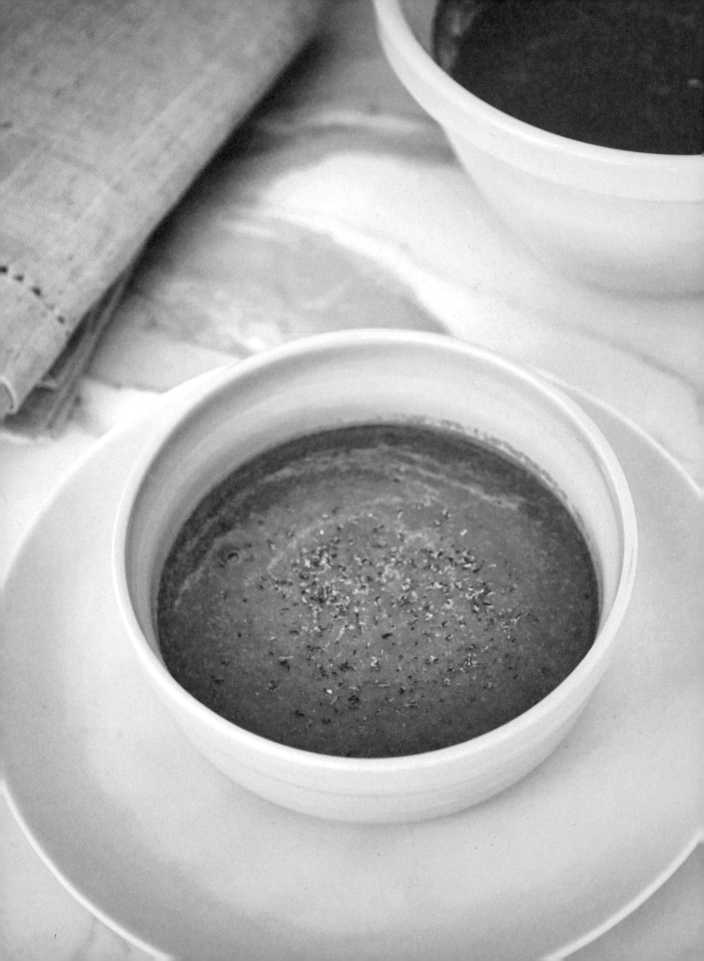

SPINACH & NUTMEG SOUP

Serves 4

Popeye sold me on spinach as a small child and I've adored it ever since. Such a divinely colored jewel green soup, the nutmeg completes it by adding some warmth and exoticism to what could otherwise be bland. We love growing New Zealand spinach at the Ranch, as it fares better in the hot California sun and its succulent leaves work well in soups.

1 tablespoon olive oil

1 white or yellow onion, finely chopped

1 quart chicken stock or vegetable stock

1 pound spinach

½ teaspoon freshly grated nutmeg or ground ginger, plus more for garnish

In a saucepan over medium-high heat, heat the olive oil. Add the onion and cook, stirring, until soft, 3 to 5 minutes.

Pour in the stock and bring to a simmer. Slowly add the spinach by the handful until all of it is wilted. Add the nutmeg or ginger and remove from the heat.

Let cool slightly, then transfer the soup to a blender, working in batches if necessary. Carefully (it's hot!) whizz the soup until smooth and creamy.

Ladle into bowls, sprinkle with a little more nutmeg or ginger, and serve hot.

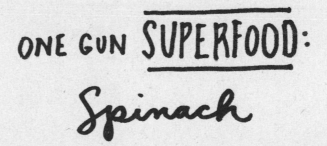

ONE GUN **SUPERFOOD:**

Spinach

Highly alkaline, spinach is high in antioxidants, vitamins C and K, and beta-carotene, and is also a great vegetarian source of iron.

ARUGULA,
FENNEL & ORANGE SALAD

Serves 4 to 6

This delightful summer salad perfectly balances peppery arugula with the sweet, aniseed flavor of fennel—and looks beautiful on the plate to boot. If I'm serving it to guests, I also like to add finely grated orange peel to garnish.

5 ounces baby arugula (if you are able to buy some stems with flowers attached at the farmers' market, reserve for garnish)

1 fennel bulb, cored and very thinly sliced or shaved on a mandoline; finely chop a few of the feathery fronds for garnish

1 orange, peeled and segmented

Juice of 1 orange

2 tablespoons Dijon Vinaigrette (page 294)

Put the arugula in a serving bowl or on a large platter. Arrange the shaved fennel and orange segments on top of the arugula.

In a small bowl, whisk together the orange juice and vinaigrette. Drizzle the orange vinaigrette over the salad. Garnish with the fennel fronds and arugula flowers, if you have them.

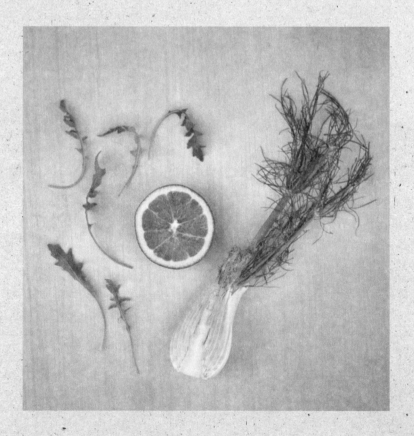

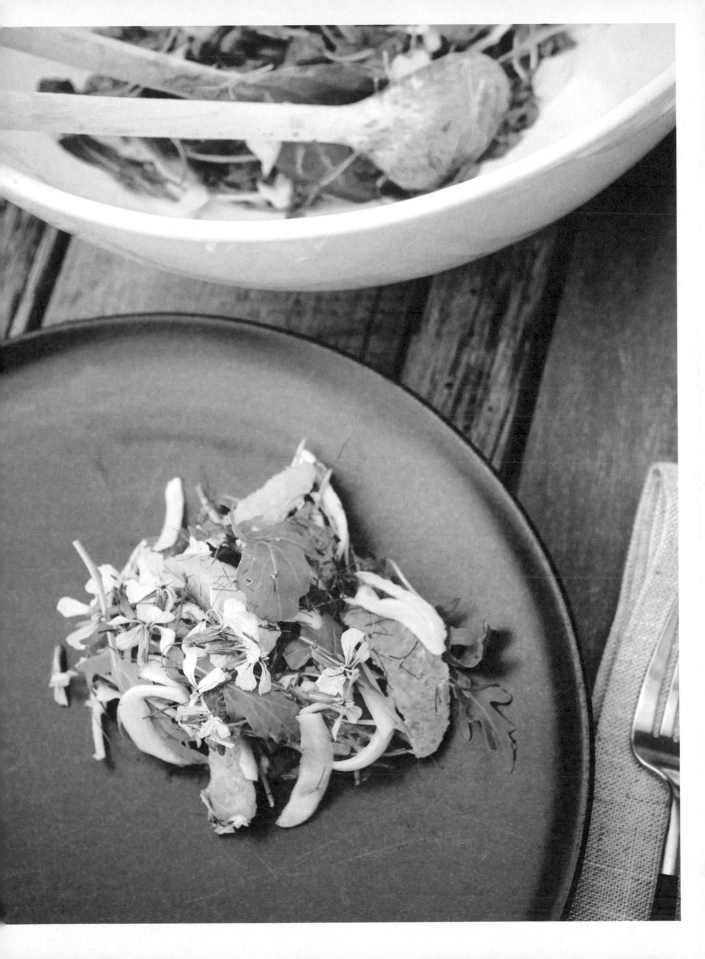

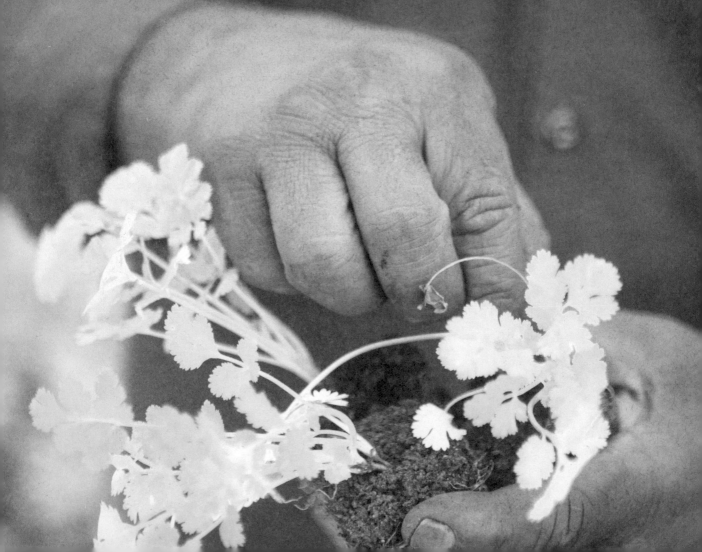

Flower Days

While edible flowers such as nasturtium, pea shoots, and borage and herbs such as chives, basil, and cilantro are undeniably delicious and add color and flavor to a dish, rest assured that broccoli, cauliflower, and artichokes are all examples of flowering vegetables that should be eaten on Flower Days. Feel free to add a dish from the protein recipes on a Flower Day or a grain like quinoa to round out the menu.

GRILLED
BROCCOLI
WITH JALAPEÑO

Serves 4 to 6

This Italian-influenced side dish can also be made with the more traditional red pepper flakes. Serve with Salt-Baked Fish (page 248) or Spaghetti Squash Arrabiata (page 193) for a little taste of the Mediterranean.

1 large head broccoli, cut into long, thin spears

2 tablespoons olive oil

2 teaspoons balsamic vinegar

2 teaspoons Meyer lemon juice, plus zest for garnish

2 jalapeño chiles, seeded and coarsely chopped

Build a hot fire in a charcoal grill or preheat a gas grill to high.

In a large bowl, toss the broccoli with the olive oil, vinegar, lemon juice, and jalapeños.

Arrange the broccoli on the grill rack and grill until tender-crisp and nicely grill-marked, about 5 minutes. Garnish with the lemon zest and serve immediately.

ONE GUN SUPERFOOD:

Jalapeño Chiles

Jalapeños are packed with vitamin C and antioxidants. Capsaicin—the compound that makes chiles spicy—acts as an anti-inflammatory and also kick-starts the metabolism.

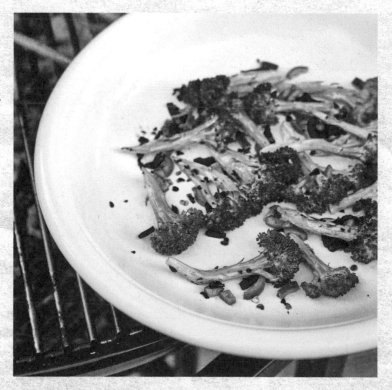

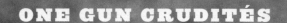

ONE GUN CRUDITÉS

WITH RAW-NASTURTIUM PESTO

Serves 4 to 6

For the crudités, use any vegetables that are ready to pick in the garden or are in season at the farmers' market. All you need to do is clean, peel, and slice them into sticks or bite-size pieces. In winter, we might serve a combination of deliciously crunchy carrots, radishes, cauliflower, and celery; in summer, cucumbers, tomatoes, and peppers fill the platter. Nasturtium grows wildly and abundantly at the Ranch. It's wonderfully peppery and, combined in a raw pesto with rich, sharp pecorino cheese, it lends a perfect zing to fresh, crunchy vegetables.

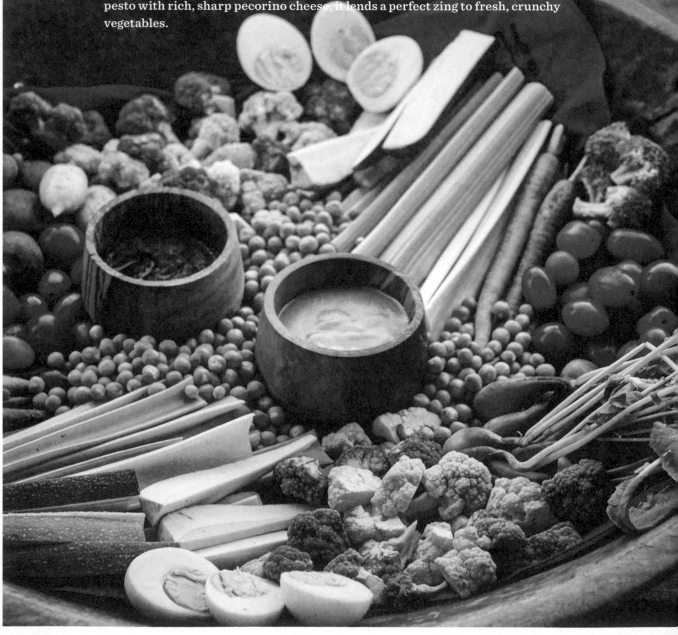

4 cups nasturtium leaves

2 cups nasturtium flowers

2 cloves garlic, roughly chopped

2 tablespoons raw pine nuts, walnuts, or almonds

1 cup freshly grated pecorino cheese

1 cup olive oil

A selection of raw vegetables (see recipe introduction)

Tear the leaves in half and put in a blender. Add the flowers, garlic, pine nuts, pecorino, and olive oil. Blend until smooth, scraping down the sides of the blender jar as needed.

Transfer to a small serving bowl and refrigerate until ready to serve with your crudités.

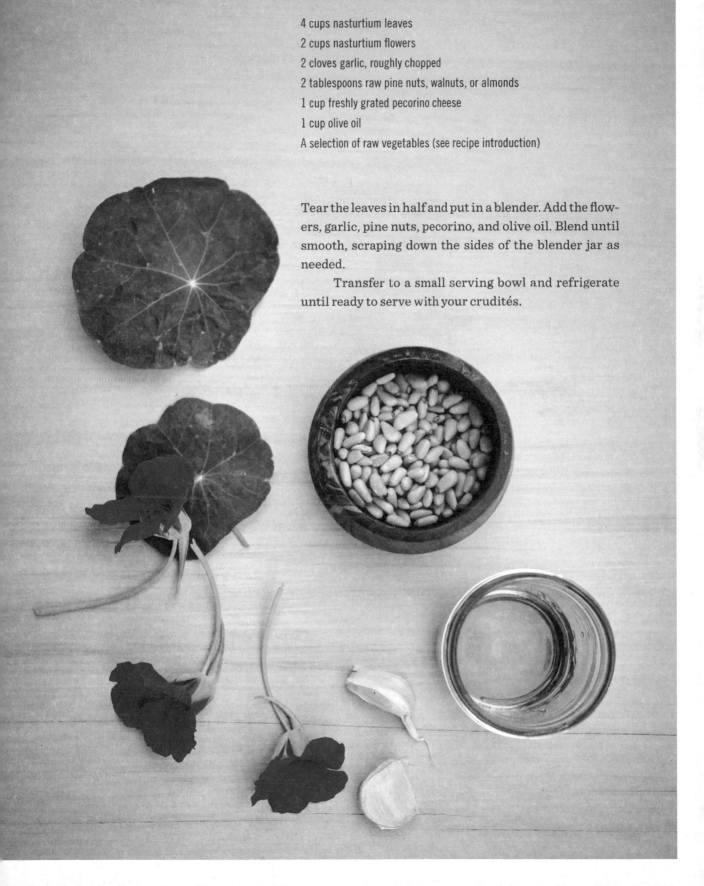

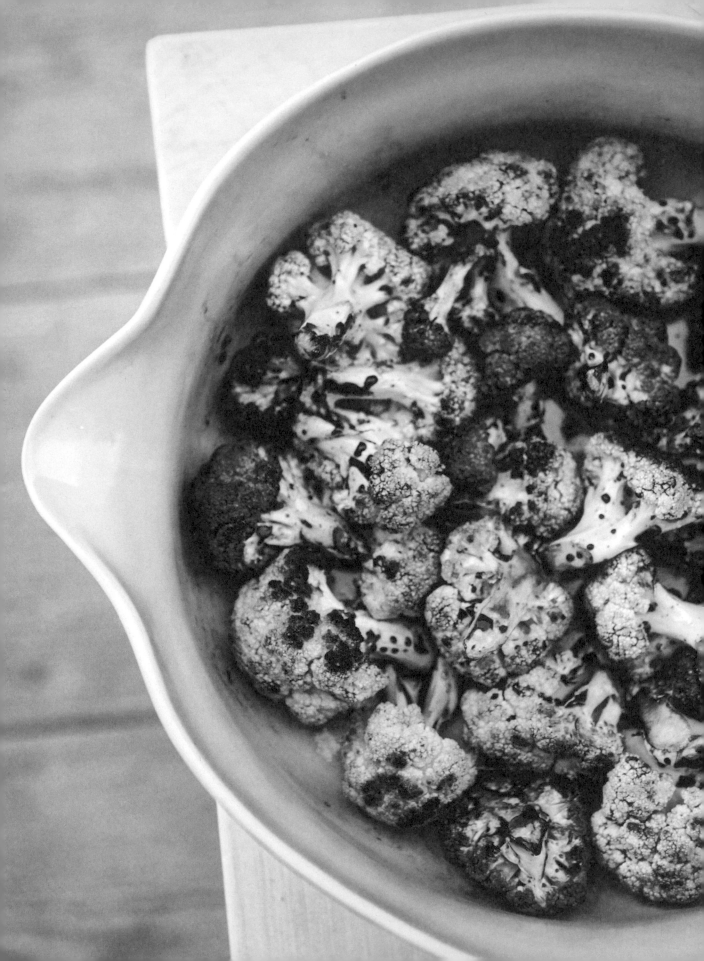

— GRILLED
THREE-COLOR CAULIFLOWER
WITH BALSAMIC

Serves 4

Purple, orange, white: We love cauliflower so much that we grow all of these types at One Gun Ranch. While all three have the same delicious, nutty flavor, the purple hue is a result of the naturally occurring antioxidant anthocyanin (which is also found in red cabbage and red wine), while the orange hue is a result of an excess of beta-carotene (which also gives this cauliflower 25 percent more vitamin A than the more common white variety). If you like, you can also use the green variety, sometimes called broccoflower or romanesco broccoli.

3 halves of different colored cauliflower heads (depending on the season, you'll see white, green, purple, and saffron colored heads at your farmers' market or green grocer), cored cut into large florets

2 tablespoons olive oil

2 tablespoons balsamic vinegar

Build a medium-hot fire in a charcoal grill or preheat a gas grill to medium-high.

In a large bowl, toss the cauliflower with the olive oil and vinegar.

Arrange the cauliflower on the grill rack and grill, turning as needed, until tender and a little charred, about 5 minutes total. Serve immediately.

ONE GUN SUPERFOOD:
Cauliflower

Cauliflower is rich with vitamins C, K, and choline (a B vitamin vital to brain development) and contains a wealth of anti-inflammatory nutrients. Cauliflower also contains a compound called sulforaphane, which has been shown in studies to protect against cancer.

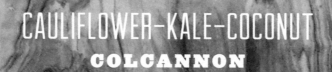

CAULIFLOWER-KALE-COCONUT
COLCANNON

Serves 4

A dairy-free version of a hearty Irish staple, this makes for a fantastic side dish for a hearty Sunday lunch.

2 cups chopped cauliflower

1 clove garlic, minced

1 tablespoon coconut oil

Pinch of sea salt

2 young kale leaves

Bring about ½ inch of water to a boil in a saucepan and fit a steamer basket into the pan. Add the cauliflower to the basket and steam until tender, about 8 minutes.

Let cool, then transfer the cauliflower to a blender. Add the garlic, coconut oil, and salt. Blend until creamy.

Tear the kale leaves into pieces and add to the blender for a quick whizz until it's chopped. Serve immediately.

MASHED
CAULIFLOWER & BROCCOLI

Serves 4

Classic nursery food, this comforting dish makes for a healthy, dairy-free alternative to mashed potatoes made with cream and butter.

1 head cauliflower, cored and cut into chunks

1 head, broccoli, trimmed and cut into chunks

3 tablespoons olive oil

Almond milk (optional)

Freshly ground black pepper

Bring about ½ inch of water to a boil in a saucepan and fit a steamer basket into the pan. Add the broccoli and cauliflower to the basket and steam until tender, about 8 minutes.

Let cool, then transfer the vegetables to a blender. Add the olive oil and blend to a coarse purée. If you're using almond milk, add a little at a time here, to taste. Season with black pepper.

Serve immediately.

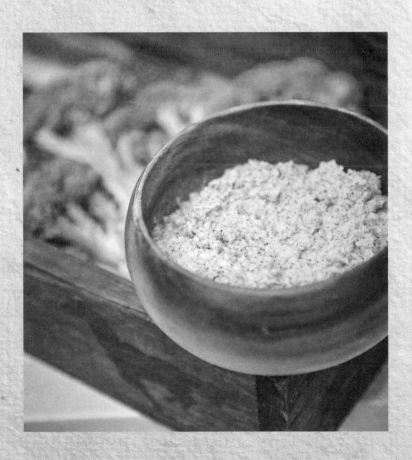

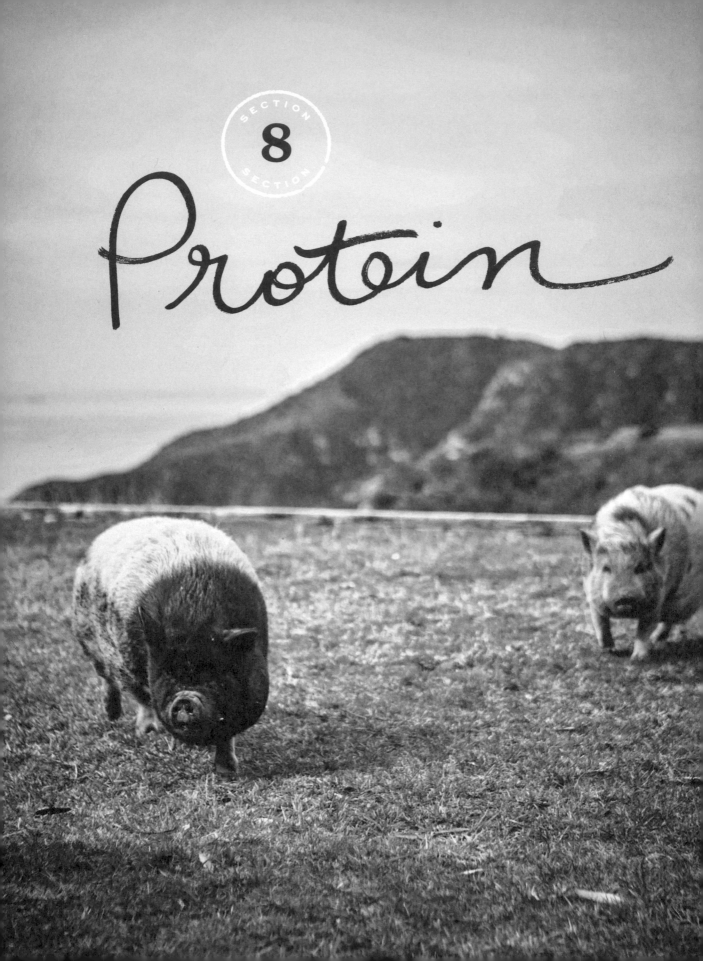

Protein

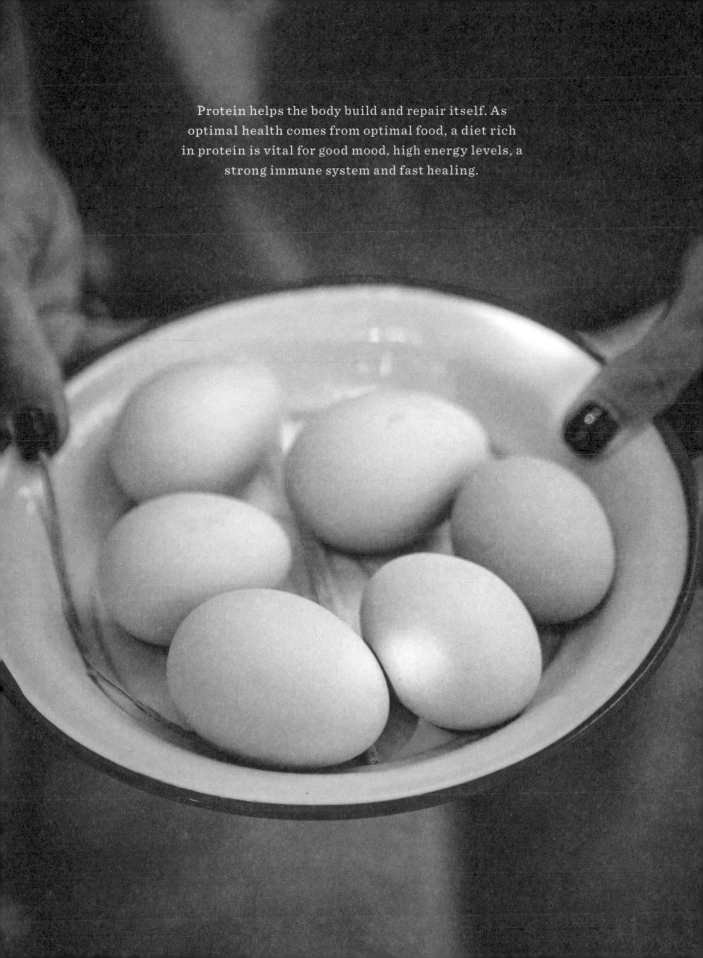

Protein helps the body build and repair itself. As optimal health comes from optimal food, a diet rich in protein is vital for good mood, high energy levels, a strong immune system and fast healing.

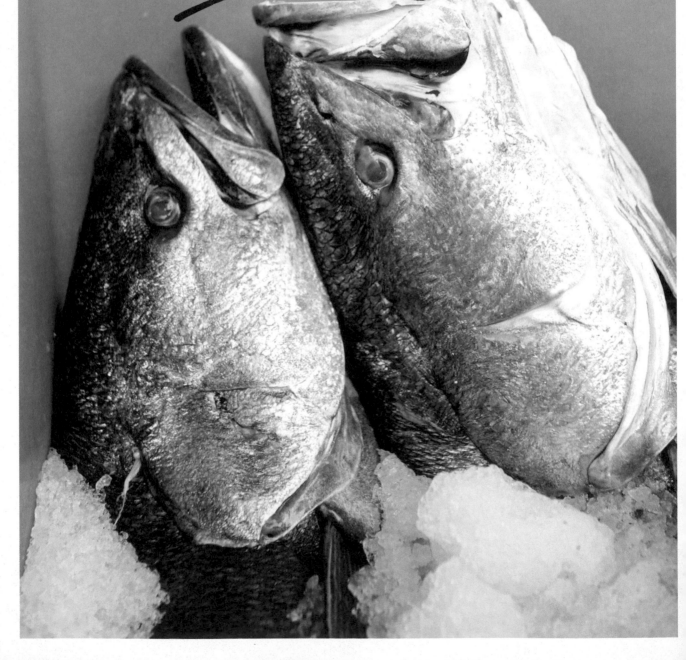

GRILLED
YELLOW TAIL
WITH PONZU

Serves 1 or 2

**I fell in love with this dish while in Japan. The collar is the most succulent part
of the fish and a real delicacy. When we are lucky enough to catch a yellowtail
off Malibu, this simple dish is a great way to make the most of every part of
the fish.**

1 tablespoon ponzu sauce

1 small jalapeño chile, finely diced

½ tablespoon peeled and finely
  diced fresh ginger

1 (6 to 8–ounce) yellowtail steak

Chopped fresh cilantro and lime
  wedges for serving

In a zippered plastic bag, combine the ponzu, jalapeño, and ginger. Add the yellowtail and seal tightly. Let marinate for 1 hour
in the refrigerator.

Build a medium-hot fire in a charcoal grill or preheat a gas
grill to medium-high.

Remove the fish from the marinade and place on the grill
rack. Grill, turning once, until crispy and charred on both sides,
about 5 minutes per side. Serve with the cilantro and a squeeze
of lime.

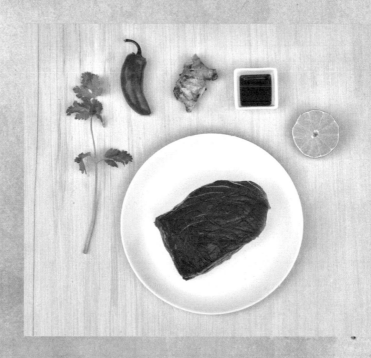

CIOPPINO

Serves 6

This is my biodynamic spin on cioppino, a delicious seafood stew packed with plenty of freshly picked One Gun Ranch herbs and greens and perfectly ripe heritage tomatoes, when in season. I love the history of this dish, which was conceived in the 1800s in San Francisco by Italian fishermen—they used leftover cuts from the catch of the day to make this rich stew, to be devoured with huge hunks of bread. I've found that the more diverse the mixture of fish, the better this dish works. It is wonderful the next day as a leftover; reheat gently and toss in some fresh greens or other vegetables and some fresh salmon, if needed.

¼ cup olive oil

1 white onion, chopped

2 cloves garlic

1 small jalapeño chile, chopped

2-inch piece fresh ginger, peeled and chopped (optional)

1 bunch fresh parsley, chopped, a handful reserved for garnish

2 (18-ounce) jars organic tomato passata (I like Yellow Barn biodynamic, but you can use any organic or biodynamic brand) or 1 (28-ounce) can organic chopped tomatoes

1 fennel bulb, cored and thinly sliced

1 quart chicken stock

6 leaves fresh basil

2 bay leaves

1 bunch fresh cilantro, chopped, a handful reserved for garnish

½ teaspoon dried thyme

½ teaspoon dried oregano

½ teaspoon red pepper flakes

USE A VARIETY OF ANY OF THESE FISH, AT LEAST 4:

1½ pounds Chilean sea bass

1½ pounds squid (optional)

16 mussels or clams, scrubbed

1½ pounds tilapia

1½ pounds shrimp, peeled and deveined

1½ pounds shucked sea scallops

1½ pounds salmon

2 handfuls curly or Tuscan kale leaves, roughly chopped

Sea salt and freshly ground black pepper

In a large pot over medium heat, heat the olive oil. Add onion, garlic, jalapeño, ginger (if using), and parsley. Cook, stirring, until the onion is soft, about 5 minutes. Add the tomatoes and fennel and stir to coat, then add the stock, basil, bay leaves, cilantro, thyme, oregano, and red pepper flakes. Stir to mix well.

Reduce the heat to medium-low and simmer gently for about 45 minutes.

Cut your fish and squid, if using, into approximately 2-inch cubes and set aside. First add any mussels or clams you're using to the pot. Next add any thicker fish like the sea bass, along with the kale. If using, add the squid. Stir constantly. Follow with softer fish like tiliapia and shrimp and/or scallops. If using salmon, add that last. Cook until all the seafood is just cooked through, about 6 minutes from the time the softer types went into the pot. Season with salt and pepper.

Using a large ladle, scoop into bowls. Garnish with cilantro and parsley and serve hot.

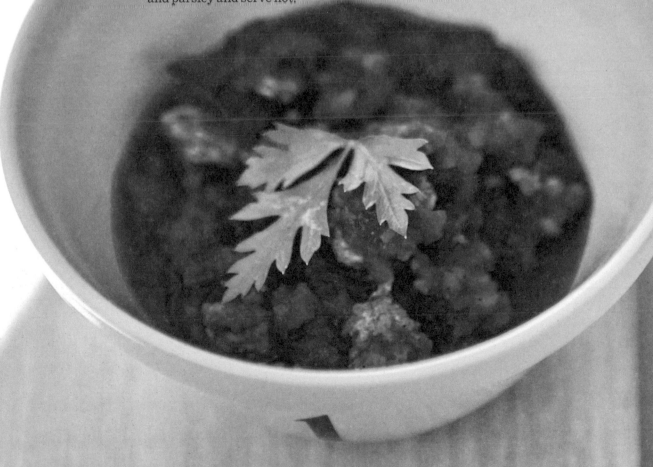

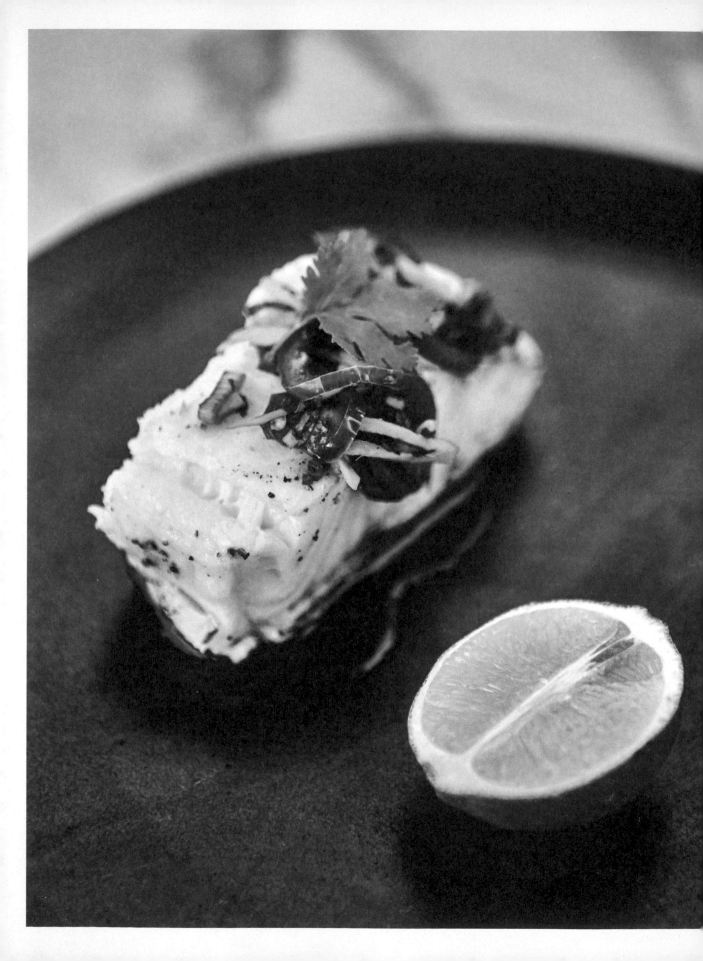

SPICY STEAMED
SEA BASS
WITH GINGER & CHILES

Serves 4

I discovered this dish in Thailand and have adapted it to make with our local fish. We are lucky enough to be able to catch white sea bass in the waters off Malibu, but sustainable Chilean sea bass is just as good. The steaming is most easily done in a stainless-steel fish-poaching pan with the tray propped over water that's seasoned with a few lemon halves.

1 pound sea bass fillets

Freshly ground black pepper

3 green onions, white and tender green parts only, thinly sliced

2 red or jalapeño chiles, thinly sliced, a few pinches reserved for garnish

1 clove garlic, minced

1 tablespoon peeled and grated fresh ginger

¼ cup tamari

¼ cup Chinese wine

1 tablespoon chopped fresh cilantro

Prepare a large steamer that will hold the fillets comfortably (see recipe introduction).

Season the fish with lots of pepper and let sit for 2 or 3 minutes.

In a bowl, combine the green onions, chiles, garlic, ginger, tamari, and wine and stir to mix well. Place the fish in the steamer and spoon the sauce all over it. Steam until cooked through, about 5 minutes.

Carefully remove the fillets from the steamer and transfer to a serving platter or individual plates. Sprinkle with the cilantro and reserved chile and serve immediately.

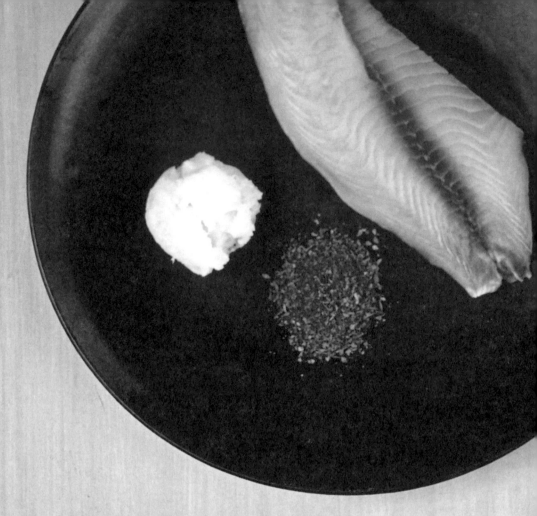

BLACKENED FISH

Serves 2

This is a dish that I grew up with at my family's house in Barbados, where it's eaten for breakfast, lunch, and dinner. It's a great, healthy way to get your daily protein.

2 (8-ounce) snapper or tilapia
   steaks

1 tablespoon blackening spice mix
   (or 1 teaspoon each paprika,
   dried thyme, cayenne pepper,
   ground black pepper, ground
   white pepper, and garlic powder,
   mixed well)

1 teaspoon coconut oil

Fresh lime wedges and hot sauce
   for serving

Thoroughly coat the fish steaks with the blackening spice. In a
large skillet over medium-high heat, melt the oil. When the oil
is hot, sear the fish, turning once, until cooked through, 3 or 4
minutes per side.

Serve with a squeeze of fresh lime and hot sauce.

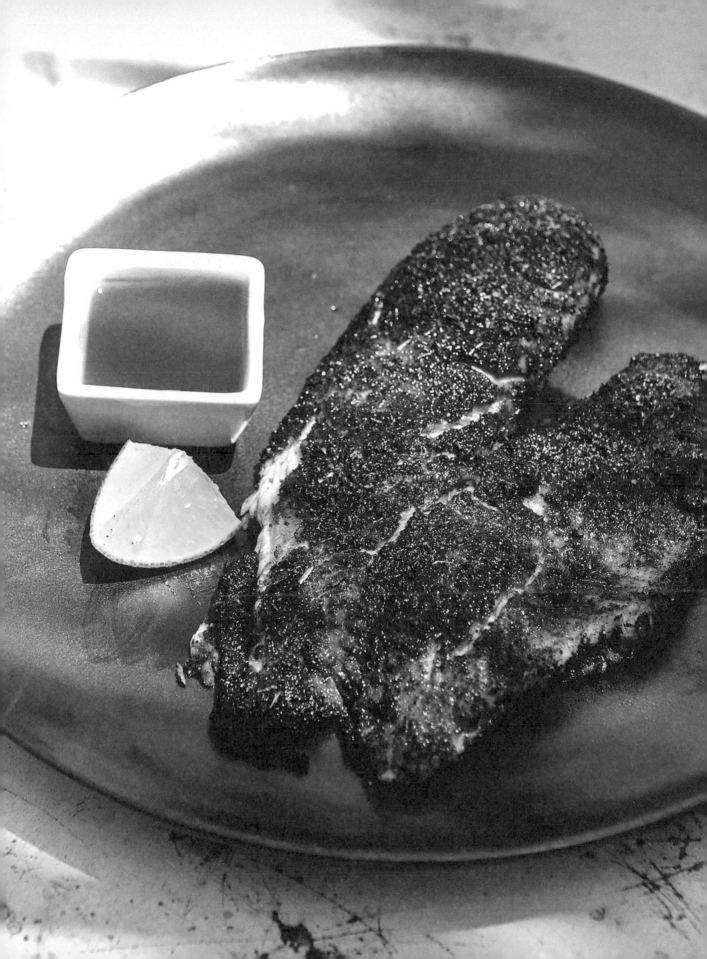

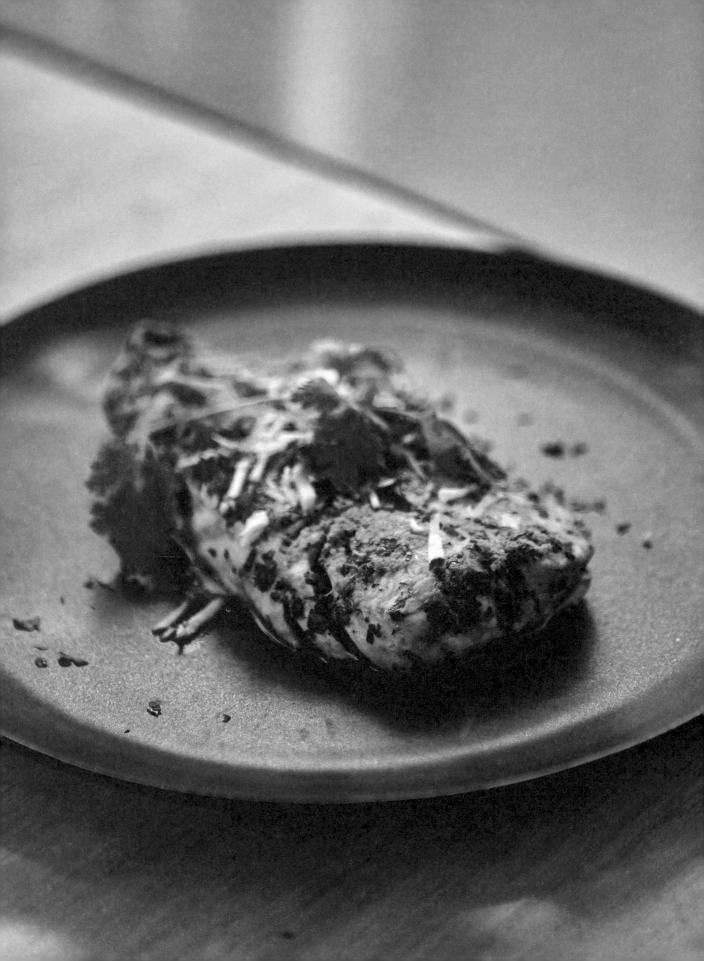

TURMERIC POACHED HALIBUT

Serves 2 to 4

I love turmeric: the taste, the color, and its anti-inflammatory and antioxidant properties. Therefore, I try to include it in as many dishes as I can. California halibut is a delicious, delicate white fish that is plentiful in the waters off of Malibu in the late spring. Unlike Atlantic halibut, Pacific halibut has the best eco-rating from the EDF Seafood Selector, so make sure that's what you are buying.

1 tablespoon peeled and grated fresh turmeric

1 tablespoon peeled and grated fresh ginger, plus extra, thinly sliced, for garnish

1 clove garlic

1 tablespoon tamari

2 tablespoons olive oil

Juice of 1 lime

1 bunch fresh cilantro, finely chopped, a few big pinches reserved for garnish

2 (6– to 8–ounce) halibut fillets

Prepare a large steamer that will hold the fillets comfortably.

In a mortar using a pestle, combine the turmeric, grated ginger, garlic, tamari, olive oil, and lime juice. Combine and crush it until a smooth paste forms. Stir in the cilantro.

Spread the herb paste over the fish fillets, coating them well. Wrap each fillet individually in parchment paper, folding the edges to seal well.

Arrange the packets in the steamer and steam for 8 to 10 minutes, or until cooked through (use the tip of a knife to lift a corner of one packet to peek). Serve immediately, opening the packets at the table and garnishing with the sliced ginger and reserved cilantro.

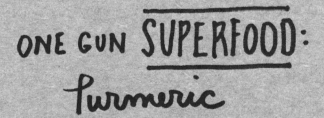

ONE GUN SUPERFOOD: Turmeric

High in curcumin, which has been shown to have anticancer effects, turmeric is also an anti-inflammatory and great for liver function.

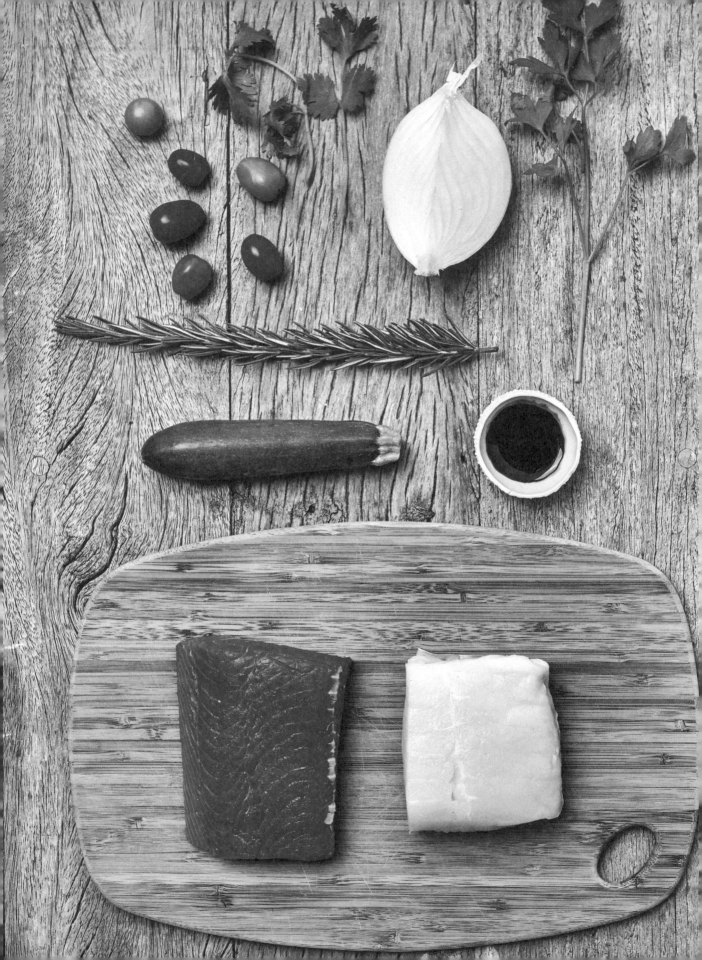

BARBECUED
FISH KEBABS

Serves 4

A Fourth of July barbecue favorite, this is a super-versatile dish, as you can use whatever the best, sustainable catch is from your fishmonger. (My only caveat is that I prefer not to mix freshwater and saltwater fish.) Perfectly sweet summer cherry tomatoes and lots of fresh One Gun Ranch herbs make this a flavorful, healthy dish. A splash of balsamic vinegar also works wonderfully to bring out the richness of the fish.

½ pound salmon

½ pound halibut

Leaves from 1 sprig fresh rosemary, finely chopped

Leaves from 1 sprig fresh parsley, finely chopped

Sea salt and freshly ground black pepper

1 white or yellow onion

1 zucchini

½ cup cherry tomatoes

Olive oil for brushing

Build a hot fire in a charcoal grill or preheat a gas grill to high.

Cut the fish into 1-inch cubes and transfer to a bowl. Add the rosemary, parsley, and salt and pepper to taste to the bowl with the fish and stir to coat.

Cut the onion and zucchini into 1-inch cubes.

Thread the fish, onion, zucchini, and cherry tomatoes on the skewers, alternating fish and vegetables. Brush with the olive oil. Arrange the skewers on the grill rack and grill, turning as needed, until the vegetables are tender and nicely grill-marked and the fish is cooked through, about 10 minutes total.

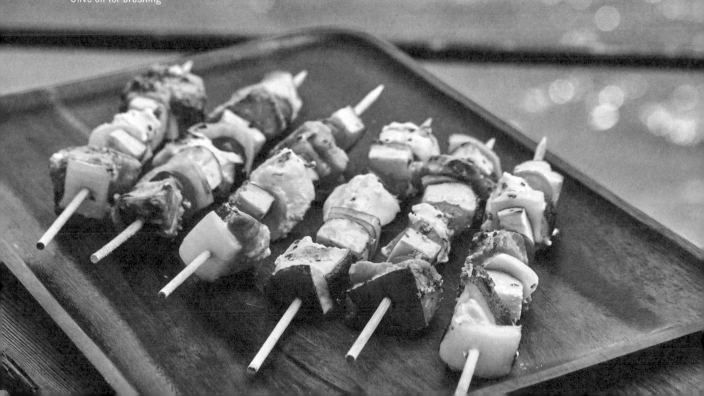

SALT-BAKED FISH

Serves 4

For me, this dish is the epitome of a Mediterranean summer meal. A simple showpiece of a dish, the theatrics of cracking the salt open to reveal the most perfectly cooked, juicy fish is always a crowd-pleaser. When buying fish, go to a reputable fishmonger who knows what has been responsibly caught. Sablefish, also known as black cod, or barramundi are good options here.

1 (2-pound) whole white fish

1 Meyer lemon, thinly sliced

10 fresh herb sprigs such as rosemary, thyme, fennel, marjoram, parsley, or tarragon, or a mixture

Olive oil for brushing

6 to 8 cups sea salt

2 or 3 large organic free-range egg whites

Extra-virgin olive oil, lemon juice and lemon slices for serving

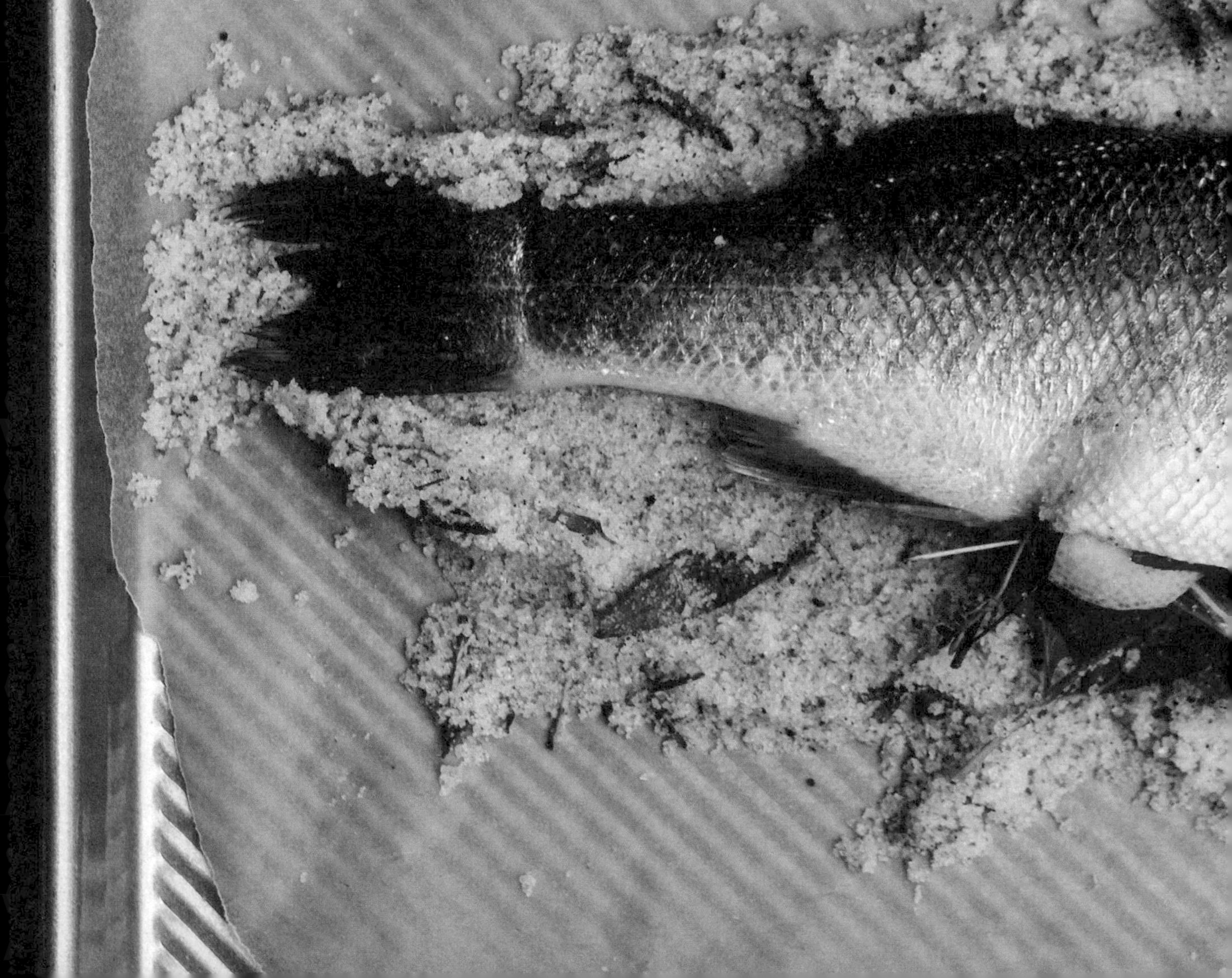

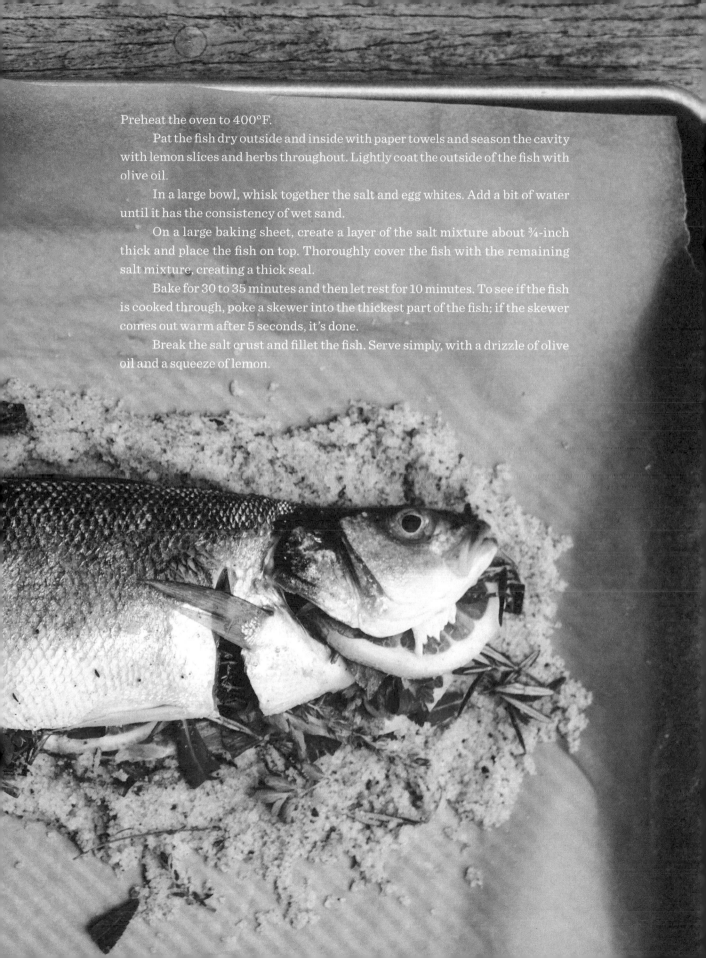

Preheat the oven to 400°F.

Pat the fish dry outside and inside with paper towels and season the cavity with lemon slices and herbs throughout. Lightly coat the outside of the fish with olive oil.

In a large bowl, whisk together the salt and egg whites. Add a bit of water until it has the consistency of wet sand.

On a large baking sheet, create a layer of the salt mixture about ¾-inch thick and place the fish on top. Thoroughly cover the fish with the remaining salt mixture, creating a thick seal.

Bake for 30 to 35 minutes and then let rest for 10 minutes. To see if the fish is cooked through, poke a skewer into the thickest part of the fish; if the skewer comes out warm after 5 seconds, it's done.

Break the salt crust and fillet the fish. Serve simply, with a drizzle of olive oil and a squeeze of lemon.

FLATTENED
SWORDFISH STEAK
WITH PEPPERCORNS

Serves 2

This swordfish with pink peppercorns makes quite a presentation, brilliantly flavored to melt in the mouth and beautiful to look at. We enjoy this served with an arugula salad dressed with a lemon vinaigrette. Look for US Atlantic swordfish when shopping for this dish.

2 (8–ounce) swordfish steaks

Olive oil or melted coconut oil for drizzling, plus 1 tablespoon

Juice of 1 Meyer lemon, plus finely grated zest for garnish

1 tablespoon pink peppercorns, dried or toasted, plus more for garnish

One at a time, place the swordfish steaks between two large pieces of plastic wrap. Using the flat side of a meat pounder, pound to a thickness of about ⅓ inch. Put the fish in a large shallow bowl or baking dish and drizzle liberally with olive or coconut oil to cover. Add the lemon juice and scatter the 1 tablespoon peppercorns on top.

In a sauté pan over medium-high heat, heat the tablespoon of olive oil. Add the fish and sear until lightly cooked, 4 or 5 minutes.

Transfer to plates and drizzle on a little more olive or coconut oil. Garnish with more peppercorns and the lemon zest and serve immediately.

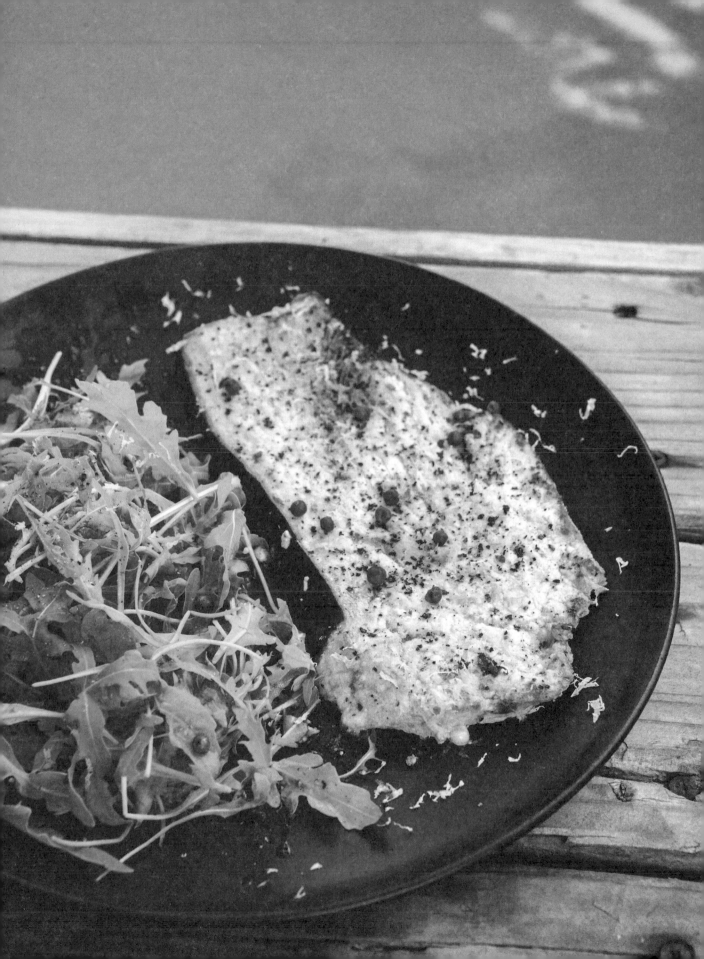

GRAPEFRUIT
SASHIMI

Serves 4

I discovered this dish in a Japanese restaurant in Palm Springs. It looks and tastes great, and the acids in the grapefruit quickly "cook" the fish like a light ceviche. If you have had a successful day of fishing, this is a perfect way to eat your catch; otherwise, when shopping look for fresh, sushi-grade fish that has not been previously frozen.

1 grapefruit, halved

1 pound super-fresh sushi-grade fish, preferably a mixture, such as salmon, bream, halibut, and/ or tuna, cut into 1-inch cubes

A few fresh shiso leaves, minced, for garnish

Segment the grapefruit flesh, reserving the grapefruit shells.

Squeeze the juice of half of the grapefruit segments into a small bowl and set aside. Cut the remaining segments into 1-inch cubes.

In a large bowl, combine the grapefruit cubes and fish cubes and gently toss together. Divide the mixture between the grapefruit shells.

Drizzle the reserved grapefruit juice over each half, garnish with the shiso, and serve.

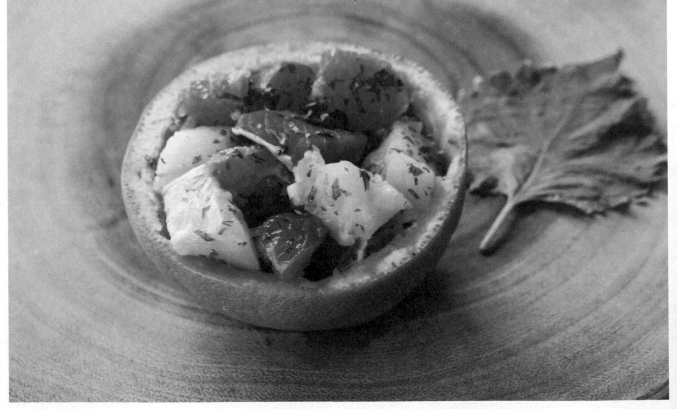

TUNA & WHITE BEAN
SALAD

Serves 4

This is one of my parents' favorite dishes and I have fond memories of eating this Italian-influenced salad on summer holidays. It's easy to throw together and packed with protein. I adore sage, so, for me, some freshly gathered One Gun Ranch sage is the finishing note here.

1 tablespoon olive oil if using oil-packed tuna, 2½ tablespoons if not

3 tablespoons fresh lemon juice

Freshly ground black pepper

2 (5-ounce) cans tuna (I prefer olive oil–packed but salt is fine)

2 (15-ounce) cans cannellini beans, rinsed and drained

½ small red onion, finely chopped

1 clove garlic, minced

2 tablespoons finely chopped fresh basil or sage

In a large bowl, whisk together the olive oil, lemon juice, and pepper to taste.

Add the tuna, beans, onion, garlic, and herbs and toss gently to mix well. Serve immediately.

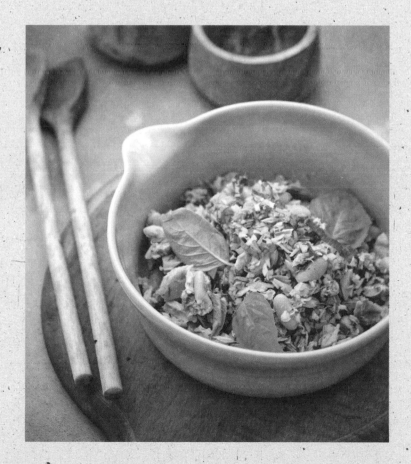

SESAME-CILANTRO
PRAWNS

Serves 4

I always make this dish for our beach barbecues. It's a serious favorite among friends. When buying prawns or shrimp, US-farmed shellfish produced under strict environmental laws are the most sustainable; wild shrimp from the Gulf of Mexico are another good option.

1 tablespoon sesame oil

1 small bunch fresh cilantro, chopped, a few big pinches reserved for garnish

1 tablespoon peeled and finely chopped fresh ginger

1 tablespoon tamari

Juice of 1 lime, plus wedges for garnish

About 12 large prawns (PC or SM Seafood), peeled and deveined

1 teaspoon coconut oil

In a bowl, combine the sesame oil, cilantro, ginger, tamari, and lime juice. Add the prawns and toss to thoroughly coat. Cover and put in the fridge to marinate for a few hours.

In a large skillet over medium-high heat, melt the coconut oil. When the oil is hot, add the prawns and cook until just opaque throughout and pink, about 2 minutes.

Alternatively, build a hot fire in a charcoal grill or preheat a gas grill to high. Arrange the prawns on the grill rack and grill until just opaque throughout and pink, about 2 minutes.

Serve immediately, with fresh chopped cilantro and a squeeze of lime.

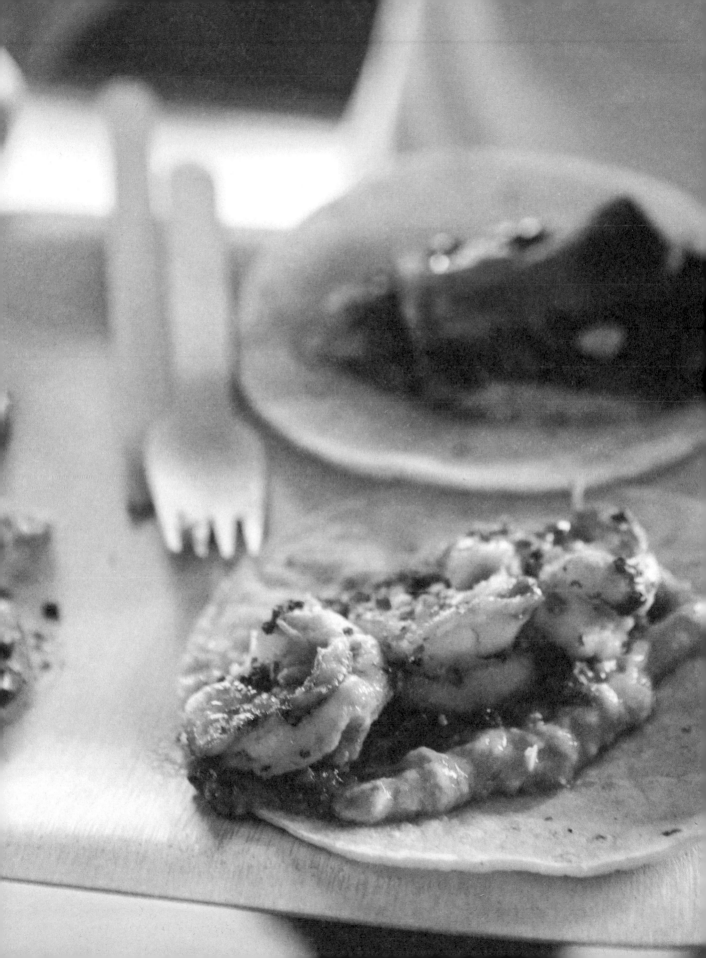

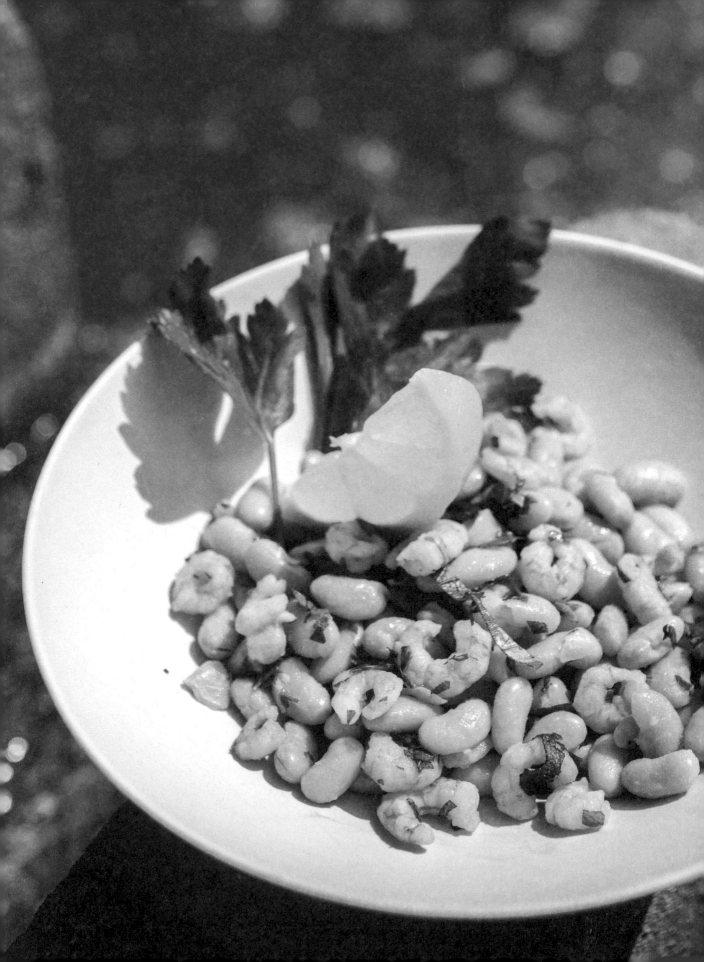

FRESH
SANTA BARBARA SHRIMP
WITH WHITE BEANS & SAGE

Serves 2

Wherever I am, I love to eat local, and sticking to local seafood is the best way to make sure it's fresh and sustainable. These delicious rock shrimp, which are native to the Santa Barbara Channel, are really sweet and tender in texture, so we take every opportunity to eat them when they are in season, November through spring. This is a dish that I adapted from the Ivy at the Shore restaurant in Santa Monica after a particularly happy lunch with my mama.

1½ pounds small Santa Barbara shrimp, peeled and deveined

3 tablespoons olive oil, plus more for drizzling

1 tablespoon fresh lemon juice

2 cloves garlic, minced

1 tablespoon chopped fresh parsley, plus more for garnish

1½ tablespoons chopped fresh sage

1 (15-ounce) can cannellini beans, rinsed and drained

In a bowl, toss the shrimp with 1 tablespoon of the olive oil and the lemon juice and set aside.

In a large sauté pan over medium-high heat, heat 1 tablespoon of the olive oil. Add the garlic and cook until it begins to brown, 1 or 2 minutes. Add the shrimp and sear in the pan with the browned garlic until just opaque throughout and pink, about 2 minutes.

Transfer to a bowl or plate and toss with the lemon juice, parsley, and half of the sage.

In a small saucepan over medium-high heat, warm the beans with enough water to cover them, the remaining 1 tablespoon olive oil, and the remaining sage. Bring to a simmer and cook gently until heated through, about 3 minutes.

Divide the beans between 2 plates, drizzling on some cold olive oil. Arrange the shrimp on top, dividing it evenly, and garnish with the parsley. Serve immediately.

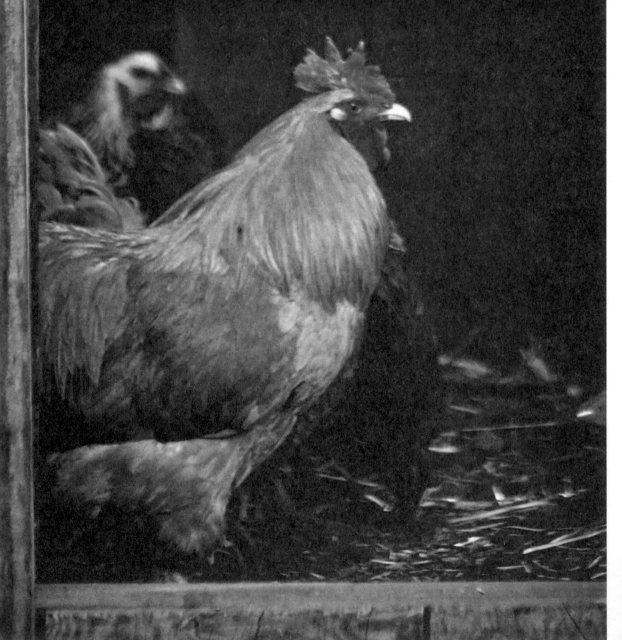

POULTRY

SIMPLE
CHICKEN STOCK

Makes about 6 cups; serves 4 to 6

Learning how to make your own chicken stock is so easy, and once mastered, this nourishing soup can be eaten on its own, used in place of oil to sauté vegetables, as a base for other soups, or in place of water to add a richness to quinoa or rice. Above all, it is the absolute best cure for the flu, colds, and general aches and pains.

2 pounds organic chicken wings

1 white onion

1 clove garlic

Pinch of sea salt

Dash of organic apple cider vinegar

Put the ingredients in a large stockpot or slow-cooker, together with enough cold, filtered water to cover by 1 inches. Bring to a gentle simmer, then reduce the heat to the lowest possible setting to maintain a very gentle simmer and cook for about 5 hours. You don't need to do anything more than languorously skim any rising scum off the surface when the mood takes you.

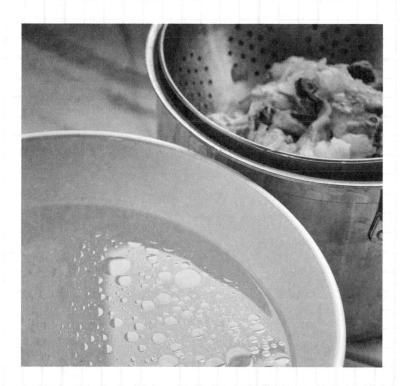

DOUBLE-COOKED
CHICKEN STOCK

Makes about 6 cups; serves 4 to 6

This is a more hearty, umami version of the Simple Chicken Stock (see previous page). The addition of the tamari and ginger lends the soup more richness and the chicken an amazing succulence that will elevate any number of dishes you choose to use this stock in.

1 quart Simple Chicken Stock (page 259) or other plain organic chicken stock

1 whole organic chicken

½ cup tamari

3 tablespoons apple cider vinegar

1 bunch green onions (it makes life easier to tie these together with kitchen string)

Thumb-sized piece fresh ginger, sliced (don't bother to peel it for this recipe, life is too short)

Put all of the ingredients in a large stockpot. Top with water as needed to cover the chicken and then bring to a gentle simmer and cook for 15 minutes. Skim the surface of any rising scum.

One traditional way to make an especially silky stock is to turn off the heat, cover your pot tightly, and leave overnight—your unheated oven is a good place. The residual heat will cook the chicken through, as long as you definitely brought the chicken up to a simmer for 15 minutes first. The chicken cooks slowly, and the proteins don't tighten with shock. The tamari and ginger make the chicken gently fragrant.

Alternatively, bring your stock to a gentle simmer, very slowly—not a rolling boil—and let the chicken poach for about 45 minutes. Don't let it overcook, and definitely let it cool in its poaching liquid. This will give you a succulent, umami-rich chicken with an utterly delicious broth.

Save the cooled chicken for a salad and shredded chicken tacos (see pages 262 and 263) the following day.

ASIAN
CHICKEN SOUP

Serves 4 to 6

You'll note that this recipe has no set amounts for ingredients. This is by design, as it's a whatever-you-have-on-hand kind of a recipe. Asian vegetables could include pak choy, Chinese cabbage, eggplant, and mushrooms.

Double-Cooked Chicken Stock (opposite page)

Peeled and grated fresh ginger

Thinly sliced jalapeño chiles or red pepper flakes

Grated carrots, diced onion, bean sprouts, and your choice of Asian vegetables

Cooked chicken (optional)

Seasonal herbs to flavor and garnish

Warm the chicken stock in a big soup pot over medium heat. Add the ginger and jalapeño or red pepper flakes to taste. Pile in the carrots, onion, bean sprouts, and any other Asian vegetables you like. Shred any leftover cooked chicken you have on hand (or make some fresh just for this soup) and throw it in the pot. Cook gently until the vegetables are tender and everything is warmed through.

Flavor and garnish with fresh herbs of your choice. Ladle into bowls and enjoy.

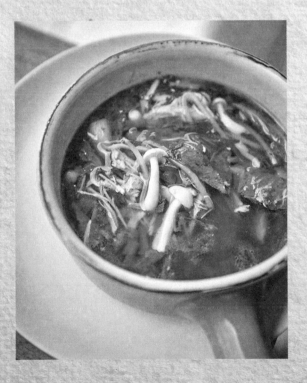

THAI
CHICKEN SALAD

Serves 4

This fresh and bright summer salad is a fun way to use large lettuce—varieties like romaine, leaf, and butter head varieties work best. A perfect lunch dish.

Juice of 1 Meyer lemon

2 teaspoons apple concentrate or 1 teaspoon honey

1 teaspoon tamari

2 cloves garlic, crushed

3 ripe tomatoes

2 stalks celery

1 white or yellow onion

4 green onions, white and tender green parts only, thinly sliced

1 bunch fresh cilantro, roughly chopped, a few big pinches reserved for garnish

1 jalapeño chile, seeded and finely sliced

1 pound organic boneless, skinless chicken breast, poached and shredded

8 large lettuce leaves

In a small bowl, whisk together the lemon juice, apple concentrate or honey, tamari, and crushed garlic. Set aside.

Halve the tomatoes and remove the seeds. Cut the tomatoes, celery, and white or yellow onion into matchsticks.

In a large bowl, combine the tomatoes, celery, onion, green onions, cilantro, jalapeño, and chicken. Drizzle in the tamari mixture and toss to coat and mix well. Serve the salad on lettuce garnished with cilantro.

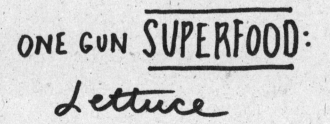

ONE GUN SUPERFOOD:

Lettuce

High in folic acid, vitamins A and K, and omega-3s, romaine and leaf lettuces are actually more nutrient-dense than kale.

SHREDDED
CHICKEN LETTUCE CUP TACOS

Serves 4

This is my homage to the cult Malibu taqueria Howdy's and Chef Benjamin. Now sadly closed, their delicious, healthy tacos and burritos were beloved by locals and fueled many a long day out on the water surfing or paddle boarding. I have swapped out tortillas for lettuce cups, but don't skimp on a good hot sauce and liberal squeezes of lime.

Large lettuce leaves

Leftover cooked chicken, shredded

1 bunch chopped fresh cilantro

Juice of 1 or 2 limes

Hot sauce

Make simple wraps by filling each lettuce leaf with shredded chicken and lots of chopped cilantro. Sprinkle with lime juice and hot sauce, roll up, and serve.

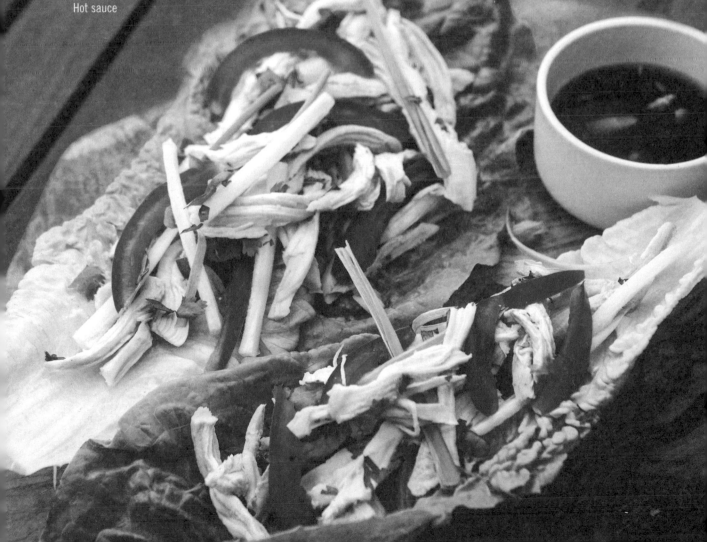

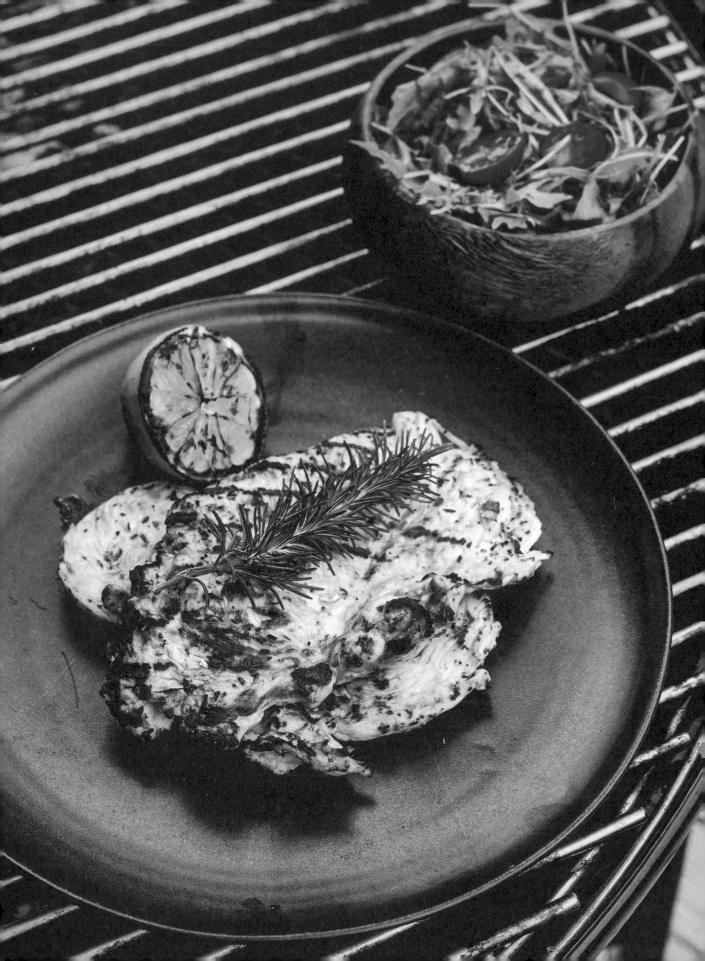

CHICKEN PAILLARD

WITH LEMON & HERBS

Serves 2

A classic French dish, *paillard* simply means the chicken has been pounded flat and grilled. Clean and tasty, the one "must" when preparing this super-easy meal is to use good-quality organic free-range chicken. Serve with an arugula and tomato salad dressed with a simple vinaigrette.

2 (6-ounce) organic boneless, skinless chicken breasts

1 tablespoon olive oil

1½ teaspoons balsamic vinegar

Juice of ½ Meyer lemon

Leaves from 1 sprig fresh rosemary, finely chopped

One at a time, place the chicken breasts between two large pieces of plastic wrap. Using the flat side of a meat pounder, pound to a thickness of about a ½ inch.

In a large, shallow nonreactive bowl, whisk together the olive oil, vinegar, lemon juice, and rosemary. Add the chicken and turn to coat. Let marinate in the refrigerator for an hour or so.

Build a hot fire in a charcoal grill or preheat a gas grill to high.

Arrange the chicken on the rack and grill until golden brown, 2 to 3 minutes per side. Serve immediately.

TURKEY & SAGE
BURGERS

Makes 8; serves 4

No summer barbecue is complete without a great burger, so we devised this super-healthy, lean recipe and even swapped out the buns for lettuce cups. The addition of sage and jalapeño add a kick of flavor.

½ pound organic ground turkey

1 tablespoon olive oil

Leaves from 1 sprig fresh sage, finely chopped

1 jalapeño chile, finely chopped

8 medium or 16 small cup-shaped lettuce leaves

2 large pickles, sliced or chopped

Chopped onion for topping

Chopped mozzarella cheese for topping (optional)

Carrot-Beet Ketchup (page 298) for serving

Build a hot fire in a charcoal grill or preheat a gas grill to 400°F.

Put the ground turkey in a bowl and drizzle in the olive oil. Add the sage and jalapeño and mix with your hands just until well blended; do not overmix.

Divide the mixture into eight 2-inch patties. Arrange the patties on the grill rack and grill until nicely browned, about 5 minutes per side.

Tuck each pattie into a lettuce cup, either 1 leaf or 2 nested together, and top with the pickles and onions. Sprinkle with the mozzarella, if using. Serve immediately, with the Carrot-Beet Ketchup on the side.

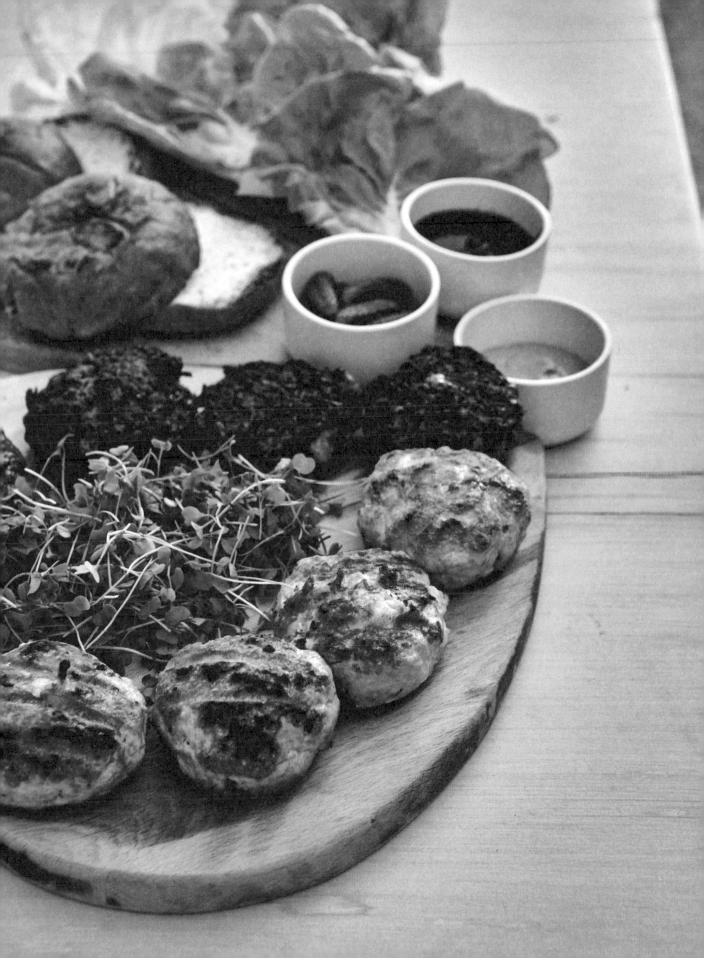

TURKEY GINGER
BROTH

Serves 6

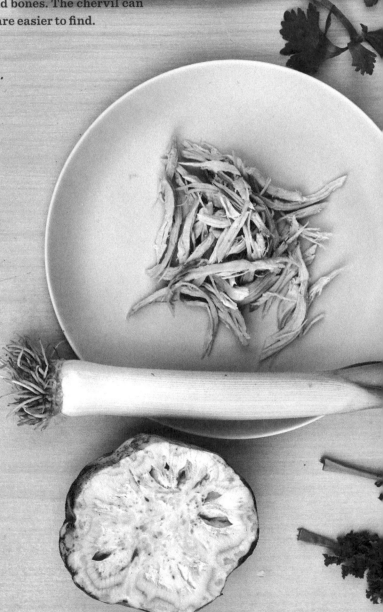

A Daylesford favorite, this hearty detox soup is the best way to use leftover Thanksgiving and Christmas turkey. Do make your own stock using the Simple Chicken Stock recipe (page 259), which can also be made using turkey wings and bones. The chervil can be replaced with fennel fronds, if those are easier to find.

2½ quarts good-quality chicken or turkey stock

1⅔ cups mixture of equal parts shredded red onion, carrots, cabbage, leeks, celery, and kale

1-inch piece fresh ginger, peeled and finely chopped

2 cups cooked organic turkey meat, shredded

Sea salt and freshly ground black pepper

3 tablespoons chopped fresh flat-leaf parsley

2 tablespoons chopped fresh chervil

In a large stockpot, bring the stock to a boil. Add the shredded vegetables and the ginger and simmer until all the vegetables are soft, about 5 minutes. Add the turkey and return to a boil, then remove from the heat.

Season with salt and pepper. Ladle into bowls, sprinkle with the parsley and chervil, and serve hot.

TURKEY CHILI

Serves 4

This warming, winter dish is a firm favorite at the Ranch. Organic turkey (a mix of white and dark meat makes for a better flavor) is low in fat and high in tryptophan, an amino acid that produces serotonin in the brain and is essential for healthy sleep.

1½ teaspoons coconut or olive oil

1 white onion, finely chopped

1 tablespoon minced garlic

1 jalapeño chile, finely chopped

1 pound organic ground turkey

2 cups water

1 (24-ounce) can crushed tomatoes

3 stalks celery, finely chopped

3 carrots, peeled and finely chopped

1 (15-ounce) can kidney beans (optional; I prefer it without!)

1 tablespoon chili powder

1 teaspoon ground cayenne pepper

½ teaspoon dried oregano

½ teaspoon ground cumin

½ teaspoon paprika

½ tablespoon freshly ground black pepper

Large pinch of sea salt

A few sprigs fresh parsley for garnish

In a large pot over medium-high heat, melt the coconut or olive oil. Add the onion, garlic, and jalapeño and cook until softened, 2 to 3 minutes. Add the turkey and cook until browned, using a wooden spoon to break up the meat, 5 to 7 minutes.

Add 2 cups water to the pot and stir in the tomatoes, celery, carrots, and kidney beans, if using. Add the chili powder, cayenne, oregano, cumin, paprika, black pepper, and salt and bring to a boil. Reduce the heat to maintain a gentle simmer and cook, stirring occasionally, for about 30 minutes.

Scoop into large individual bowls, garnish with small sprigs of parsley, and serve immediately.

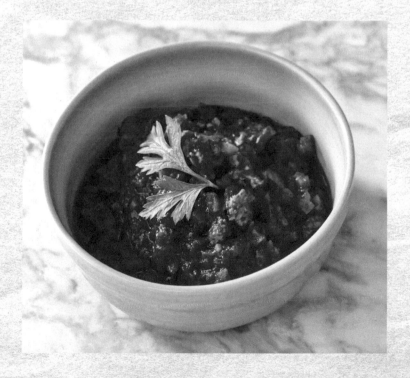

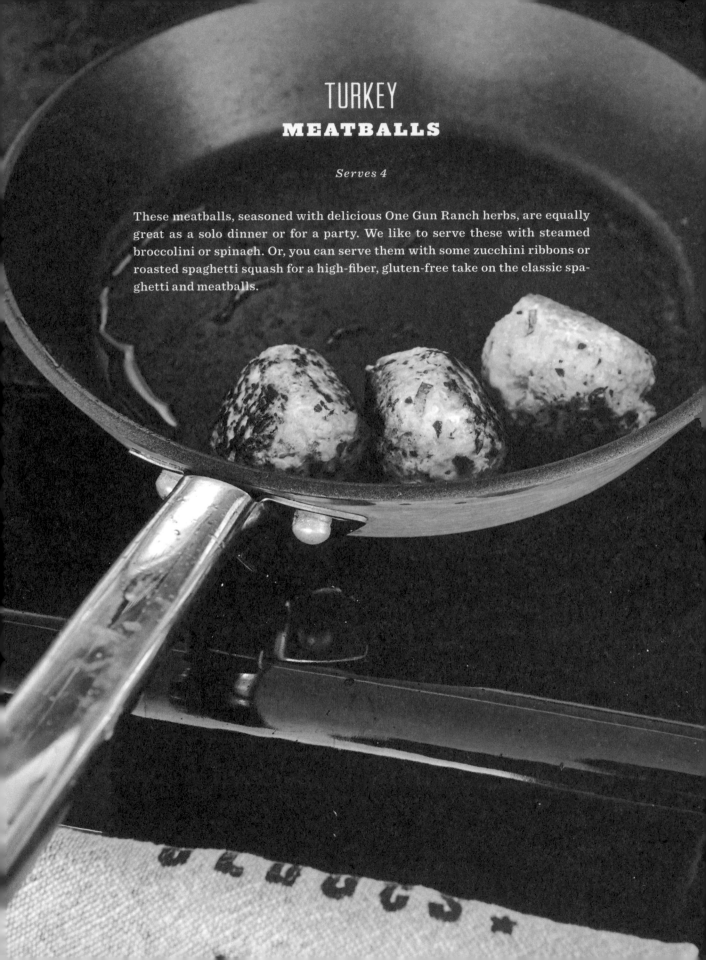

TURKEY
MEATBALLS

Serves 4

These meatballs, seasoned with delicious One Gun Ranch herbs, are equally great as a solo dinner or for a party. We like to serve these with steamed broccolini or spinach. Or, you can serve them with some zucchini ribbons or roasted spaghetti squash for a high-fiber, gluten-free take on the classic spaghetti and meatballs.

1 pound organic ground turkey

½ white onion, finely chopped

1 bunch fresh flat-leaf parsley,
  finely chopped

1 tablespoon finely chopped
  fresh rosemary

1 tablespoon finely chopped
  fresh sage

1½ teaspoons minced garlic

1 tablespoon olive oil

Arrabiata Sauce (page 193)

1 tablespoon chopped fresh basil

In a large bowl, combine the turkey, onion, parsley, rosemary, sage, and garlic. Using your hands, mix just until well blended; do not overmix. Roll the mixture into 1- to 2-inch-diameter meatballs.

In a sauté pan over medium-high heat, heat the olive oil. Arrange the meatballs in the pan ;and cook, turning as needed to brown on all sides, until the meatballs are cooked through, about 10 minutes.

Alternatively, preheat the oven to 300°F. Spread the meatballs on a baking sheet and bake until cooked through, 20 to 30 minutes.

Serve with the Arrabiata sauce, garnish with the basil.

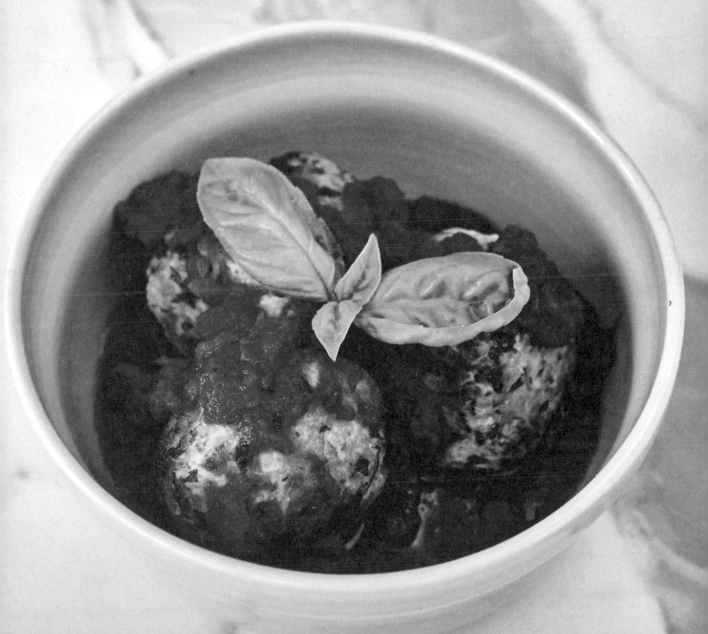

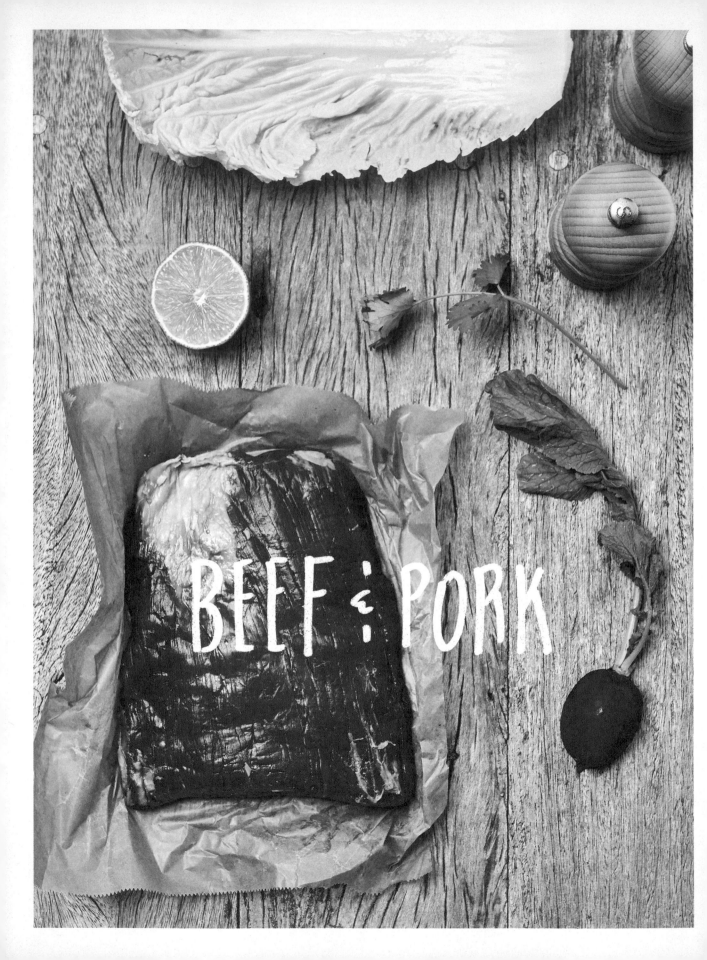

BEEF & PORK

BEEF
CONSOMMÉ
WITH GINGER

Serves 6

This classic-with-a-twist nourishing soup is one that we love to take in a thermos as sustenance during a hike along the mountain trails—just as much as we love to serve it as a first course at a dinner party. Ask your butcher for organic grass-fed beef and some nice bones when shopping for this recipe.

Note, you need to start this recipe at least a day in advance.

1½ pounds lean organic grass-fed beef stew meat, cubed

A few beef bones

1 white or yellow onion, halved

1 carrot, scrubbed and halved

1 leek, halved and rinsed

1 stalk celery, halved

3 sprigs fresh parsley

1 bay leaf

8 black peppercorns

½ pound organic grass-fed ground beef

Sea salt and freshly ground black pepper

1 tablespoon peeled and thinly sliced fresh ginger

6 green onions, white and tender green parts only, cut into slivers (reserve a few slivers for garnish)

The day before you are planning to serve, in a deep soup pot, combine the beef stew meat with the bones, onion, carrot, leek, celery, parsley, bay leaf, and peppercorns. Add cold water to cover and slowly bring to boil, skimming off any scum that rises to the surface frequently as the mixture nears boiling point. When the surface is clear, cover and simmer gently for 2½ to 3 hours.

Next, add the ground beef and a pinch of salt and pepper, return to a boil, and skim again. Reduce the heat to maintain a low simmer and cook for 20 minutes, then remove from the heat. Let cool slightly, then strain the stock into another pot or a large bowl and set aside to cool completely. Discard the solids. Cover the stock and chill overnight.

The next day, remove the fat from the surface and discard. Bring the stock to a boil and cook until reduced to 4 cups of well-flavored consommé, about 30 minutes.

Before serving, reheat the consommé to a boil, if necessary. When it comes to a boil, add the ginger and season with salt and pepper. Remove from the heat and leave covered for 5 minutes, then remove the ginger and add the green onions. Return to a boil, then remove from the heat again and let stand covered for another 5 minutes.

Ladle the consommé into bowls, garnish each with slivers of green onion, and serve hot.

CARNE ASADA

Serves 6

Try this Mexican party favorite that we've cleaned up and made super healthy. Look for organic grass-fed beef. The more time you have to marinate it, the better.

Juice of 3 limes

2 bunches fresh cilantro, chopped

Pinch of sea salt and freshly ground black pepper

1 pound organic, grass-fed skirt or flank steak

6 large or 12 smaller whole leaves of napa cabbage or sturdy lettuce

1 bunch radishes, trimmed and sliced

One Gun Salsa (page 293) for serving

Guacamole for serving

In a zippered plastic bag, combine the lime juice, cilantro, and salt and pepper. Add the steak, close tightly, and turn to coat. Let marinate in the refrigerate for at least 1 hour.

Build a hot fire in a charcoal grill or preheat a gas grill to high. Remove the steak from the marinade, place on the grill rack, and grill, turning once, until nicely grill-marked, 3 or 4 minutes per side for medium-rare. Transfer to a cutting board, cover lightly with aluminum foil, and let rest for 5 minutes.

Slice the steak thinly across grain on the diagonal. Divide into the cabbage or lettuce leaves and tuck some sliced radishes on top. Serve immediately with the salsa and guacamole.

ONE GUN SUPERFOOD: Cabbage

High in fiber, cabbage is also packed with vitamin C, antioxidants, calcium, and iron. It has also been shown to lower cholesterol levels.

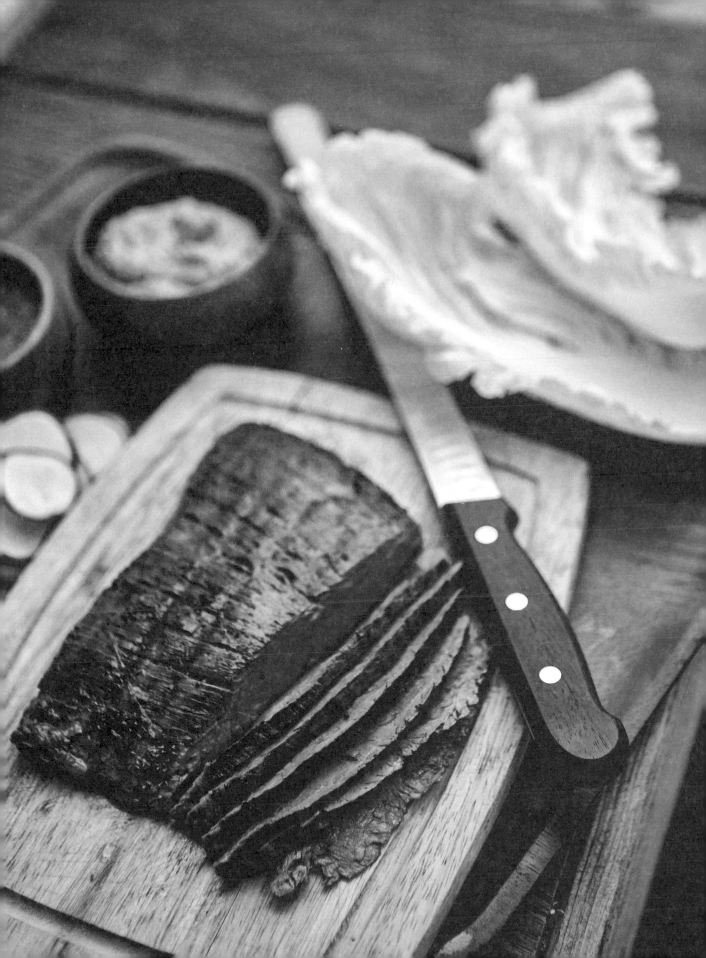

CORNED BEEF
HASH

Serves 1 or 2

For my brothers and me, this is remembered as a firm favorite of ours growing up. We always asked for it to be made on our birthdays. I have made a lighter version of this very hearty dish by using gluten-free flour and sweet potatoes. I love the crust that forms on the outside combined with the warm hash, topped with a fresh, golden One Gun egg. Perfect for St. Patrick's Day.

1 pound corned beef, chopped

½ pound potatoes or sweet potatoes, peeled and diced

1 medium white or yellow onion, diced

1 tablespoon Worcestershire sauce

Dash of Tabasco sauce, plus more for serving

½ jalapeño chile, diced

Freshly ground black pepper

1 tablespoon chopped fresh parsley

2 tablespoons all-purpose flour (plain or gluten-free)

2 tablespoons olive oil

1 large organic free-range egg, poached

Ketchup and hot sauce for serving

In a large bowl, combine the corned beef, potatoes, onion, Worcestershire, Tabasco, jalapeño, black pepper, parsley, and flour. Stir to blend well.

Heat the olive oil in a sauté pan over medium-low heat. Add the beef mixture to the pan and press into an even layer. Brown the hash on one side over a low heat, 2 to 3 minutes.

Carefully turn the hash out of the pan onto an oiled plate and then slide it back into the pan to brown the second side. Continue to turn from side to side, transferring from plate to pan, until cooked through, 5 minutes total.

Serve with a poached egg on top and ketchup and hot sauce on the side.

BEEF BURGERS

WITH JALAPEÑO & CILANTRO

Makes eight 2-inch burgers;
serves 4 to 8 depending on hunger levels!

For those who insist on their burgers being 100 percent beef, look for grass-fed organic meat, which is leaner than conventionally raised beef and contains more healthy omega-3 fatty acids.

1 teaspoon olive oil

½ pound organic, grass-fed ground beef

1 jalapeño chile, finely chopped

1 sprig fresh cilantro, chopped

8 medium or 16 small sturdy lettuce leaves, such as romaine

Freshly grated pecorino cheese (optional)

Carrot-Beet Ketchup (page 298)

Build a hot fire in a charcoal grill or preheat a gas grill to 400°F.

Put the olive oil in a bowl and add the ground beef, jalapeño, and cilantro and mix with your hands just until well blended; do not overmix.

Divide the mixture into eight 2-inch patties. Arrange the patties on the grill rack and grill until nicely browned, about 5 minutes per side.

Tuck each pattie into a lettuce cup, either 1 leaf or 2 nested together, and top with the pecorino, if using. Serve immediately, with the Carrot-Beet Ketchup on the side.

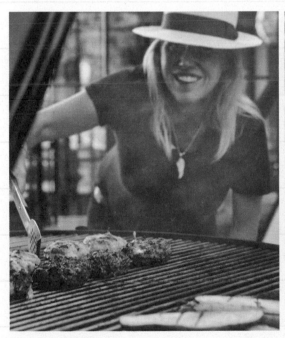
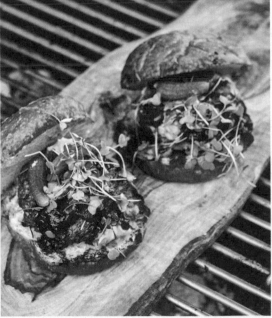

PROPER
ZUCCHINI BOLOGNESE

Serves 4

Here's another very healthy, gluten-free alternative to regular pasta, this time served with a hearty, no-holds-barred, meaty Bolognese sauce. You can substitute spaghetti squash for the zucchini, roasted and then shredded with a fork into "noodles." When buying the beef, look for organic grass-fed meat, as it is lower in saturated fat and higher in heart-healthy omega-3 fats. Grass-fed beef production is more biodynamic in its closed loop approach, wherein the grazing animals fertilize the pasture as they eat the grass. Studies have also shown increased biodiversity of pasture ecosystems and improved quality of run-off water in grass-fed beef production.

2 tablespoons olive oil

1 medium white or yellow onion, finely diced

2 cloves garlic, minced

2 small carrots, peeled and chopped

1 stalk celery, chopped

1 pound organic grass-fed ground beef

1 (28-ounce) can organic crushed tomatoes

⅓ cup red wine (optional)

1 tablespoon finely chopped fresh basil or 1 teaspoon dried basil

½ teaspoon finely chopped fresh thyme

Sea salt and freshly ground black pepper

4 to 6 medium zucchini

In a large saucepan over medium-high heat, heat 1 tablespoon of the oil. Add the onion, garlic, carrots, and celery and sauté until golden, 2 to 3 minutes. Add the ground beef and sauté until the beef is evenly browned, using a wooden spoon to break up the meat, about 5 minutes.

Add the tomatoes and wine, if using. Stir well and bring to a boil. Reduce the heat to low and let simmer for 45 minutes, stirring occasionally. Add the herbs and season with salt and pepper.

Meanwhile, using a vegetable peeler or a spiralizer, shave the zucchini very thinly into long ribbons. In a skillet over medium high heat, heat the remaining 1 tablespoon olive oil and the zucchini pasta and cook until soft, about 5 to 10 minutes.

Divide the zucchini pasta among 4 plates and liberally cover with the bolognese. Serve immediately.

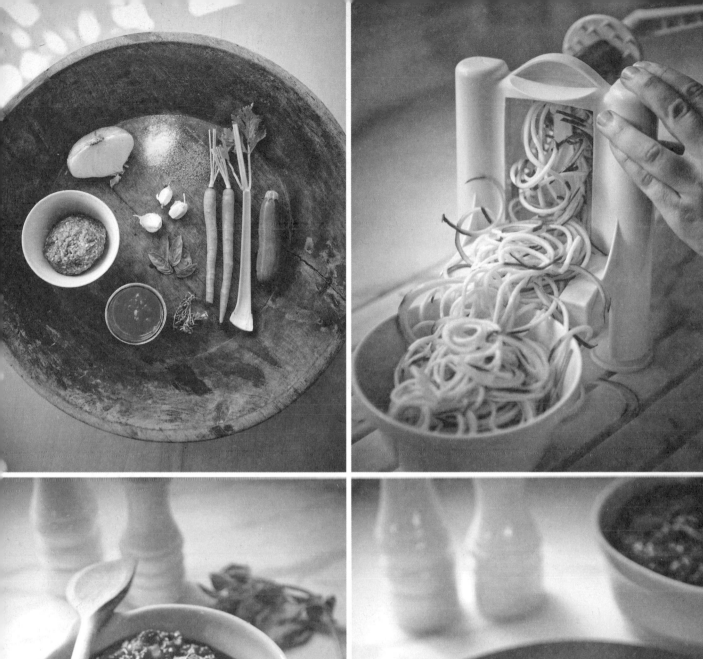
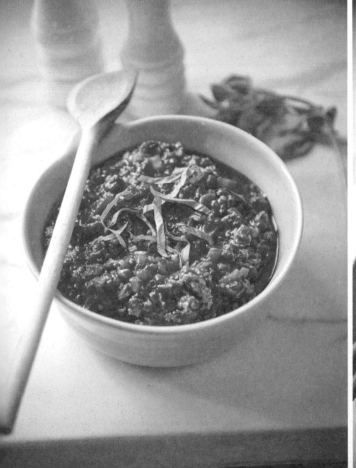
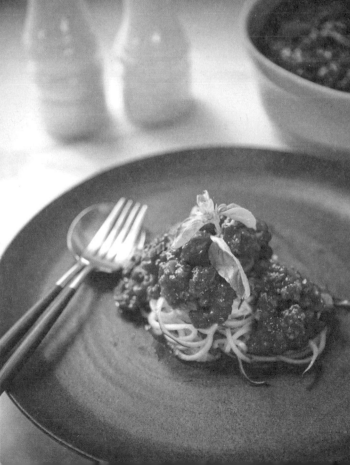

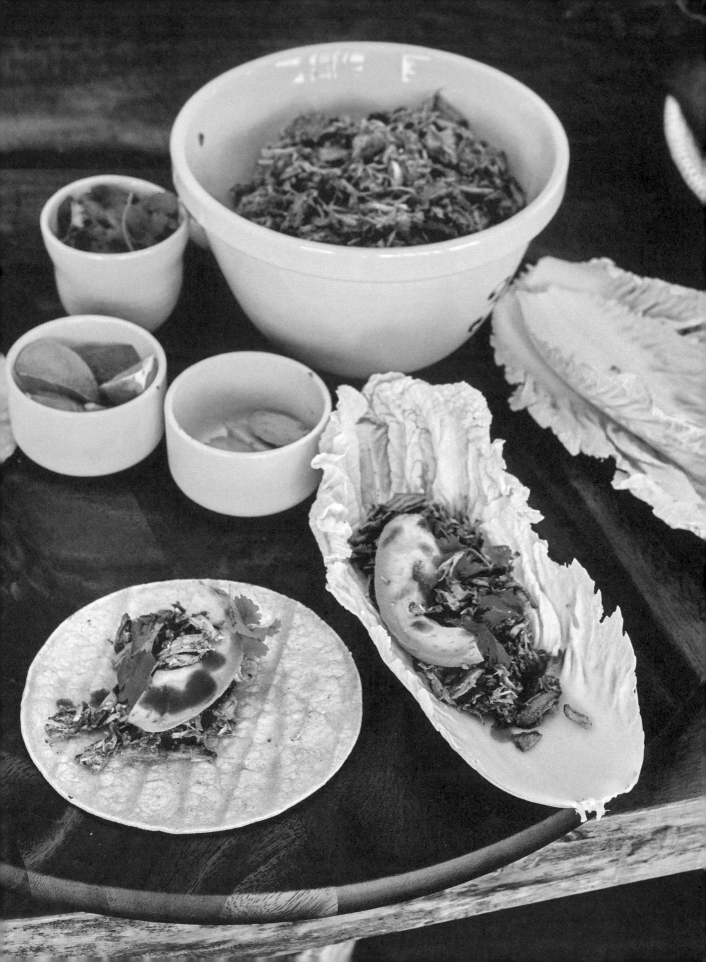

HEALTHY
CARNITAS

Serves 6

Another great party dish—we cut out the lard and opted for a leaner cut of pork but kept all of the delicious flavor. Look for organic, humanely raised pigs that have grazed on open pastures and in oak forests.

1½ tablespoons ancho chile powder

2 teaspoons ground cumin

1 teaspoon garlic powder

1 teaspoon ground ginger

1 teaspoon sea salt

3 pounds boneless pork loin, cut into 3- to 4-inch pieces

2 tablespoons coconut oil

1½ cups chicken stock

½ cup fresh orange juice

1 package (6-inch) fresh corn tortillas

6 large or 12 smaller whole leaves of napa cabbage or sturdy lettuce such as romaine

FOR THE TOPPINGS:

One Gun Salsa (page 293)

1 or 2 ripe avocados, pitted, peeled, and sliced

Lime wedges

Hot sauce

Chopped fresh cilantro

Preheat the oven to 350°F.

In a small bowl, combine the chile powder, cumin, garlic powder, ground ginger, and salt. Dry rub the pork with the spice mixture.

In a large, heavy-bottomed Dutch oven or other ovenproof pot with a tight-fitting lid, over medium heat, melt the coconut oil. When the oil is hot, add the pork and sear until browned on all sides, about 1 minute. Depending on how large your pot is, you may need to work in batches.

Transfer the pork to a plate and pour in the chicken stock to deglaze, scraping any browned bits of pork from the bottom of the pan to mix in. Add the orange juice and bring the mixture to a boil. Return the pork to the pot, cover, and transfer to the oven. Bake for 30 minutes.

Remove the pot from the oven, uncover, and turn the pork, giving it a good stir. Return to the oven and cook, uncovered, until the pork is tender, about 1 to 1½ hours longer. Give the pork a good stir and turn it over in the pot 1 or 2 times during the cooking time.

When the pork is meltingly tender, remove from the oven and let cool slightly. Using two forks, shred the pork into the sauce.

Serve in both corn and lettuce tacos with the toppings on the side for everyone to choose from as they like. Enjoy!

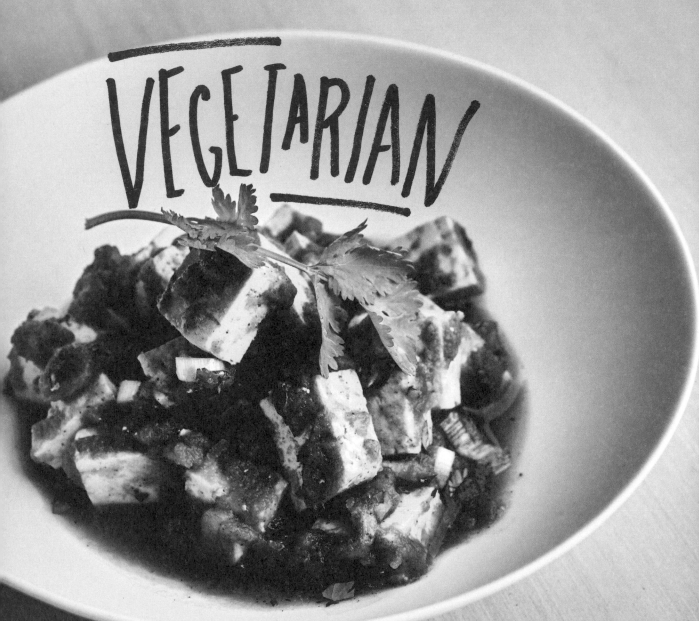

VEGETARIAN

TURMERIC
TOFU CURRY

Serves 4

I love a good curry and this vegan version is simply delicious, although you could also use two 6-ounce breasts of organic free-range chicken cut into cubes instead of tofu, if you wish. It tastes even better the next day, as the flavors have had time to develop. You may also make this with coconut milk for a richer curry. Simply heat a 12-ounce can of coconut milk in a saucepan, add the purée from the blender, and stir well to incorporate, then add the tofu, cilantro, and green onions.

½ cup vegetable stock

1 tablespoon coconut oil

1 medium white or yellow onion, cut into small dice

1 tablespoon minced garlic (2 or 3 cloves)

1 tablespoon peeled and minced fresh ginger

2 teaspoons ground turmeric

1 teaspoon curry powder

¾ teaspoon ground cumin

¼ teaspoon ancho chile powder

1 (14-ounce) package firm or extra-firm tofu, cut into cubes (about 2½ cups)

½ cup chopped fresh cilantro

3 green onions, white and tender green parts only, chopped

Steamed brown rice and/or steamed green vegetables for serving

Heat the stock in a small saucepan until it reaches a simmer and set aside.

In a saucepan over medium-high heat, melt the coconut oil. When the oil is hot, add onion, garlic, and ginger. Cook until the onion is soft, 2 to 3 minutes. Reduce the heat to medium-low and add the turmeric, curry powder, cumin, and chile powder and cook for another 3 to 5 minutes, adding a little of the stock, up to ¼ cup if needed, to help incorporate the spices, stirring often. Make sure that your heat is not too high or your spices will burn, and they will taste bitter!

Put the onion and spice mixture in a blender and blend to a smooth purée. Add a little more of the hot stock if the purée seems a bit too dry.

Add the purée to the remaining stock over medium heat and stir well to combine. Add the tofu and mix well. Simmer for 3 to 4 minutes, or until the tofu takes on the turmeric color and is heated through. Add the cilantro and green onions.

Serve immediately, with the steamed brown rice or steamed green vegetables.

TURMERIC
CHIA SEED CRACKERS

Serves 4

Eat your seeds! These nutrition-packed crackers are the perfect on-the-go snack. I always make sure to make a batch to take on long road trips or flights. They are also a perfect accompaniment to soup. You can find brown linseed in natural-food stores and online.

¼ cup chia seeds

3 tablespoons brown linseed

1½ tablespoons sunflower seeds

1½ tablespoons pumpkin seeds

1 teaspoon bee pollen

½ teaspoon sea salt

⅔ cup water

1½ tablespoons olive oil

1 teaspoon turmeric powder

½ teaspoon curry powder

¼ teaspoon chili powder

In a bowl, combine the chia seeds, linseed, sunflower seeds, pumpkin seeds, bee pollen, and salt and stir to mix. Stir in the water and let stand for 30 minutes, to allow the chia seeds to absorb some of the moisture and form a thick dough.

Stir in the spices and let stand for 1 minute longer.

Preheat the oven to 300°F.

Spread the dough out on a piece of parchment paper fitted in a baking sheet and place a second piece of parchment on top. Roll the dough as thinly as possible, using a rolling pin or even just by pressing out with your hand. When the dough is rolled out, remove the top layer of paper carefully to avoid damaging the thin dough.

Bake until golden brown and crisp, about 45 minutes. Alternatively, the crackers can be dehydrated at 100°F for 12 to 16 hours.

Snap the crackers into pieces and enjoy.

HEALTHY
MEXICAN BEANS

Serves 4

These beans are a mandatory side dish to accompany either the Carnitas (page 281) or Carne Asada (page 274) . Again we've cut out the lard to make it guilt-free yet delicious.

2 (15-ounce) cans black beans, half drained

1 small white onion, diced

1 clove garlic, minced

¼ teaspoon cayenne pepper, or to taste

2 tablespoons minced fresh cilantro

In a medium saucepan over medium-high heat, stir together the beans, onion, garlic, and cayenne. Bring the mixture to a boil, stirring, then reduce the heat medium-low. Stir in the cilantro. Simmer for 5 minutes and serve.

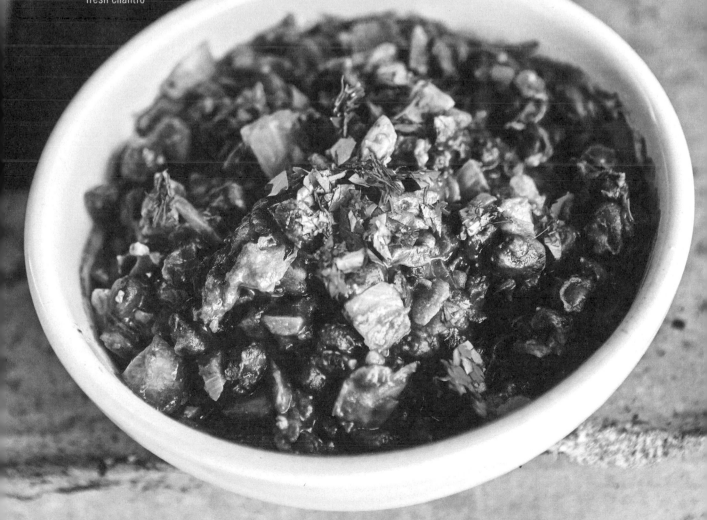

YELLOW
DAL

Serves 4

Heaven in a bowl, this vegan dish is a regular supper at the Ranch, especially on cold, foggy days when it evokes memories of my time living in India. Lentils are a great source of fiber, lean protein, and iron, making them a perfect substitute for meat.

1 cup red lentils (or ½ cup red lentils and ½ cup yellow moong dal—split mung beans—if you can find them!)

3 cups water

2 teaspoons coconut oil

1 large red or white onion, finely chopped

3 cloves garlic, minced

1 teaspoon peeled and minced fresh ginger or 1 teaspoon ground ginger

1 teaspoon cumin seeds

½ teaspoon ground turmeric

½ teaspoon red pepper flakes

2 large or 3 small ripe tomatoes, chopped

½ teaspoon garam masala

1 tablespoon chopped fresh cilantro

1 cup spinach or chard leaves, tough stems removed

Cucumber, Mint & Cumin Yogurt (opposite page) for serving

In a bowl, soak the lentils in 3 cups water.

Melt the coconut oil in a large saucepan over medium-high heat. When the oil is hot, add the onion and garlic and cook, stirring, until the onion is browned, about 5 minutes. Add the ginger, cumin, turmeric, and red pepper flakes. Cook all together, stirring, for 1 minute. Add the tomatoes and cook until the sauce thickens, about 15 minutes longer.

Rinse the lentils and drain well, then add to the sauce with enough water to cover. Stir all together and cook until softened and well blended, about 35 minutes.

Add the garam masala and stir vigorously to make sure the lentils are creamy; add a little water if they seem too thick. Cook for another 10 minutes or so, then stir in the cilantro and spinach. Cooking for about 10 minutes longer, or until the spinach is wilted.

Ladle into bowls and dollop the yogurt on top. Serve immediately.

Cucumber, Mint & Cumin Yogurt

Makes about 1 cup

Our spin on a traditional Indian raita. The cooling yogurt beautifully offsets the heat of curries.

¼ cucumber, peeled, seeded, and finely chopped

1 cup lactose-free yogurt

2 teaspoons ground cumin

Leaves from 1 sprig fresh mint, finely chopped

Sea salt and freshly ground black pepper

Pinch of finely chopped fresh cilantro for garnish (optional)

Combine the cucumber, yogurt, cumin, and mint in a bowl and mix well. Season with salt and pepper. Serve with a pinch of finely chopped cilantro, if you like.

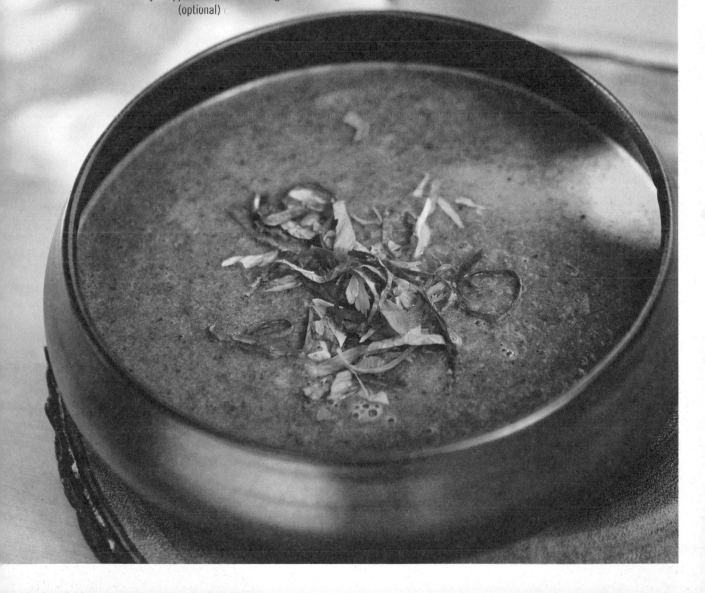

Teas, Tonics, and Tipples

MAUVIEL 18

HOT TODDY

Serves 6 to 8

We have a large pot of this warming winter brew sitting on top of the Aga oven anytime the mercury drops, to fend off any hint of a sniffle or sore throat.

Juice of 10 Meyer lemons

Juice of 2 oranges

2 tablespoons raw local honey or maple syrup, or more to taste

1 tablespoon ground ginger or 3-inch piece fresh ginger, peeled and finely chopped

1 teaspoon ground turmeric or 1-inch piece fresh turmeric, peeled and finely chopped

Big pinch of cayenne pepper

In a medium or large saucepan, combine the lemon and orange juices. Add the honey or maple syrup, ginger, turmeric, and cayenne. Fill the pot three-fourths full with water and bring to a boil. Reduce to a simmer and cook until the flavors have concentrated nicely, about 30 minutes. Add a little more honey or maple syrup, if desired.

Leave the pot to cool and warm it up whenever necessary, or leave on top of the Aga or heat storage oven for an instant pick-me-up.

TURMERIC TONIC

Serves 2

Turmeric is a fabulous superfood to include in your diet. The fresh root, which looks similar to ginger, can be found in whole foods and Asian markets and the dried powder in most spice sections of your local market. This healthful tonic is a wonderful way to start the day. Highly anti-inflammatory, the addition of coconut oil also supplies a boost of energy.

4-inch piece fresh turmeric

2-inch piece fresh ginger or 2 teaspoons ground ginger

Zest of 2 small organic Meyer lemons

⅓ cup raw local honey

½ teaspoon freshly ground black pepper

Coconut oil (optional)

Grate the turmeric and ginger root into a bowl. Add the zest, honey, and pepper and mash into a paste. Put 2 teaspoons of the paste into each of the 2 mugs and add 1 cup hot water to each. Stir well and serve. For extra energy, add 1 teaspoon of coconut oil to each serving.

THE ONE GUN

Serves 1

We love to serve this cocktail in the evening whilst sitting outside, watching the sun set over the mountains at the Ranch.

3 leaves fresh basil

2 slices jalapeño chile, with seeds

Squeeze of lime juice

2 ounces Prairie Organic vodka, or other organic vodka

Seaworth Coconut Simple Syrup, or any coconut-sugar syrup

Muddle the basil, jalapeño, and lime juice in a mortar using a pestle. Transfer to a chilled cocktail shaker and add the vodka and simple syrup, to taste. Fill the shaker with ice, shake vigorously, then strain into a chilled martini glass.

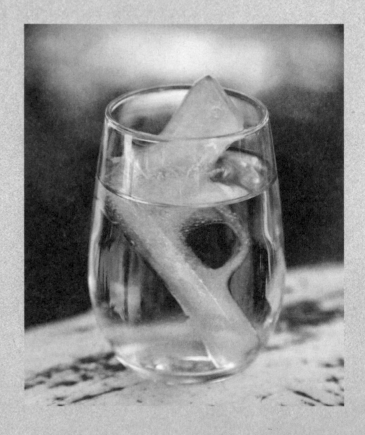

HIGH NOON

Serves 6 to 8

This is our biodynamic spin on the traditional British summertime tipple, the Pimm's Cup. We always use Leoube Rose, which is grown using biodynamic methods at our family vineyard in the South of France (and I swear is headache-free). If there are other berries at the farmers' market that look appealing, you can add those or swap out the strawberries.

1 (750-ml) bottle organic rosé wine

1 (750-ml) bottle sparkling water

Fresh mint sprigs

½ cucumber, peeled, seeded, and chopped or thinly sliced

12 strawberries, hulled and thinly sliced

Grated or julienned zest of 1 organic Meyer lemon

In a large pitcher, mix the wine and sparkling water. Add sprigs of fresh mint, to taste, the cucumber, strawberries, and lemon zest. Stir gently. Serve in tall glasses over ice.

ONE GUN BIODYNAMIC TEA

Serves 6 to 8

This calming tea is based on the biodynamic preparations we make to spray on the compost pile. To make the herbal tea blend, we simply gather bunches of each while out hiking (remember to wear gloves when picking that stinging nettle) and hang them to dry in the rafters of the Edible Saloon down by the horse corral. Once dried, we crumble the stalks between our hands to separate the buds, flowers, and leaves from the stems and store the mixture in a Mason jar.

3 tablespoons dried chamomile

3 tablespoons dried valerian

3 tablespoons dried stinging nettle

3 tablespoons dried dandelion

3 tablespoons dried yarrow

In a bowl, mix all the dried herbs together.

Warm a tea pot. Put 1 tablespoon of the herb mix per cup in the pot and fill with freshly boiled water. Allow to steep for 5 minutes before pouring.

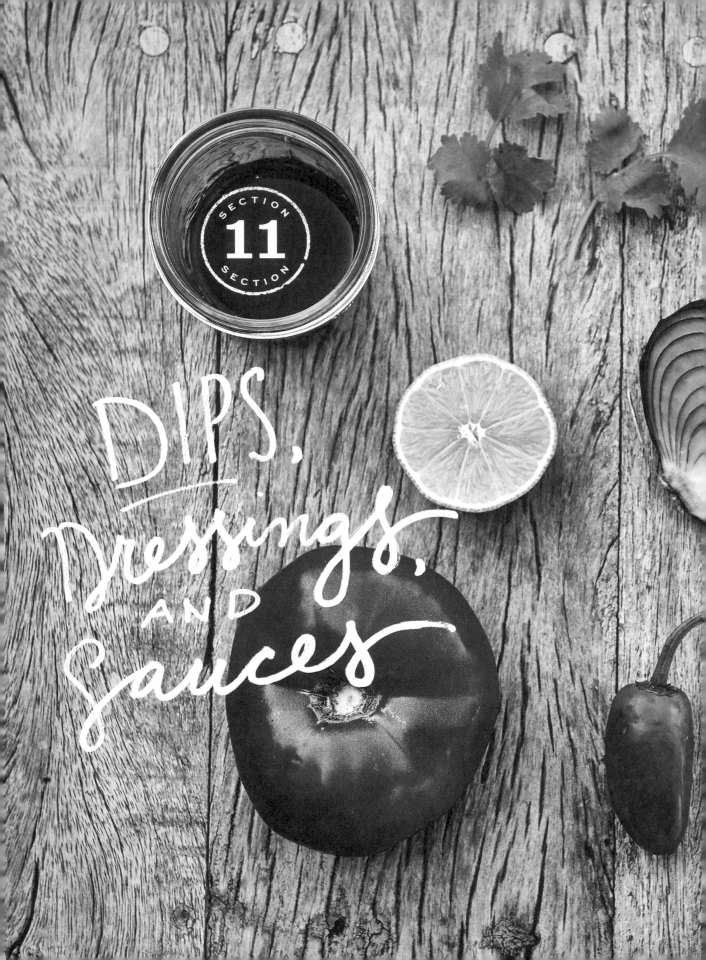

SECTION
11
SECTION

DIPS,
Dressings,
AND
Sauces

ONE GUN
SALSA

Makes about 2 cups

3 to 4 pounds ripe organic tomatoes

½ small red onion

3 small jalapeño chiles, seeded

Large handful of fresh cilantro leaves

Juice of ½ lime, plus more if needed

2 splashes red wine vinegar, plus more if needed

Roughly chop the tomatoes, onion, and jalapeños. Transfer to a blender and add the cilantro, lime, and vinegar. Pulse until the salsa reaches the desired consistency. Taste for flavor and add additional vinegar or lime juice, if needed.

VINAIGRETTES

I have always have a supply of these simple dressings on hand, stored in Mason jars in the fridge, to brighten up our micro green mix or any lettuces that have been picked that day.

Dijon Vinaigrette

Makes about ⅓ cup

2 tablespoons Dijon mustard

1 tablespoon red wine vinegar

3 tablespoons olive oil

Sea salt and freshly ground black pepper

Combine the mustard and vinegar in a bowl or a small Mason jar. Whisk in the olive oil, cover, and shake until nicely emulsified. Season with salt and pepper.

Meyer Lemon Vinaigrette

Makes about ⅓ cup

When citrus is in season, we like to make the most of our lemon crop, so in this dressing we have swapped out vinegar for fresh lemon juice.

2 tablespoons Dijon mustard

1 tablespoon fresh lemon juice

2 teaspoons raw local honey

3 tablespoons olive oil

Sea salt and freshly ground black pepper

Combine the mustard, lemon juice, and honey in a bowl or a small Mason jar. Whisk in the olive oil or cover and shake until nicely emulsified. Season with salt and pepper.

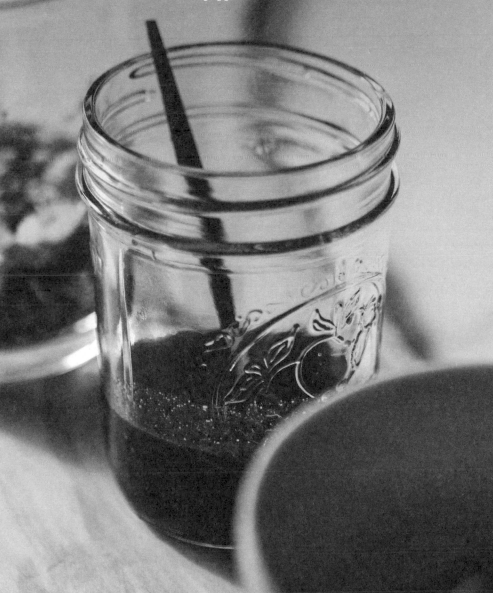

Balsamic Vinaigrette

Makes about ⅓ cup

2 tablespoons Dijon mustard

1 tablespoon balsamic vinegar

3 tablespoons olive oil

Sea salt and freshly ground black pepper

Combine the mustard and vinegar in a bowl or a small Mason jar. Whisk in the olive oil, cover, and shake until nicely emulsified. Season with salt and pepper.

GINGER–TURMERIC–ORANGE
DRESSING

Makes about 1¼ cups

I would never smother the fresh, vibrant biodynamic salad mixes we grow at the Ranch with a store-bought salad dressing full of stabilizers and preservatives. This delicious homemade dressing packs a superfood punch thanks to the addition of anti-inflammatory turmeric and ginger, and vitamin C–packed orange juice. The avocado also provides a lovely creaminess to offset the bite of the ginger.

1 cup good-quality olive, hemp, or flaxseed oil

Juice of 1 orange

½ ripe avocado

1 teaspoon peeled and chopped fresh ginger

1 teaspoon peeled and chopped fresh turmeric

¼ teaspoon red pepper flakes or sweet paprika

Good pinch of sea salt

Juice of ½ lemon or apple cider vinegar to taste (optional)

In a blender, combine the olive oil, orange juice, avocado, ginger, turmeric, red pepper flakes, and salt and blend until smooth. Taste and adjust the seasoning, if necessary. If it needs more sharpness or brightness to contrast with the sweetness of the orange juice, add in a splash of lemon juice or apple cider vinegar.

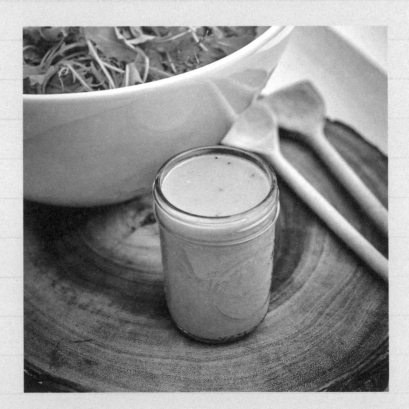

JALAPEÑO
HOT SAUCE

Makes about 2 cups

The One Gun version of Tabasco, this sauce adds a wonderfully clean, hot kick to accompany anything from avocados and eggs to tacos. You may want to have all your windows open when preparing this!

2 cups (about 1 pound) green jalapeño chiles, roughly diced

⅔ cup apple cider vinegar

⅓ cup white vinegar

2 teaspoons salt

In a blender, combine the chiles, vinegars, and salt and blend to a smooth purée. Strain through a fine-mesh strainer into a bowl or Mason jar.

Serve immediately, or store in the refrigerator for up to 6 months.

VARIATIONS

ROASTED JALAPEÑO HOT SAUCE
Roast the whole peppers in a 350°F oven for 45 minutes or on a well-oiled grill until the skins are nicely charred and the peppers are fragrant. Remove the stems and chop the peppers in half. Continue with the recipe as directed.

RED JALAPEÑO HOT SAUCE
Use red jalapeño chiles, and reduce the apple cider vinegar to ½ cup and the white vinegar to ¼ cup. Continue with the recipe as directed.

CARROT-BEET KETCHUP

Makes about 1 cup

The color of this healthy, biodynamic ketchup is divine. Much higher in fiber and lower in sugar than traditional ketchup, we've swapped out tomatoes for these nutritious root veggies and, we think, improved on the taste in the process.

1 beet (about 4 ounces), trimmed and scrubbed but not peeled

1 pound carrots, peeled and cut into ½-inch dice

⅓ cup water

2½ tablespoons apple cider vinegar

2 tablespoons grade B maple syrup

Pinch of ground cloves

Pinch of sea salt

⅛ teaspoon chili powder (optional)

Preheat the oven to 400°F.

On a small baking sheet or in a small baking dish, roast the beet until tender, about 1 hour. Set aside to cool slightly, then peel and roughly chop.

Meanwhile, bring about ½ inch of water to a boil in a saucepan and fit a steamer basket into the pan. Add the carrots to the basket and steam until they are soft but not mushy, 8 to 10 minutes.

In a blender, combine the carrots and beets with the water, vinegar, maple syrup, cloves, and salt and blend until you have a thick, smooth purée. Pulse in the chili powder, if using. Taste and adjust the seasoning.

PINK PEPPERCORN SYRUP

Makes about 1 cup

The combination of sweet maple syrup and spicy peppercorns is a real winner, and a great way to use the abundance of peppercorns at the Ranch. Pink peppercorns are not true peppercorns but a berry that grows wild on Peruvian Pepper trees throughout California. This sauce is perfect with everything from pancakes to sorbets and ice cream. It looks beautiful in a bottle and makes a great gift for friends, as do our infused olive oils.

1 tablespoon pink peppercorns

1 cup grade B maple syrup

In a small saucepan over low heat, combine the peppercorns and maple syrup and bring to a simmer. Remove the syrup from the heat and set aside to cool for about 1 hour.

Strain the syrup through a fine-mesh strainer, reserving about a teaspoon or so of the peppercorns to store in your syrup.

Serve immediately or refrigerate in an airtight container for up to 6 months.

ONE GUN RANCH
Infused Oils

WE LOVE USING THE herbs and spices we grow at the Ranch to infuse olive oils that we can then use when cooking or dressing vegetables and salads. If you are lucky enough to live in an area that produces olives, use a locally sourced oil. Otherwise, go for a good, imported organic olive oil.

PINK PEPPERCORN & ROSEMARY–INFUSED OLIVE OIL

Place 2 sprigs of fresh rosemary and 20 peppercorns into a 24-ounce Mason jar, cruet, or bottle and fill with good-quality organic olive oil or locally sourced olive oil, leaving 1 inch of room at the top. Leave to infuse for a month in a cool dry pantry or cupboard before using.

DRIED JALAPEÑO–INFUSED OLIVE OIL

Place 1 dried jalapeño chile in a 24-ounce Mason jar, cruet, or bottle and fill with good-quality organic olive oil or locally sourced olive oil, leaving 1 inch of room at the top. A little goes a long a way with these! Leave to infuse for a month in a cool dry pantry or cupboard before using.

MEYER LEMON, SAGE & THYME–INFUSED OLIVE OIL

Slice 1 Meyer Lemon, leaving the rind on, and pack into a 24-ounce Mason jar, cruet, or bottle along with 1 sprig fresh sage and 1 sprig fresh thyme. Fill with good-quality organic olive oil or locally sourced olive oil, leaving 1 inch of room at the top. Leave to infuse for a month in a cool dry pantry or cupboard before using.

Desserts

We love to indulge once in a while, but we also want to avoid high-glycemic, sugary foods. Most of these recipes use honey and maple syrup, beets, and fruit for sweetness. A couple of squares of dark chocolate also make for a superfood treat.

POACHED FIGS

Serves 4

This is a decadent use of the glut of figs we grow at One Gun Ranch each summer, evoking the flavors of Italy.

8 ripe figs

½ cup sheep's-milk ricotta

Zest and juice of 2 Meyer lemons

1 teaspoon balsamic vinegar

2 teaspoons honey

Handful of almonds, roughly chopped

Preheat the oven to 400°F.

Cut a deep X into the top of each fig and place on a baking sheet.

In a bowl, whisk together the ricotta, lemon zest, vinegar, and 1 teaspoon of the honey. Spoon a little of the ricotta mixture into each fig, dividing it evenly. In a small bowl, stir together the remaining 1 teaspoon honey with the lemon juice, then pour over the figs. Sprinkle the almonds on top.

Bake until the almonds are golden and the figs are soft and collapsing, about 20 minutes.

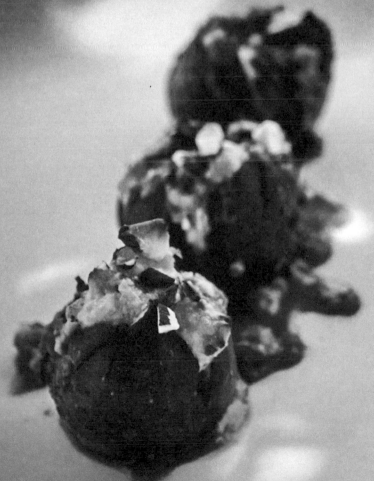

ONE GUN
SUPERFOOD:

Figs

Figs are high in fiber and vitamins A, K, and E; they are also an excellent plant-based source of calcium and potassium.

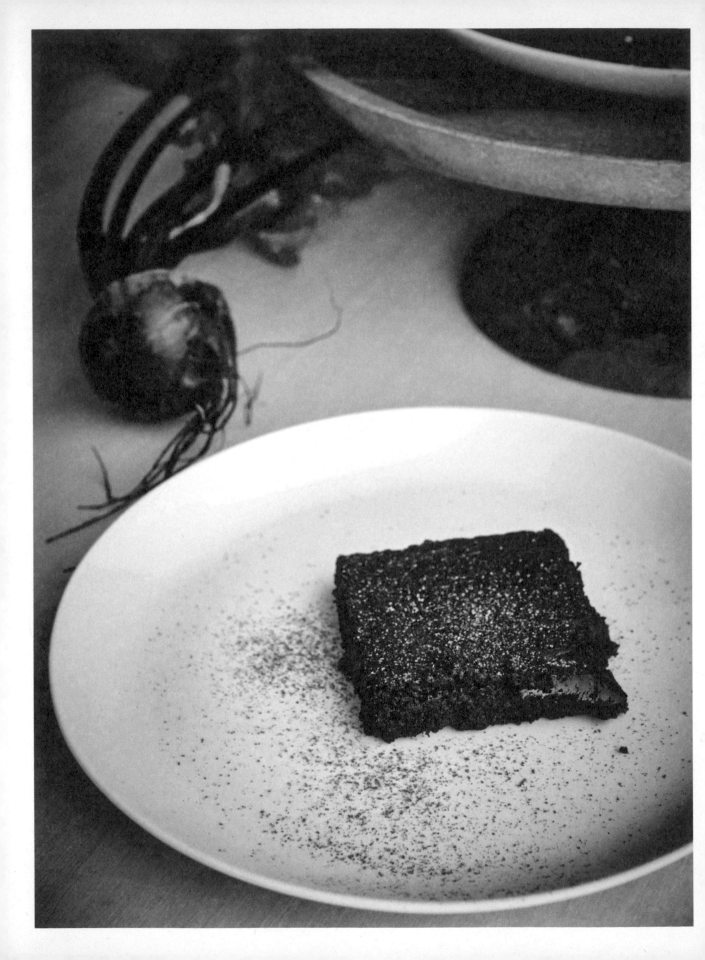

DARK CHOCOLATE & BEET
BROWNIES

Serves 4 to 6

Pure indulgence, this is a heavenly yet healthy treat. The beets keep the brownies incredibly moist, cutting out the need for the usual stick of butter. I lived on these during the last weeks of pregnancy.

1 pound beets, trimmed, peeled, and cut into ½-inch dice

7 ounces dark chocolate (best quality, at least 75 percent cacao)

½ cup coconut oil

¼ cup unsweetened cocoa powder (good quality), plus more for dusting

¼ cup all-purpose gluten-free flour or rice flour

1 heaping teaspoon baking powder

3 large organic free-range eggs

1 cup coconut sugar

¼ cup ground almonds

OPTIONAL ADD-INS:

Handful of sour cherries

1 tablespoon shredded unsweetened coconut

1 tablespoon peeled and grated fresh ginger

Juice of 1 ripe passion fruit

Ginger powder for dusting (optional)

Preheat the oven to 350°F.

Meanwhile, bring about ½ inch of water to a boil in a saucepan and fit a steamer basket into the pan. Add the beets to the basket and steam until tender, about 10 minutes. Let cool to room temperature, then put in a blender and process to a smooth and silky purée. Set aside.

Bring about 1 inch of water to a gentle boil in the bottom of a double boiler. Break up the chocolate into the top pan and add the coconut oil. Nest the top pan in the bottom pan over but not touching the boiling water. Stir until the chocolate melts. Once the chocolate has melted, stir well. (Alternatively, bring 1 inch water to a boil in a saucepan and melt the chocolate in a glass or metal bowl that nests into the saucepan without touching the water.)

Sift together the cocoa, flour, and baking powder into a medium bowl.

In large bowl, beat the eggs with the coconut sugar until pale and fluffy. Fold the melted chocolate mixture into the egg mixture, then fold in the flour mixture and the ground almonds.

Finally, add the beet purée and fold to combine well. Gently stir in any of the optional ingredients you like.

Pour the batter into a lightly coconut oil–greased 9-inch round or square baking pan. Bake until the edges begin to pull away from the sides, 40 to 45 minutes.

Let cool. Dust with the cocoa powder and the ground ginger, if you like. Cut into squares and enjoy!

DARK CHOCOLATE
CORNFLAKE CAKES

Serves 4 to 6

¼ cup coconut oil

¼ cup raw local honey or golden syrup

½ cup best-quality dark chocolate, at least 75 percent cacao

1 (18-ounce) box cornflakes

In a large saucepan over low heat, gently melt the coconut oil, honey, and chocolate together. Fold in the cornflakes until completely covered.

Pour into a large, well-oiled 9-inch square baking pan or a small baking sheet. Refrigerate or freeze until completely set, 3 to 4 hours. Cut into squares and serve.

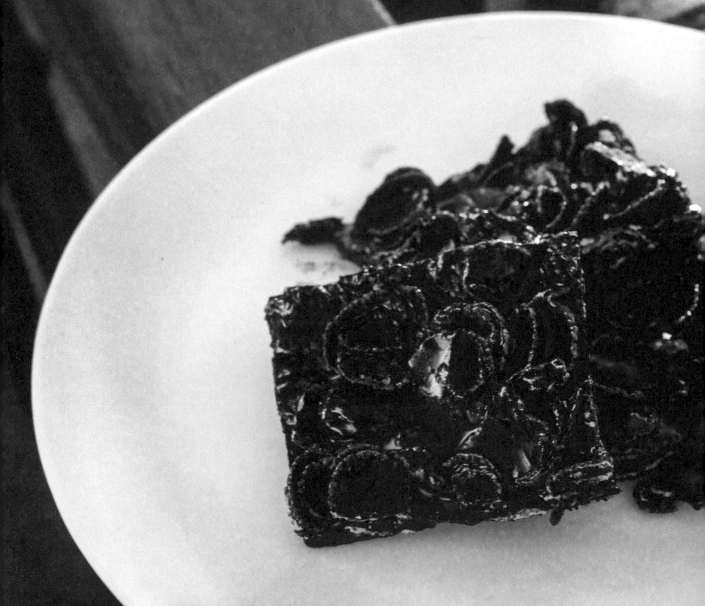

GLUTEN-FREE
JAMAICAN GINGER LOAF

Makes one 4-inch loaf; serves 4

Annie and I adore ginger and add it to everything and anything. This is seriously one of our favorite treats, perfect for dessert on a weekend served with a ginger lemon syrup or just straight up.

½ cup brown rice flour

½ cup buckwheat flour

2 teaspoons ground ginger

⅛ teaspoon ground cloves

Pinch of sea salt

1 teaspoon gluten-free baking powder

½ teaspoon gluten-free baking soda

2 large organic free-range eggs

3 tablespoons golden syrup

½ cup almond milk or buttermilk

3 tablespoons coconut oil, melted

½ cup chopped crystallized ginger

Finely grated zest of ½ orange

Preheat the oven to 350°F. Grease and flour a 9 x 5-inch loaf pan.

In a large bowl, whisk together the flours, ground ginger, cloves, salt, baking powder, and baking soda.

In another large bowl, stir together the eggs, syrup, almond milk or buttermilk, and coconut oil.

Gently fold the dry ingredients into the wet ingredients, until just incorporated, then add in the crystallized ginger and the zest.

Pour everything into the loaf pan and bake until a knife inserted into the center comes out clean, about 35 minutes.

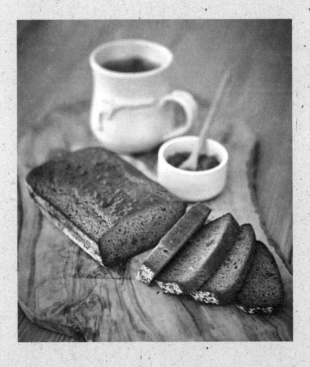

SORBETS & JELLOS

These two desserts are not terribly fashionable. In fact, they are very old-fashioned, but they deserve a place on a contemporary table, as there is a real purity to their flavors. Sorbets and jellies take the essence of a fruit and suspend that freshly picked taste perfectly without any distraction. They appeal to both adults, as they are elegant and refined, and children, as they're fun and easy, with uncomplicated flavors, and so make for a perfect party treat. Fruit served three ways—fresh, jellied, and in a sorbet—makes for an especially chic dish that looks fantastic on the plate. And I love the sensation of the different textures in your mouth.

sorbet

SORBET IS A FAVORITE OF MINE, as it makes for such a wonderful flavor explosion of seasonal fruit and flowers and are the perfect way to use a glut of summer fruit and cool off on sweltering afternoons—plus, eating sorbet releases endorphins! These recipes are very adaptable, so use anything that is in season—from blood oranges and elderflower to mango, apples, or pears.

To make the base: Combine all of the ingredients in a blender and blend until smooth. Strain the base through a fine-mesh strainer into a baking dish or bowl.

To make the sorbet in a blender: Cover the base and freeze overnight, or until completely frozen. Remove from the freezer, carefully break the sorbet up into large pieces, and quickly add to a blender. Give it a quick whizz in the blender until it has a soft, creamy, texture. Transfer to an airtight container and return to the freezer for another 1 to 2 hours, or until the sorbet is completely frozen.

To make the sorbet in an ice-cream maker: Freeze the ice-cream maker freezer bowl overnight. Cover the base and refrigerate until well-chilled, 2 to 3 hours, or overnight. Freeze in the ice-cream maker according to the manufacturer's instructions. The sorbet will have a soft, creamy texture. Serve right away, or for a more frozen consistency, transfer to an airtight container and freeze for up to 2 hours longer.

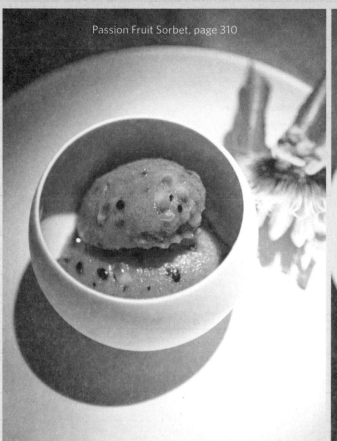

Passion Fruit Sorbet, page 310

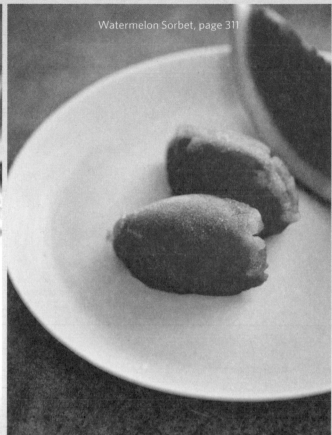

Watermelon Sorbet, page 311

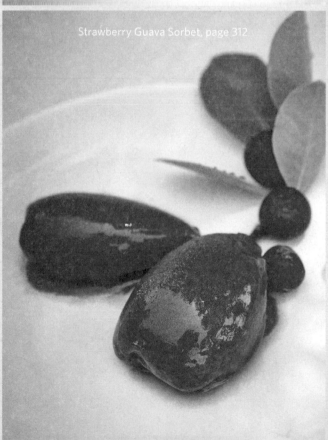

Strawberry Guava Sorbet, page 312

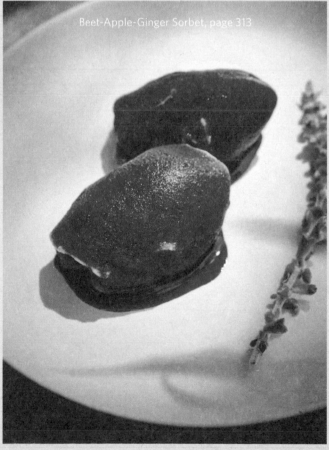

Beet-Apple-Ginger Sorbet, page 313

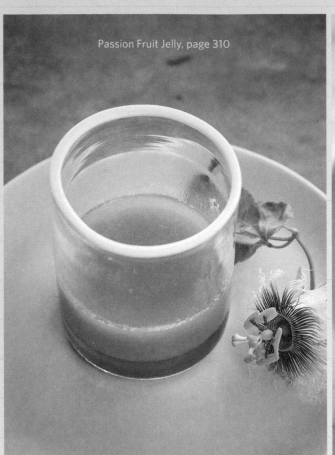
Passion Fruit Jelly, page 310

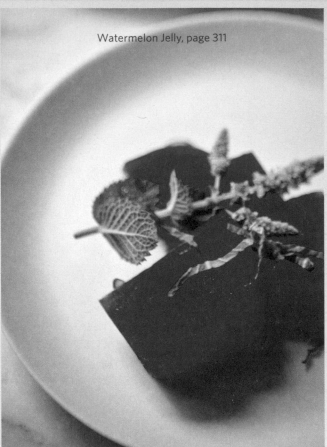
Watermelon Jelly, page 311

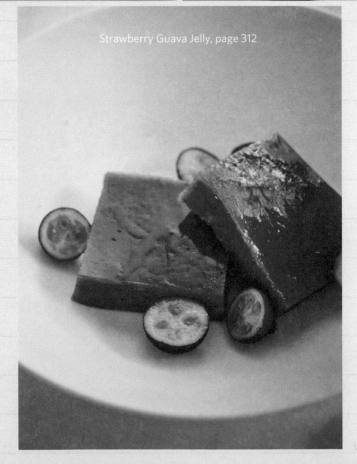
Strawberry Guava Jelly, page 312

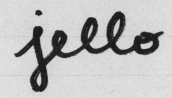

jello

I GREW UP WITH JELLO, or "jelly," as it is know in England, where it is a very traditional dessert. The Victorians used to make several jellies for dinner parties using elaborate molds, and would display them as table centerpieces. The perfect jelly should hold its shape but wobble alluringly when anyone knocks against the table.

USING GELATIN One envelope of Knox gelatin contains 2¼ to 2½ teaspoons powdered gelatin, which is the equivalent of 6 leaves of gelatin. This amount sets 2 cups total liquid.

To use powdered gelatin: Sprinkle 1 envelope gelatin over ¼ cup of cold liquid. Let stand for 5 to 10 minutes. Warm the remaining 1¾ cups liquid, and add the cold gelatin mixture, and stir gently until all of the gelatin has dissolved.

To use gelatin leaves: Soak 6 gelatin leaves in a bowl of ice-cold water for 5 to 10 minutes. The water must be very cold or the gelatin will dissolve. Use about 1 cup of ice water per leaf.

When the leaves are soft, lift thom from the water and squeeze to remove the excess water. Warm 2 cups of liquid over low heat, then add the softened gelatin leaves and stir until completely melted. Do not let boil.

ONE GUN SUPERFOODS:

Passion Fruit

A good source of potassium and folate, passion fruit is also high in vitamins A and C.

Strawberry Guava

This beautiful fruit is high in fiber and antioxidants, vitamins A and C, folic acid, and lycopene.

PASSION FRUIT SORBET

Serves 4 to 6

Passion fruit grows abundantly at One Gun Ranch, offering much needed shade and fractured light for our raised vegetable beds, while the beautiful flowers act as a deterrent to some insects. The fruit is incredibly delicious and one of our best sellers at the farmers' market. Everyone loves the sharp, sweet flavor. Della, the pastry chef at the famed LA restaurant Spago, also frequently travels up to the Ranch to buy a bag and uses them for all types of desserts.

13 to 15 passion fruits (to make about 1 cup strained juice)

½ cup water

¼ cup light-colored honey, such as acacia or wildflower

Juice and zest of 1 lemon

Scoop the pulp from the passion fruit into a fine-mesh strainer nested over a bowl to separate the juice from the seeds.

Combine the passion fruit juice with the water, honey, and lemon juice and zest in a blender. Blend until smooth. Strain the sorbet base through a fine-mesh strainer into a glass or metal container. Discard the solids.

Freeze the sorbet base according to your preferred method in the Master Recipe (page 306). Remove the sorbet from the freezer about 15 minutes before serving. Scoop into bowls and serve. The sorbet will keep, frozen in an airtight container, for up to 8 weeks.

PASSION FRUIT JELLY

Serves 4

13 to 15 passion fruits (to make about 1 cup strained juice)

½ cup water

2 tablespoons light-colored honey, such as acacia or wildflower

12 gelatin leaves or 2 packets powdered gelatin (this jelly needs a bit more gelatin to set)

Scoop the pulp from the passion fruits into a large fine-mesh strainer nested over a bowl to separate the juice from the seeds.

In a small saucepan over high heat, heat the water with the honey and bring to a boil. Pass through a fine-mesh strainer into a suitable container.

Sprinkle gelatin over ¼ cup of the cold water. Let stand for 5 to 10 minutes.

Warm the remaining liquid, and add to cold liquid, stirring gently until all of the gelatin has dissolved. Pour into a glass or metal container and cover.

Refrigerate until set, about 12 hours.

WATERMELON SORBET

A perfect Californian dessert served either as a sorbet or a jelly. That combination of the sweet melon and sharp lime is something we at One Gun Ranch come back to again and again.

4 cups cubed watermelon, plus more for serving

Juice of 1 lime

¼ cup water

2 tablespoons light-colored honey, such as acacia or wildflower

Minced fresh mint leaves for serving

Put the watermelon in a blender and process until smooth. Pass the purée through a fine-mesh strainer. Measure out 2½ cups watermelon juice.

Combine the watermelon juice, lime juice, water, and honey in a blender and blend until smooth. Strain the sorbet base through a fine-mesh strainer into a glass or metal container.

Freeze the base according to the Master Recipe (page 306). Remove the sorbet from the freezer about 15 minutes before serving. Scoop into bowls and serve garnished with fresh cubes of watermelon and minced mint leaves. The sorbet will keep, frozen in an airtight container, for up to 8 weeks.

WATERMELON JELLY

Serves 4

4 cups watermelon, cubed

Juice of 1 lime

1 tablespoon raw local honey

2 packets powdered gelatin

Put the watermelon in a

blender and process until smooth. Pass the purée through a fine-mesh strainer. Measure out 2½ cups watermelon juice and set aside.

Heat the juice with the honey and bring to a boil.

Bloom the gelatin in the watermelon juice and allow to sit for 5 to 10 minutes, or if using packets, stir to combine well for 1 to 2 minutes.

Stir in the hot liquid. Pour into a metal or glass container and cover.

Refrigerate until set, 6 to 8 hours.

STRAWBERRY GUAVA SORBET

Serves 4 to 6

Our strawberry guavas come into season in late August, early September, and the air at the Ranch becomes heavy with their scent. Follow your nose when choosing guavas and pick only the sweetest, plumpest specimens—if you're with me, they'll still be warm from the sun—and I promise this sorbet will not disappoint.

2 cups whole fresh strawberry guavas, peeled

⅔ cup water

½ cup apple juice

Juice of 1 lemon

¼ cup honey

In a blender, purée the strawberry guavas. Drain through cheese-cloth; you should have about 1¼ cups purée.

Combine the purée, water, apple juice, lemon juice, and honey in the blender and blend until smooth. Strain the base through a fine-mesh strainer into a glass or metal container.

Freeze the base according to your preferred method in the Master Recipe (page 306). Remove the sorbet from the freezer about 15 minutes before serving. Scoop into bowls and serve. The sorbet will keep, frozen in an airtight container, for up to 8 weeks.

STRAWBERRY GUAVA JELLY

Serves 4

You can substitute apple juice for the water in this recipe, taste for sweetness, and adjust the amount of honey accordingly.

2 cups whole fresh strawberry guavas, peeled

1 cup water

2 tablespoons raw wildflower honey

2 packets gelatin or 5 to 6 gelatin leaves

In a blender, purée the strawberry guavas. Drain through cheese-cloth; you should have about 1 cup purée.

In a small saucepan over high heat, heat the water with the honey and bring to a boil.

Follow the Master Recipe for jelly instructions (page 309). Cover and refrigerate until set, 6 to 8 hours.

BEET-APPLE-GINGER SORBET

Serves 4 to 6

This zesty, seasonal sorbet is another great way to use beets to surprising effect. The super refreshing balance of flavors is also gorgeous looking.

1 cup apple juice

½ cup fresh beet juice

½ teaspoon peeled and minced fresh ginger

¼ cup honey

Juice of 1 lime

Combine all the ingredients in a blender. Blend until smooth. Strain the base through a fine-mesh strainer into a glass or metal container.

Freeze the base according to your preferred method in the Master Recipe (page 306). Remove the sorbet from the freezer about 15 minutes before serving. Scoop into bowls and serve. The sorbet will keep, frozen in an airtight container, for up to 8 weeks.

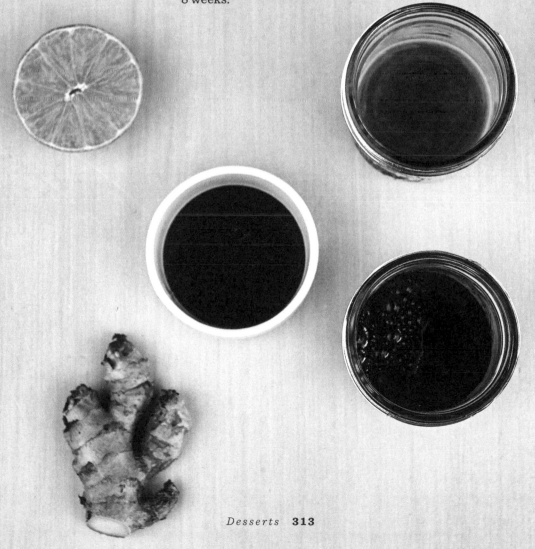

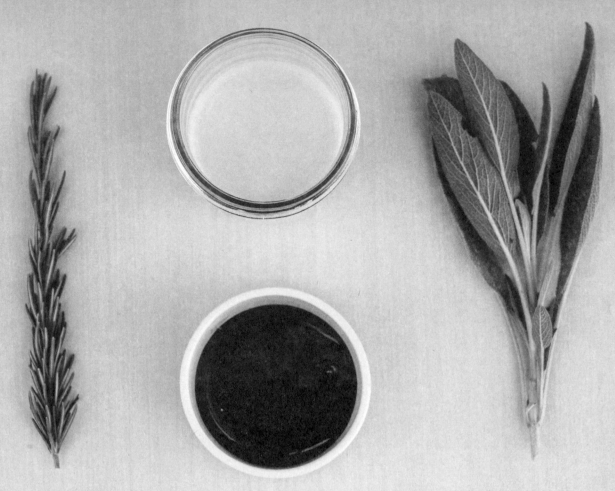

HONEY, SAGE & ROSEMARY ICE CREAM

Serves 4 to 6

The flavors of One Gun in an ice cream.

Sprig fresh sage, plus ½ teaspoon minced sage

Sprig fresh rosemary, plus ½ teaspoon minced rosemary

½ cup unsweetened almond milk

¼ to ½ cup honey

Place the herb sprigs in a pot of 1 cup very warm water for 1 to 2 minutes. The infusion should still be clear. Strain the herbs from the water.

Combine ½ cup of the herbal infusion, the almond milk, and the honey in a blender and blend until smooth.

Pour into a glass or metal dish. Stir in the minced herbs. Cover and freeze.

Freeze the base according to the Master Recipe for sorbet made in an ice-cream maker (page 306). Remove the ice cream from the freezer about 15 minutes before serving. Scoop into bowls and serve. The ice cream will keep, frozen in an airtight container, for up to 2 weeks.

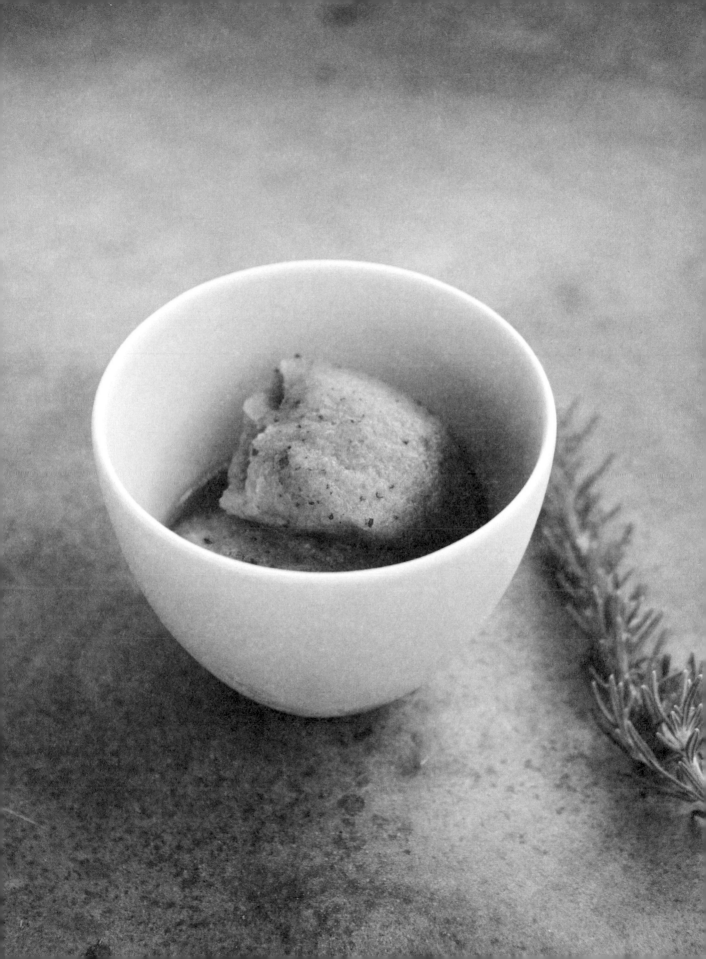

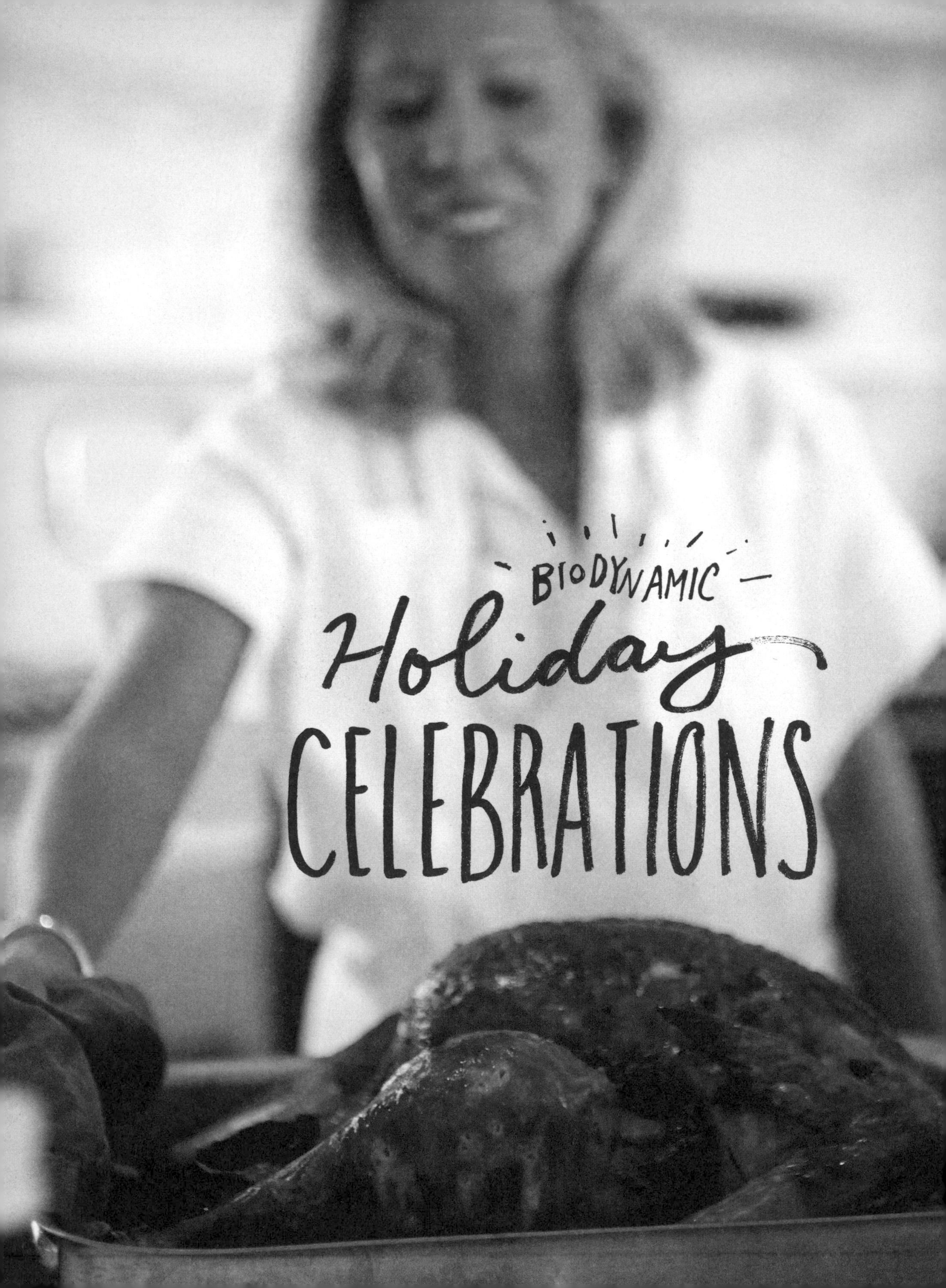

- BIODYNAMIC -

Holiday

CELEBRATIONS

I grew up celebrating both Easter and Christmas in Barbados, so the traditional holiday meals always had a Bajan twist to them, with the spices and exquisite flavors used in Caribbean cooking. You can buy Bajan spice mix in markets that stock Caribbean goods or online, or make your own.

The lovely Rita, who cooks for my family in Barbados, is a legend; these are my takes on her mouthwatering recipes, which I've tweaked to make the perfect roast chicken or Thanksgiving Turkey. Always look for free-range, organic birds.

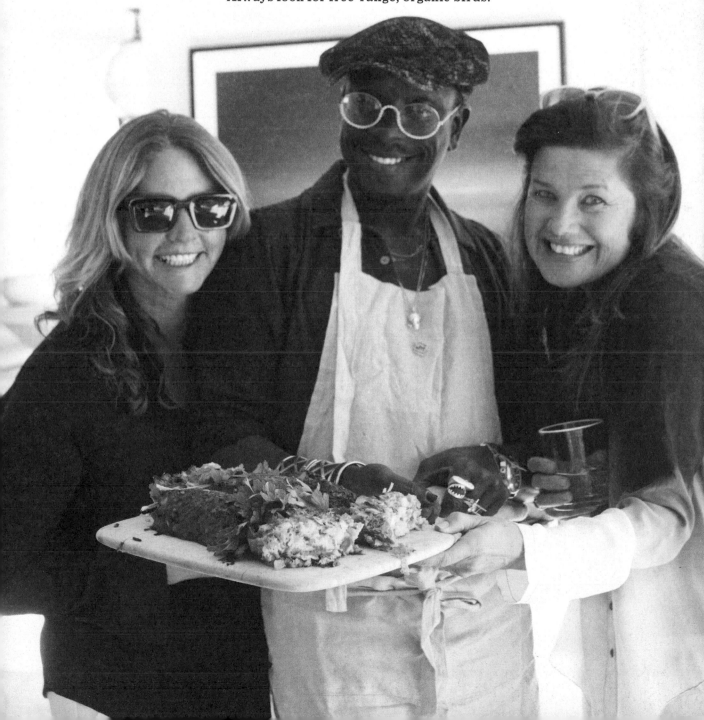

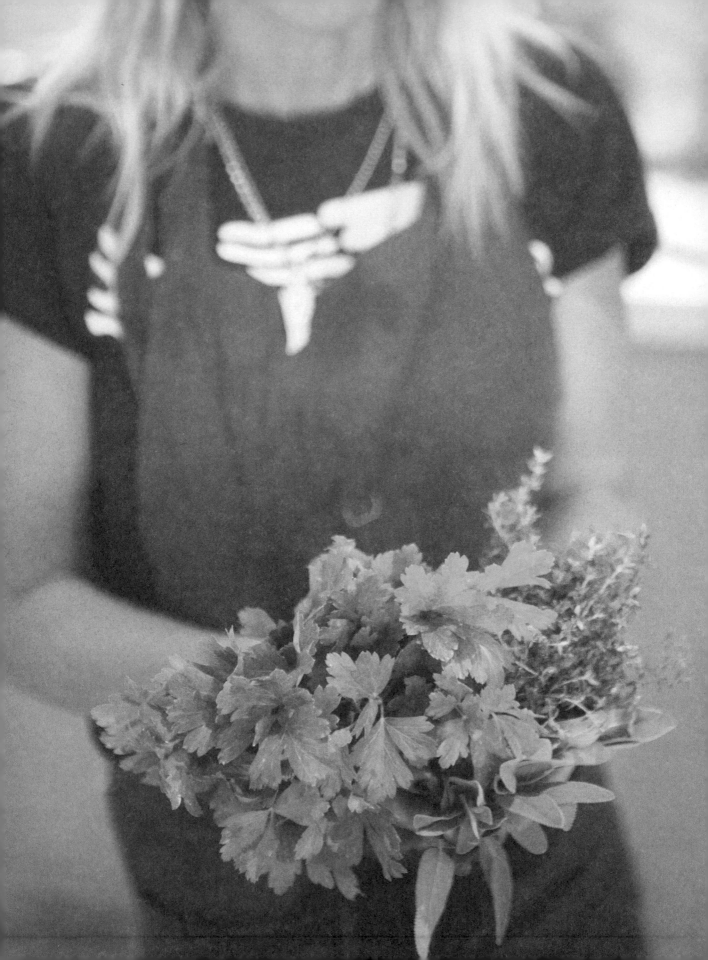

RITA'S
GRAVY

Makes 8

1 tablespoon olive oil

1 white or yellow onion

4 ripe tomatoes, chopped

Leaves from 2 sprigs fresh thyme

1 tablespoon tomato paste

1 cube organic chicken bouillon or
   1 cup chicken stock

½ tablespoon Gravy Browning
   (below)

3 cups water

Sea salt and freshly ground
   black pepper

In a saucepan over medium heat, heat the olive oil. Add the onion, tomatoes, thyme, tomato paste, and chicken cube or stock. Sauté the ingredients until nicely browned and fragrant, 5 to 10 minutes. Add the Gravy Browning and 3 cups water. Bring to a simmer and cook for 20 minutes. Remove from the heat and let cool slightly.

Pass the gravy through a fine-mesh strainer, rubbing out and lumps with a wooden spoon. Season to taste with salt and pepper.

To make a proper, flavorful gravy, follow the recipe below.

Gravy Browning

½ cup sugar

1 cup hot water

1 cup beef stock

In a small saucepan over medium-low heat, stir together the sugar and water. Cook, stirring often, until the sugar mixture is browned, 5 minutes. Stir in the beef stock and cook until the mixture reaches a syrupy, caramel texture, about 5 minutes more.

THANKSGIVING
ROAST TURKEY

Serves 8

We've both grown up with the tradition of turkey for Thanksgiving and Christmas and look forward to it every year! There's nothing better than the aromas filling the kitchen to create a sense of togetherness, with a big bird feeding family and friends for days to come.

1 (12-pound) whole organic turkey

1 cup fresh lime juice

4 tablespoons Bajan seasoning (or a mixture of equal parts ground coriander, turmeric, black pepper, cumin, allspice, cardamom, ginger, and anise; and dried marjoram, parsley, and fenugreek)

1 cup olive oil

2 white or yellow onions, cut into wedges

6 shallots, cut into wedges

8 carrots, peeled and cut into chunks

Rita's Gravy (page 319) for serving

Gluten-Free Parsley, Sage & Onion Stuffing (page 322) for serving

Preheat the oven to 350°F.

Put the turkey in a large pan and rub with the lime juice, inside the cavity and all over the outside. Let the turkey sit for about 20 minutes, then rinse thoroughly both inside and out and pat dry.

Rub the cavity and the outside of the turkey with the Bajan seasoning and the olive oil. Put the turkey in a large roasting pan and pour a little water into the bottom of the pan. Arrange all of the vegetables around the turkey in the pan to add flavor to the basting juices. Cover with aluminum foil and roast for 1 hour.

Remove the foil and continue roasting to allow the turkey to brown, basting frequently with the pan juices, about 30 minutes. Then re-cover with the foil and roast until the juices run clear when the thigh is pierced or an instant-read thermometer inserted into the thickest part of a thigh but away from the bone registers 165°F, about 15 minutes per pound longer, or 2 hours and 15 minutes for a 10- to 12-pound turkey.

Remove the turkey from the oven and let rest for 20 to 30 minutes, then carve and serve with the gravy and stuffing.

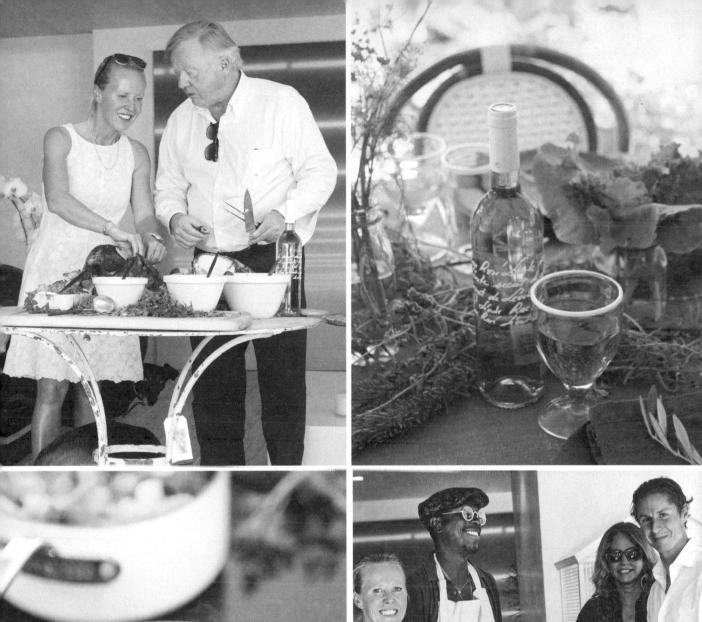

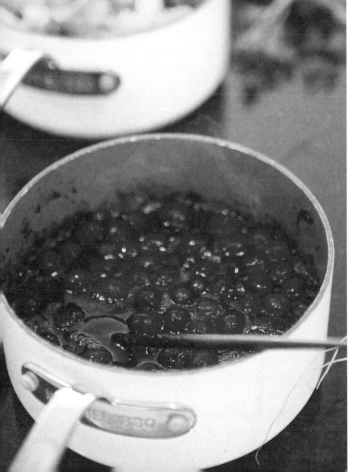

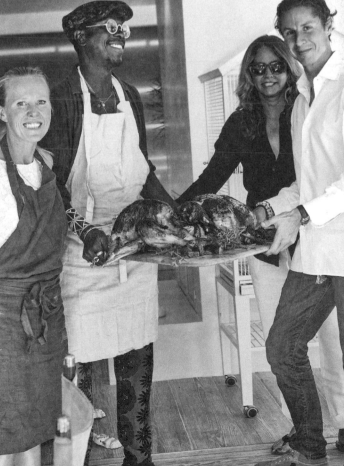

GLUTEN-FREE
PARSLEY, SAGE & ONION STUFFING

Serves 8

No roast bird is complete without a delicious stuffing like this gluten-free version.

1 tablespoon olive oil

2 white onions, finely chopped

3 stalks celery, diced

2 tablespoons finely chopped fresh sage

2 sprigs fresh parsley, finely chopped

½ teaspoon freshly grated nutmeg

Sea salt and freshly ground black pepper

6 gluten-free organic pork or chicken sausages

Zest of 1 lemon

1 large organic free-range egg

3-4 slices gluten-free bread, or torn into crumbs (optional)

Preheat the oven to 350°F.

Heat the olive oil in a large frying pan over medium heat. Add the onions and cook until browned, about 5 minutes. Stir in the celery, sage, parsley, nutmeg, and a pinch each of salt and pepper. Remove from the heat and let cool completely.

Cut the ends off the sausages and push the meat out of the casings into a bowl. Add the lemon zest, onion and herb mixture, egg, and breadcrumbs, if using. Stir to mix well.

Spoon the stuffing into a baking pan, cover, and bake for 45 minutes. Uncover and bake until the top is nicely browned, about 10 more minutes.

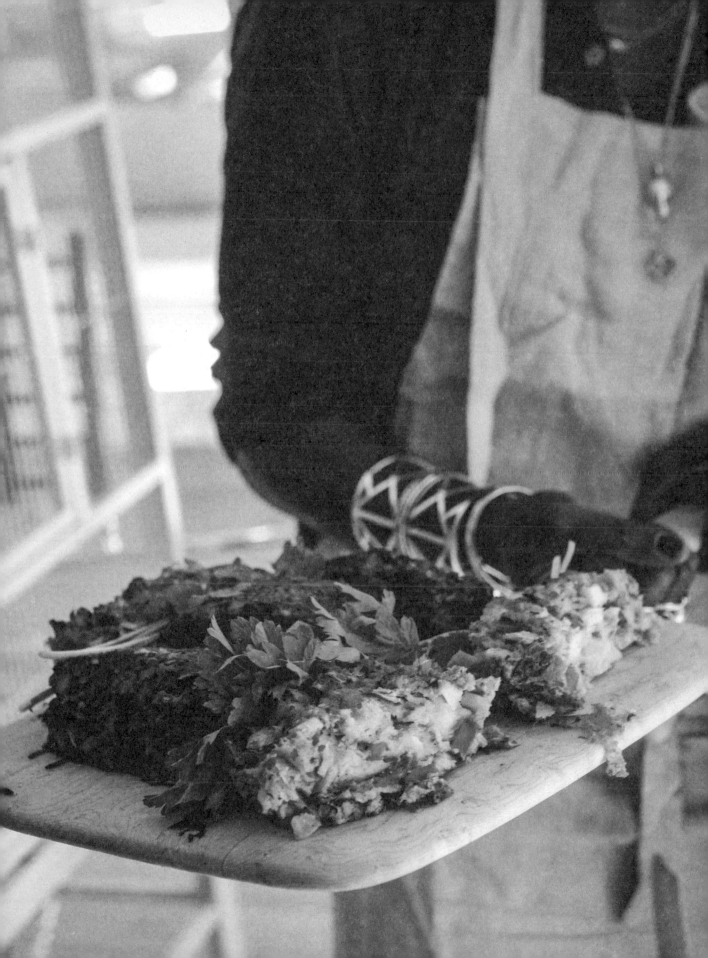

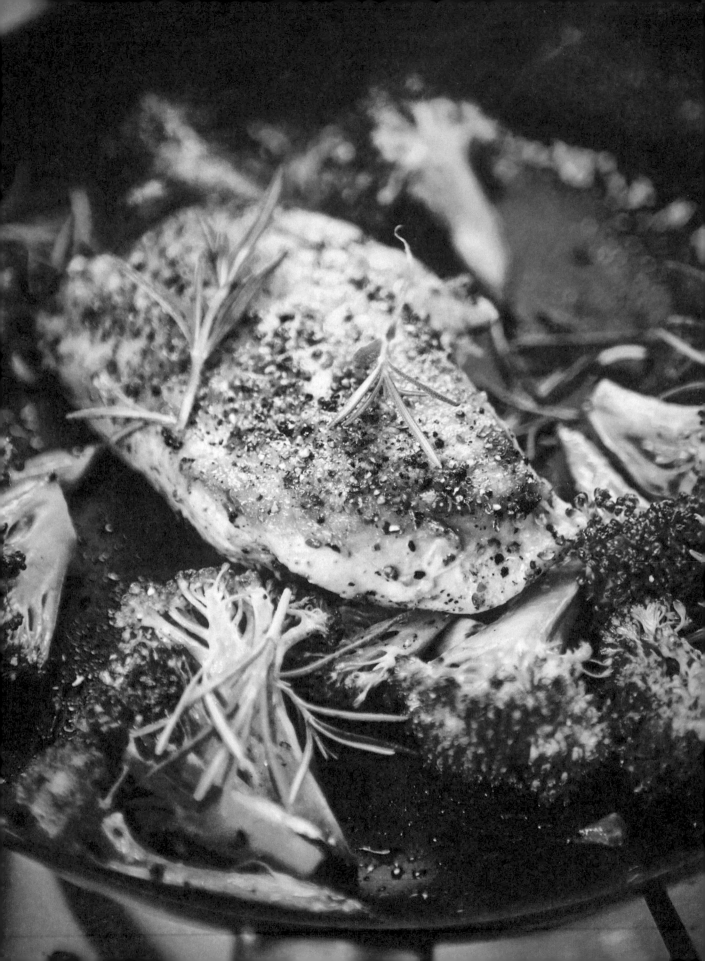

HOWARD'S
ROAST CHICKEN

Serves 6

½ cup fresh lime juice

1 tablespoon salt

1 (6-pound) whole organic chicken

2 tablespoons Bajan seasoning (see page 320)

½ cup olive oil

Preheat the oven to 350°F.

In a bowl large enough to hold the chicken, stir together the lime juice and salt.

Add the chicken to the bowl and rub the salt mixture inside the cavity and all over the outside. Let the chicken sit for about 20 minutes, then rinse thoroughly inside and out and pat dry.

Rub the cavity and the outside of the chicken with the Bajan seasoning and the olive oil. Put the chicken in a roasting pan and pour a little water into the bottom of the pan. Cover with aluminum foil and roast for 1 hour.

Remove the foil and continue roasting to allow the chicken to brown, basting frequently with the pan juices. Then re-cover with the foil and roast until the juices run clear when the thigh is pierced or an instant-read thermometer inserted into the thickest part of a thigh but away from the bone registers 165°F, about 30 minutes longer. Remove from the oven and let rest for about 15 minutes, then carve and serve.

GLUTEN-FREE
PUMPKIN PIE

Serves 4 to 6

A healthy spin on a nostalgic, childhood favorite, this pie is super-easy to make and gluten free.

FOR THE CRUST:

1½ cups all-purpose gluten-free flour

⅓ cup coconut sugar

¼ teaspoon ground ginger

⅓ cup coconut oil, melted

¾ cup water

FOR THE FILLING:

1 (15-ounce) can pumpkin purée

1 (14-ounce) can unsweetened coconut milk

1 teaspoon vanilla extract

⅓ cup coconut sugar

¼ cup gluten-free rolled oats

2 tablespoons ground flaxseed

2 teaspoons ground cinnamon, plus more for dusting

1 teaspoon pumpkin pie spice

¼ teaspoon ground ginger, plus more for dusting

Pinch of freshly grated nutmeg

Sprig of fresh Mexican sage for garnish

Honey, Sage & Rosemary Ice Cream (page 314) or Beet-Apple-Ginger Sorbet (page 313)

Preheat the oven to 200°F.

To make the crust: In a large bowl, combine the flour, sugar, and ginger. Stir in the oil. Slowly add the water, as much as needed so that the dough comes together but isn't gummy.

Press the dough evenly into a 10-inch pie pan. The crust will rise, so press down or use pie weights.

Put the crust in oven and immediately raise the oven temperature to 350°F. Bake until lightly golden brown, about 15 minutes. Transfer to a wire rack and set aside to cool.

Raise the oven temperature to 400°F.

To make the filling: In a blender, combine the pumpkin purée, coconut milk, vanilla, sugar, oats, flaxseed, cinnamon, pie spice, ginger, and nutmeg and blend until smooth. Pour the filling into the cooled pie crust.

Bake until the filling appears set and firm, 25 to 30 minutes. Transfer to a wire rack and let the pie cool slightly, then refrigerate until well-chilled, 4 or 5 hours, or until ready to serve.

When ready to serve, dust with ground ginger and cinnamon and garnish with a sprig of Mexican sage. Cut into wedges and serve with Honey, Sage & Rosemary Ice Cream or Beet-Apple-Ginger Sorbet (or both!).

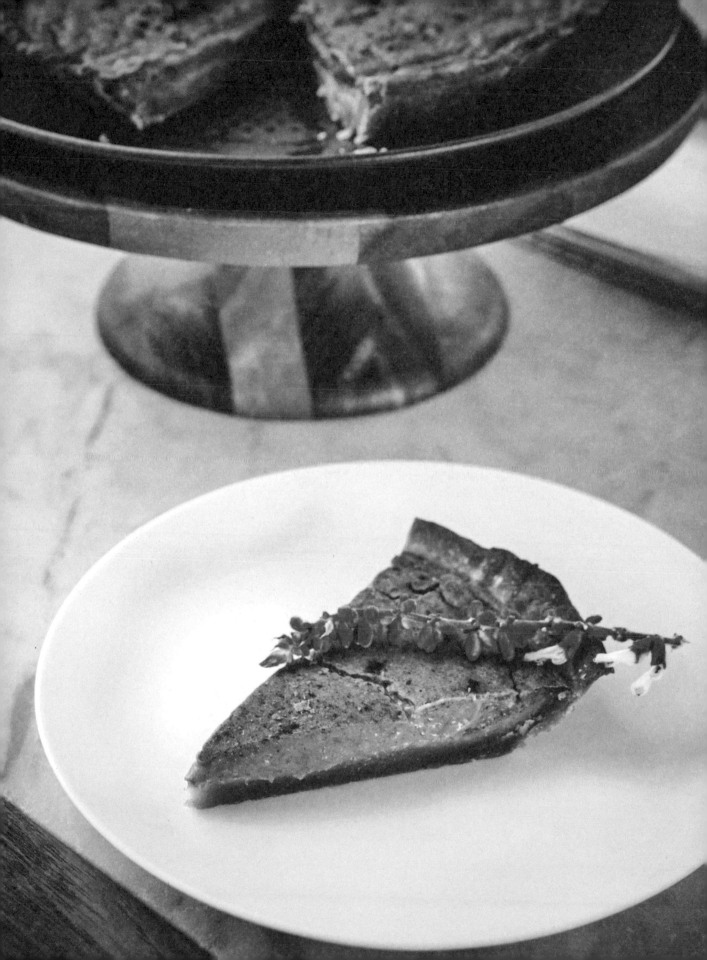

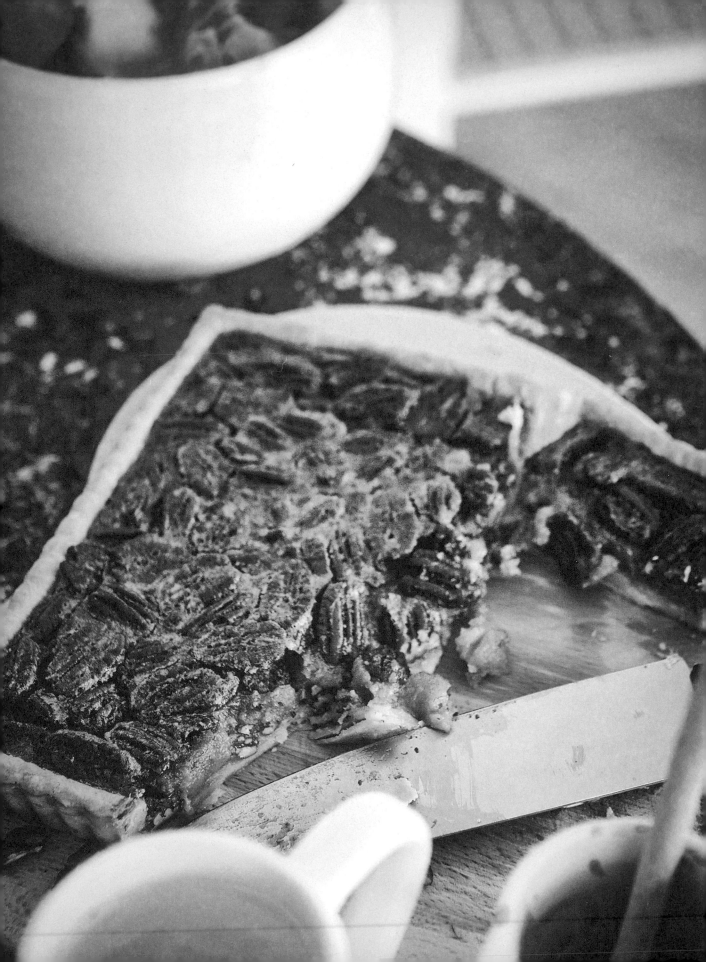

PECAN PIE

Serves 6 to 8

FOR THE CRUST:

1 cup almonds

1 cup buckwheat flour

2 tablespoons coconut sugar

2 tablespoons cinnamon

4 Medjool dates, pitted

3 tablespoons coconut oil, plus more for pan

1 pinch sea salt or Himalayan pink salt

2 pinches nutmeg

FOR THE FILLING:

1 cup whole pecans

1 16-oz jar almond butter (you can also use cashew or Brazil nut butter)

2 tablespoons maple syrup

2 tablespoons honey

10 Medjool dates

¼ cup water

FOR THE TOPPING:

1 cup whole pecans

2 tablespoons maple syrup

1 teaspoon cinnamon

Preheat the oven to 356°F.

To make the crust: Pour the almonds into a food processor and blend on high for about a minute until they resemble flour.

Add buckwheat, coconut sugar, cinnamon, dates, coconut oil, sea salt, and nutmeg, and blend until fully combined (mixture will be sticky).

Grease the bottom of your pie dish with coconut oil.

Add the mixture to the dish, spreading evenly across the base and sides. Bake for 15 minutes until the crust browns and hardens.

To make the filling: Pour the pecans into the food processor and blend for about 30 seconds until they are finely ground.

Add the almond butter and blend until combined.

Add the maple syrup, honey, and dates, slowly adding the water while blending.

For the topping: Toss the pecans with maple syrup and cinnamon.

Transfer to a baking tray and bake for approximately 4 minutes until pecans are golden brown and crunchy. Set aside to cool.

Once the crust has cooled, spread filling evenly over the crust. Sprinkle over the pecan topping.

To serve, warm the pie in the oven for about 2 minutes, or refrigerate immediately and serve cold.

The best accompaniments are warm, 100 percent pure maple syrup (warm up 6 tablespoons in a pan and pour over) or Honey Sage Ice Cream (page 314).

APPLE TART

Serves 6 to 8

Nothing signals that the holidays have arrived like the tantalizing aroma of a warm apple tart wafting through the house. This is a staple at One Gun holidays and is gluten free, dairy free, and vegan so all your friends and family can enjoy it!

FOR THE CRUST:

1½ cups almond flour (I like Bob's Red Mill)

1 cup gluten-free oat flour

¼ teaspoon salt

3 tablespoons maple syrup

¼ cup coconut oil, plus more for pan

FOR THE FILLING:

1¼ pounds of apples (I like Granny Smith, Honey Crisp, or Cox)

1 tablespoon lemon juice

¼ teaspoon cinnamon

1 tablespoon maple syrup

2 teaspoons apricot jam/conserve

2 tablespoons Calvados, cognac, or water

Preheat oven to 350°F.

Use a little coconut oil to lightly grease a 9-inch tart pan.

For the crust: Mix the almond flour, oat flour, and salt in a medium bowl. Stir in maple syrup and coconut oil until thoroughly combined.

Transfer the mixture into the pan, making sure it is evenly spread across the base and sides.

Use a fork to prick holes into the base (to prevent bubbles from forming while baking).

Bake for 10 to 12 minutes until the just crust begins to turn golden and is lightly firm. Set aside.

For the filling: Peel, core, and thinly slice the apples.

Put the slices in a mixing bowl, adding the lemon juice, cinnamon, and maple syrup. Toss until evenly mixed.

Arrange the apple slices in concentric circles in the crust, reserving the leftover maple syrup and lemon juice.

Bake for 25 minutes. Remove from oven and brush the reserved maple syrup and lemon juice mixture over the apples.

Return the tart to the oven and bake for about 20 minutes until the apples are very soft and the crust is a rich golden brown.

In a small saucepan, combine the apricot jam and cognac over low heat. While the tart is still warm, brush the apricot and cognac mixture over the apples.

Allow the tart to cool for about 15 minutes before serving.

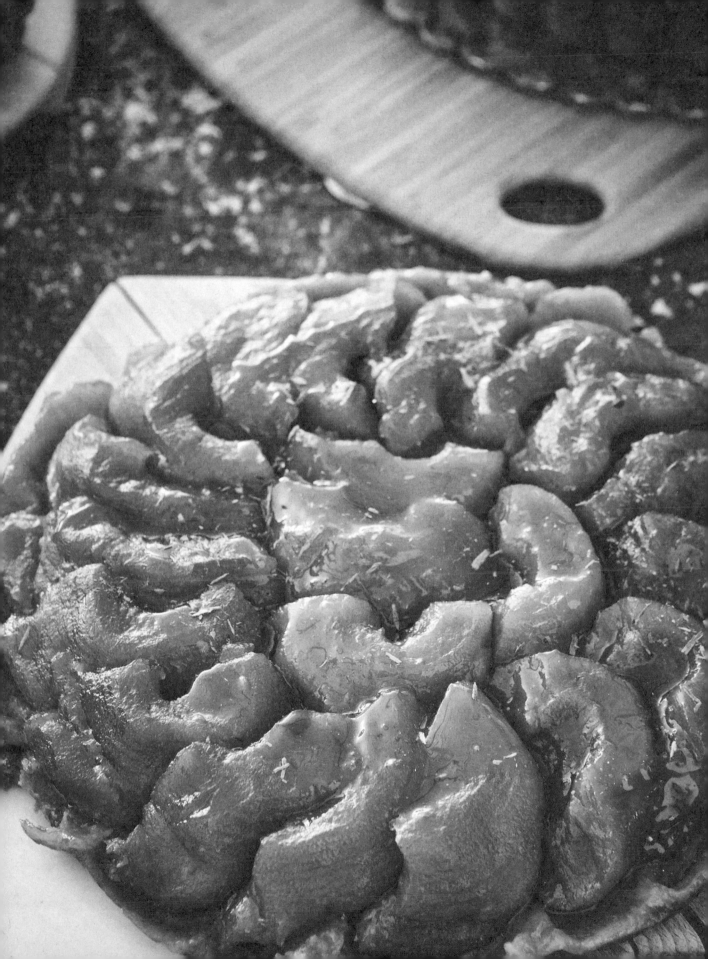

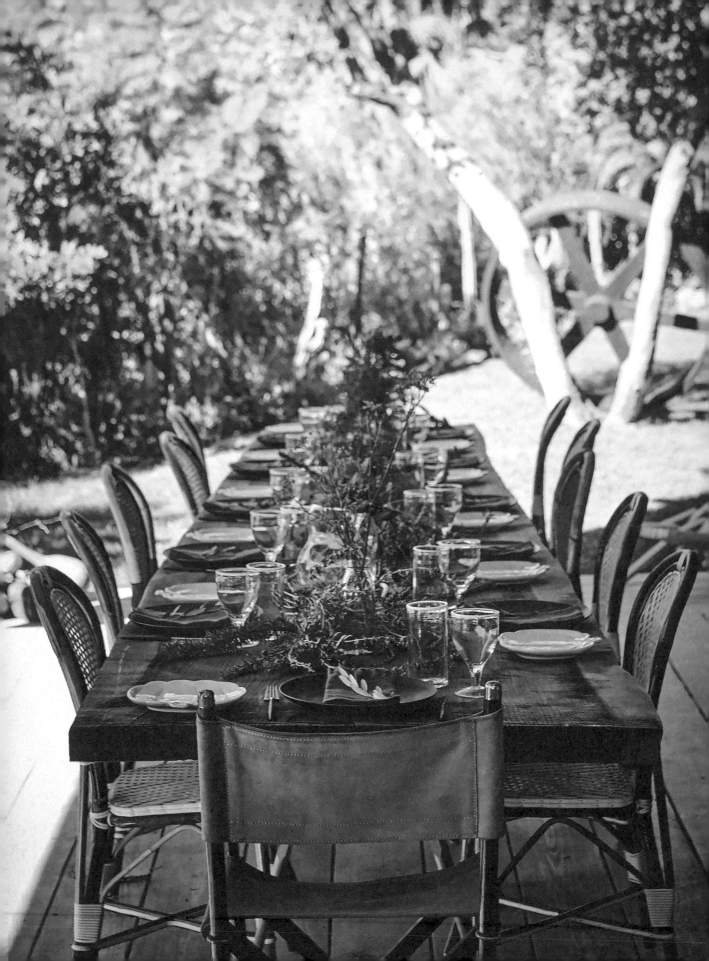

Recipe List

BIODYNAMIC BREAKFASTS

Chia Breakfast Bowl 137

Healthy Oat Pancakes 139

Banana–Bee Pollen Split 140

Steel Cut Oats with Ginger, Bee Pollen, & Goji 143

Egg White Scramble 144

Avocado Toast 146

SUPER SNACKS

Energy Balls (One Gun Bullets/Ammo) 149

Hempseed Mexican Sage Flapjacks 151

Cacao Almond Butter 152

Perfect Popcorn 153

BIODYNAMIC GLUTEN-FREE BREADS

Poppy Seed Corn Bread 156

Buckwheat, Corn & Rosemary Bread 157

Gluten-Free Banana Bread 159

ROOT DAYS

Roasted Butternut Squash & Ginger Soup 161

Beet Carpaccio with Cumin 162

Beetroot Soup 165

Celery Root Purée with Thyme, Rosemary & Lemon 166

Kale & Celery Root Soup 168

Carrot, Orange & Ginger Mash 169

Shaved Carrots with Raisins & Poppy Seeds 171

Roasted Carrots with Carrot-Top Pesto 172

Avocado, Carrot & Radish Salad 175

Balsamic-Roasted Onions 176

Ranch Veg 177

Roasted Sweet Potatoes with Turmeric 178

Parisienne Leek Vinaigrette 180

Halloween Stew, or Spiced Pumpkin Casserole 183

FRUIT DAYS

Gazpacho 185

Watermelon Gazpacho 186

Watermelon, Pineapple, & Mint 187

Barbecued Watermelon 188

Sliced Peaches with Lime & Mint 189

Roasted Beet, Squash & Pumpkin 190

Tamari Seeds 190

Spaghetti Squash Arrabiata 193

Raw Pad Thai 194

One Gun Quinoa with Tomatoes, Cilantro & Basil 197

Heritage Tomato & Basil Salad 198

Tomato Consommé with Basil Sorbet 200

Basil Sorbet 201

Chilled Tomato, Cucumber & Fennel Soup 202

Chilled Avocado & Cucumber Soup 203

Grilled Corn with Sage 205

LEAF DAYS

Grilled Tuscan Kale 207

Annie's Veggies with Quinoa 208

Raw Tabouli 211

One Gun Spinach & Pomegranate Salad 212

Fennel, Kale & Grapefruit Salad 215

Collard Wraps 216

Almond Pâté 216

Spiced Purple Cabbage with Pomegranate 219

Healthy Slaw 220

Spinach & Nutmeg Soup 223

Arugula, Fennel & Orange Salad 224

HELPFUL CONVERSIONS

DRY MEASUREMENTS

US	OUNCES	METRIC
Pinch		1 mg
½ teaspoon		2 mg
1 teaspoon	⅙ ounce	5 mg
3 teaspons	½ ounce	14 grams
½ tablespoon	¼ ounce	7 grams
1 tablespoon	½ ounce	14 grams
2 tablespoons	1 ounce	28 grams

FLUID MEASUREMENTS

US	PINT	QUART	IMPERIAL
¼ cup			
½ cup			
1 cup	½ pint		8.3 ounces
2 cups	1 pint		19.2 ounces
4	2 pints	1	40

OVEN TEMPERATURES

GAS MARK	FAHRENHEIT	CELSIUS	DESCRIPTION
¼	225°	110°	Very cool/very slow
½	250°	130°	
1	275°	140°	Cool
2	300°	150°	
3	325°	170°	Very moderate
4	350°	180°	Moderate
5	375°	190°	
6	400°	200°	Moderately hot
7	425°	220°	Hot
8	450°	230°	
9	475°	240°	Very hot

Index